AUTOPSY PRACTICES

Second Edition

Editors

Dhaneshwar Lanjewar MD
Professor and Head
Department of Pathology
Gujarat Adani Institute of Medical Sciences
Bhuj, Gujarat, India

Pradeep Vaideeswar MD
Additional Professor
Department of Pathology
Seth Gordhandas Sunderdas Medical College
Mumbai, Maharashtra, India

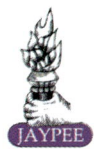

JAYPEE BROTHERS MEDICAL PUBLISHERS
The Health Sciences Publisher
New Delhi | London

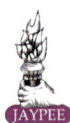 **Jaypee Brothers Medical Publishers (P) Ltd**

Headquarters

Jaypee Brothers Medical Publishers (P) Ltd
4838/24, Ansari Road, Daryaganj
New Delhi 110 002, India
Phone: +91-11-43574357
Fax: +91-11-43574314
Email: jaypee@jaypeebrothers.com

Overseas Office

J.P. Medical Ltd
83 Victoria Street, London
SW1H 0HW (UK)
Phone: +44 20 3170 8910
Fax: +44 (0)20 3008 6180
Email: info@jpmedpub.com

Website: www.jaypeebrothers.com
Website: www.jaypeedigital.com

© 2021, Jaypee Brothers Medical Publishers

The views and opinions expressed in this book are solely those of the original contributor(s)/author(s) and do not necessarily represent those of editor(s) of the book.

All rights reserved. No part of this publication may be reproduced, stored or transmitted in any form or by any means, electronic, mechanical, photocopying, recording or otherwise, without the prior permission in writing of the publishers.

All brand names and product names used in this book are trade names, service marks, trademarks or registered trademarks of their respective owners. The publisher is not associated with any product or vendor mentioned in this book.

Medical knowledge and practice change constantly. This book is designed to provide accurate, authoritative information about the subject matter in question. However, readers are advised to check the most current information available on procedures included and check information from the manufacturer of each product to be administered, to verify the recommended dose, formula, method and duration of administration, adverse effects and contraindications. It is the responsibility of the practitioner to take all appropriate safety precautions. Neither the publisher nor the author(s)/editor(s) assume any liability for any injury and/or damage to persons or property arising from or related to use of material in this book.

This book is sold on the understanding that the publisher is not engaged in providing professional medical services. If such advice or services are required, the services of a competent medical professional should be sought.

Every effort has been made where necessary to contact holders of copyright to obtain permission to reproduce copyright material. If any have been inadvertently overlooked, the publisher will be pleased to make the necessary arrangements at the first opportunity. The **CD/DVD-ROM** (if any) provided in the sealed envelope with this book is complimentary and free of cost. **Not meant for sale.**

Inquiries for bulk sales may be solicited at: jaypee@jaypeebrothers.com

Autopsy Practices / *Dhaneshwar Lanjewar, Pradeep Vaideeswar*

First Edition: 2017

Second Edition: **2021**

ISBN: 978-93-89587-04-3

Printed at Sanat Printers

Contributors

Anjali D Amarapurkar MD
Professor
Department of Pathology
Lokmanya Tilak Memorial Medical College
Mumbai, Maharashtra, India

Arvind Valand MD
Professor and Head
Department of Pathology
Vedantaa Institute of Medical Sciences
Dahanu, Maharashtra, India

Ashim Das MD
Professor
Department of Histopathology
Postgraduate Institute of Medical Education and Research
Chandigarh, India

Bhuvaneshwari Kandalkar MD
Senior Consultant - Pathology
Naryana Health
Mumbai, Maharashtra, India

Bishan Radotra MD
Professor and Head
Department of Histopathology
Postgraduate Institute of Medical Education and Research
Chandigarh, India

Daksha Prabhat MD
Professor
Department of Pathology
Seth Gordhandas Sunderdas Medical College
Mumbai, Maharashtra, India

Deepak S Joshi MD
Professor and Head
Department of Anatomy
Grant Government Medical College
Mumbai, Maharashtra, India

Dhaneshwar Lanjewar MD
Professor and Head
Department of Pathology
Gujarat Adani Institute of Medical Sciences
Bhuj, Gujarat, India

Gayathri Amonkar MD
Associate Professor
Department of Pathology
Topiwala National Medical College
Mumbai, Maharashtra, India

Jaya Deshpande MD
Former Professor and Head
Department of Pathology
Topiwala National Medical College
Mumbai, Maharashtra, India

Kusum Jashnani MD
Professor and Head
Department of Pathology
Topiwala National Medical College
Mumbai, Maharashtra, India

Pradeep Vaideeswar MD
Additional Professor
Department of Pathology
Seth Gordhandas Sunderdas Medical College
Mumbai, Maharashtra, India

Pragati Sathe MD
Associate Professor
Department of Pathology
Seth Gordhandas Sunderdas Medical College
Mumbai, Maharashtra, India

Late Ratnaprabha Ghodke MD
Former Assistant Professor
Department of Pathology
Seth Gordhandas Sunderdas Medical College
Mumbai, Maharashtra, India

Saranya Singaravel MD
Consultant Pathologist
Soleil Diagnostics
Mumbai, Maharashtra, India

Saroj Bolde MD
Associate Professor
Department of Pathology
Grant Government Medical College
Mumbai, Maharashtra, India

Shailesh Mohite MD
Professor and Head
Department of Forensic Medicine
Topiwala National Medical College
Mumbai, Maharashtra, India

Shubhangi Agale MD
Academic Professor
Department of Pathology
Grant Government Medical College
Mumbai, Maharashtra, India

Smita Divate MD
Additional Professor
Department of Pathology
Seth Gordhandas Sunderdas Medical College
Mumbai, Maharashtra, India

Subhash Yadav MD
Assistant Professor
Department of Pathology
Tata Memorial Hospital
Mumbai, Maharashtra, India

Vinaya Shah MD
Associate Professor
Department of Pathology
Hindu Hruday Samrat Balasaheb Thackeray Medical College
Mumbai, Maharashtra, India

Preface to Second Edition

In the 3.5 years since the first edition of this book was published, we have received numerous messages from readers commenting on the book and suggesting how it could be improved. We have also built up a large file of ideas based on our own experiences in reading, writing, and editing. With the aid of all this information we have revised the book. The second edition represents revision of the chapters in the first edition and a substantial enlargement through the addition of one new chapter.

Most obvious changes in this second edition are: Chapter 1 (Introduction and History) is revised and modified; Chapter 5 G (Examination of the Hemolymphatic System) is revised and expanded; Chapter 7 (Autopsy and Law) and Chapter 11 (Embalming) are also revised. A new Chapter (Chapter 12: Autopsy Guidelines in COVID-2019) has been added. In the Appendix, six additional cases of Clinicopathological conference are added.

We intend for this work to be comprehensive and helpful for those dealing with clinical and medico-legal autopsies and hope that this book will be useful to Pathology residents, Pathologists, and Forensic medicine specialists.

Dhaneshwar Lanjewar
Pradeep Vaideeswar

Preface to First Edition

The traditionally recognized contributions of the autopsy such as its role in defining new disease entities, in the quality control of patient care and in determining the cause of death, are just as relevant today as in the past. The progress of pathology in India began in 1840, and in those days, the roots of development of pathology in India were in the premier institutes. Significant contributions on neuropathology, cardiovascular and pulmonary pathology, and AIDS pathology were made from medical colleges in Mumbai; this work is known throughout the globe.

Currently, there is no autopsy book authored by Indian pathologists describing procedural details of performing autopsy. *Autopsy Practices* is a contribution by several pathologists from Mumbai and Chandigarh, and each author has performed and/or observed several thousand clinical autopsies. All the topics are written in conventional pattern and each topic is designed to offer practical guidelines that will lead pathologists to identify, interpret and correlate the autopsy findings. In addition, a topic on "Autopsy and Law" will be useful for the postgraduates in Forensic Medicine and Toxicology.

It is hoped that this first edition with its emphasis on practical procedures will be of assistance to the pathologists of developing and developed countries.

Dhaneshwar Lanjewar
Pradeep Vaideeswar

Acknowledgments

Many people have sent us extensive comments and corrections since the appearance of the first edition in 2017. To all of them, including in particular to Dr Shashank Tyagi, Assistant Professor, Department of Forensic Medicine and Toxicology, Seth GS Medical College and KEM Hospital, Parel, Mumbai.

Dhaneshwar Lanjewar
Pradeep Vaideeswar

Contents

1. **Autopsy: Introduction and History** — 1
   Dhaneshwar Lanjewar
   Types of Autopsies 1; History of Autopsy 2;
   History of Autopsy in India 5

2. **External Examination at Autopsy** — 10
   Arvind Valand, Dhaneshwar Lanjewar

3. **Utility and Techniques of Autopsy** — 15
   Jaya Deshpande
   Preliminary Skin Incisions 17; Opening of the Thoracic and Abdominal Cavities 18; Techniques of Evisceration 19

4. **In situ Examination** — 22
   Dhaneshwar Lanjewar
   Examination of Cranial Cavity 22; Pericardial Cavity 23;
   Pleural Cavity and Lungs 24; Abdominal Cavity 24

5. **Systemic Examination** — 27
   Bishan Radotra, Pradeep Vaideeswar, Gayathri Amonkar, Anjali D Amarapurkar, Ashim Das, Vinaya Shah, Daksha Prabhat, Shubhangi Agale, Subhash Yadav

   5A: Central Nervous System 27
   Bishan Radotra
   Brain Removal Procedure 28; Examination of the Brain Before Fixation 31; Fixation of the Brain 32; Removal of the Spinal Cord 32; Examination of brain After Fixation 33; Sampling for Histology 35; Spinal Cord Examination and Sampling 36

   5B: Cardiovascular System 38
   Pradeep Vaideeswar
   Separation and Fixation of the Heart 38; External Examination of the Heart 41; Opening the Heart and Heart Weight 47; Internal Examination of the Heart 48; Alterations in Dissection 53; Sampling for Histopathology 53

5C: Examination of the Respiratory System   55
Gayathri Amonkar
Importance of External and In Situ 55; Lung Dissection, Fixation and Cutting 57; Examination of the Lungs 59

5D: Gastrointestinal Tract at Autopsy   62
Anjali D Amarapurkar
In Situ Examination 63; Systemic Examination 63

5E: Approach in Autopsy of Patients with Liver-related Problems   69
Ashim Das
External Examination 69; Internal Examination 70

5F: Urogenital Tract at Autopsy   76
Vinaya Shah
External Examination of the Kidneys 76; Examination of Cut Surface of the Kidneys 79; Examination of the Ureters 83; Examination of the Urinary Bladder 84; Examination of the Testes 85; Examination of the Prostate 86; Examination of the Seminal Vesicles 86 Examination of the Female Genital Tract 86

5G: Examination of the Lymphoreticular System   88
Daksha Prabhat, Shubhangi Agale, Subhash Yadav
Spleen 88; Thymus 96

6. Autopsies in Special Situations   99
Bhuvaneshwari Kandalkar, Pragati Sathe, Late Ratnaprabha Ghodke, Kusum Jashnani

6A: Pediatric Autopsies   99
Bhuvaneshwari Kandalkar, Pragati Sathe, Late Ratnaprabha Ghodke
External Examination 100; Incisions and In Situ Examination 101; Systemic Examination 102; Postmortem Investigations 105; Sampling for Histopathology 105

6B: Autopsy in Maternal Deaths   107
Kusum Jashnani
Role of Autopsy in Maternal Deaths 108; Importance of Clinical Records 108; External Examination 108; In Situ Examination 109; Internal Systemic Examination 110

7. Autopsy and Law   118
Shailesh Mohite
Indian Law Related to Medicolegal Postmortem 122

8. Design of Autopsy Room   130
Smita Divate, Dhaneshwar Lanjewar
Basic Functional Areas 130

9. **Autopsy Safety Precautions** — 136
   Smita Divate
   General Rules for Autopsy Biosafety 137; Isolation Room for
   Specific Types of High-Risk Autopsies 138; Safe Use of
   Sharp Instruments 138; Limiting the Generation of Aerosols 138;
   Personal Protective Attire/Equipment for Autopsies 139
   Handwashing 139; Cleaning and Decontamination 139;
   Handling of Cadavers 140; Storage and Transport of Tissues 140;
   Demonstration of Organs At Meetings 141; Biowaste Disposal 141;
   Photography 141; Employee Health 141; Appendix 1 143; Appendix 2 144

10. **Autopsy Audit** — 145
    Jaya Deshpande
    Preanalytical Phase 145; Analytical Phase 146;
    Postanalytical Phase 146; Autopsy Clinical Audit Monitors 147

11. **Embalming** — 148
    Deepak S Joshi
    History 148; Modern Embalming 148; Principle of Embalming 149;
    Pre-Embalming Steps and Their Legal Aspects 150;
    Equipment Required for Embalming 150; Methods of Embalming 151;
    Packing and Transportation 152; Plastination 152

12. **Autopsy Guidelines in COVID-2019** — 154
    Dhaneshwar Lanjewar
    Guidelines and Precautions for Performing Autopsy 154;
    Recommendations for Gross Contamination and Liquids 156

Appendices — 159

Case 1: Central Nervous System 159
Bishan Radotra

Case 2: Central Nervous System 162
Bishan Radotra

Case 3: Cardiovascular System 163
Pradeep Vaideeswar

Case 4: Cardiovascular System 166
Pradeep Vaideeswar

Case 5: Gastrointestinal Tract 169
Anjali D Amarapurkar

Case 6: Urinary Tract 171
Vinaya Shah

Case 7: Autopsy In Infectious Disease 173
Dhaneshwar Lanjewar

Case 8: Maternal Mortality   176
Kusum Jashnani

Case 9: Pediatric Autopsy   179
Pragati Sathe

Case 10: Urinary System and Gastrointestinal Tract   181
Dhaneshwar Lanjewar

Case 11: Respiratory System   184
Pradeep Vaideeswar, Saranya Singaravel

Case 12: Central Nervous, Cardiovascular and Respiratory Systems   187
Bishan Radotra

Case 13: Multi-System Involvement   193
Bishan Radotra

Case 14: Gastrointestinal Tract   200
Dhaneshwar Lanjewar, Saroj Bolde

Index   **207**

CHAPTER 1

Autopsy: Introduction and History

Dhaneshwar Lanjewar

INTRODUCTION

Since the evolution, human beings have struggled for survival and knowledge. In earlier ancient time, the first systematic cadaveric dissection was performed on animals by hunters, butchers, and cooks to find edible organs. The observations of animal dissection fascinated human beings and stimulated them to know structure of human body. The work on anatomy by Andreas Vesalius (*De humani corporis fabrica*, 1543), which initiated a concept of pathologic anatomy, confirms that anatomy is the beginning of pathology; more importantly it emphasized that pathology is best studied on the autopsy table. The word "autopsy" is derived from Greek words, *autos* means oneself and *opsis* means sight or view, i.e., to see for oneself. The word "autopsy" has been used since 17th century. Necropsy (*necros* means dead, *opis* means to view) means viewing of the dead body. Necropsy is the most accurate term for the investigative dissection of the dead body, but the term autopsy is commonly used and is more popular. Other synonyms include postmortem, postmortem examination, and autopsia cadaverum. Autopsy procedure comprises thorough examination of the corpse to determine cause and manner of death and to evaluate any disease. It is considered as akin to a "surgical" operation performed by a specialized medical doctor, which is either a pathologist or a forensic medicine expert.

TYPES OF AUTOPSIES

Autopsies are classified into two types. Medicolegal or forensic or coroner's autopsy is ordered by law whenever there is violent, suspicious, or sudden death which may be a criminal matter (see Chapter 7). On the other hand, clinical, medical, or pathological autopsies are performed to know the cause of death or for research purpose and are carried out with the consent of the family of deceased person.

If the person does not have next of kin or legal heir to give consent, then information has to be given to nearest police station in whose jurisdiction the hospital is located and consent is obtained from the Investigating Officer (IO). Usually IO would conduct a police inquest. It is performed by the pathologist in tertiary care centers (ideal), but in most of the places in India, it is performed by medical officer, who may not always be a postgraduate in pathology. The aim of these autopsies is to determine, clarify, or confirm medical diagnosis that was not known prior to the death of the patient and to confirm a doubtful diagnosis. Clinical autopsies gain more insight into pathological process and determine factors that contributed to the patient's death and the extent of natural disease. It helps to identify the pathological changes that have taken place in different organs during disease processes and its progress or deterioration following treatment. It ensures the standard and care in hospital. Autopsy remains important for quality assurance of clinical work. It identifies medical error and also teaches how patient's death can be prevented in future. In autopsy, it is mandatory to carry out detailed examination of all the organs; this is called as complete autopsy. However, in reality a complete autopsy is not possible because examination of some organs/structures such as eyes, mouth, face, and the extremities are not permitted. In some cases, when the clinician is of the opinion that the patient has died due to localized disease involving one or two organs, there is a request for partial or restricted autopsy. In such situations, examination of the skull, thoracic, and/or abdominal cavities is performed. To perform partial autopsy, there is also a need of obtaining consent of the family of deceased person.

Anatomical dissection (considered by some as another type of autopsy) performed by medical students for understanding normal anatomy cannot be considered autopsy, as anatomical dissection is not carried out for knowing cause of death. Here, usually the unclaimed or unidentified dead bodies are dissected by the anatomist or the medical student to gather detail knowledge of the normal structures of different external and internal organs and structures of the human body. The consent for such autopsy is also given by the person when he was alive or his legal heir/next of kin after his death who have consented for body donation. No separate consent from any legal authority is required in such cases. Though consent is not required, permission ought to be taken from the government authority for such purpose when such donated bodies have to be transported from one place to the medical college where the body is required for dissection purpose by medical students. In some institutes, magnetic resonance imaging (MRI) and computed tomography (CT) scan of dead bodies are performed to determine lesions in various organs, a procedure termed as virtual autopsy.

HISTORY OF AUTOPSY

The beginning of autopsy was from anatomy; hence, initial history of autopsy is related to anatomical dissection. The first dissection was probably performed in ancient Babylon (Hillah-Iraq) around 3500 BC. In this time period, the organs of animals were examined to obtain messages from divine spirit. Another practice of hepatoscopy or haruspicy was also prevalent in ancient time. In this practice, examination of liver and intestine of sacrificed animals was carried out for foretelling the future. This practice has a religious background and had no relation for understanding of disease.

In the Egypt around 3000 BC, a technique of mummification was practiced, where the embalmers of ancient Egypt used to give incision on left hypochondrium and through this incision intestine, stomach, liver, spleen, pancreas, kidneys, and lungs were removed. The brain used to be removed through nostrils, but the heart used to be retained in the body. In this practice, even though organs were removed, their observations were never made and this dissection was not related for identification or understanding of any disease process. However, as time passed, the techniques of hepatoscopy or haruspicy and embalming played a major role in the progress of autopsy.

The Greek doctor, Galen of Pergamum (131-200 BC) dissected humans and animals to know pathology and he was the first to correlate the patients' symptoms and signs on the basis of findings of diseased organs. His observations eventually led to autopsy and broke an ancient barrier for progress of medicine. Herophilus and Erasistratus of Chalcedon dissected bodies (3rd century BC) of live criminals to teach anatomy and pathology. In 44 BC, an official autopsy was carried out on Julius Caesar who was murdered by rival senator. By around 150 BC, ancient Roman legal practice had established parameters for autopsies. As early as 1200, the dissection of humans used to be performed with regularity to become skillful in dissection. In England, during the 13th century, dissection of dead bodies to determine the cause of death was largely unknown. By the mid-14th century, dissections had become part of the medical curriculum in many Italian Universities. **Table 1.1** shows world leaders and their contribution in advancement in pathology through autopsy studies. Antonia Benivieni, a Florentine physician (1443-1502), used to obtain permission for postmortem from next of kin of deceased in interesting clinical cases. He performed autopsies, recorded their brief description, and correlated findings of autopsy with prior symptoms of the deceased. His autopsy records of 20 autopsies were published by his brother in 1507 as "The Hidden Causes of Disease," one of the earliest publications of autopsy work.

Andreas Vesalius (1514-1564) used to do anatomical dissection meticulously and skillfully. He moved in Padua in 1537 where he made interesting observations, therefore, understanding of anatomy became easier. His observations described in *De humani corporis fabrica* (1543) made it possible to distinguish pathologic anatomy of aortic aneurysm from the normal aorta.

Giovanni Battista Morgagni (1682-1771), a keen academician, a physician, and professor at the University of Padua, was trained under Antonio Valsalva. The autopsy examination in its modern form began in Padua with his work. He meticulously performed and described findings in 700 autopsies and produced the first exhaustive work on pathology "The Seats and Causes of Disease Investigated by Anatomy" in 1761. He was the first to correlate clinical symptoms with pathologic lesions and with him, the science of pathology reached new heights.

He convinced the physicians that if they want progress of medicine, then autopsies should be performed and clinicopathological correlation should be achieved. Morgagni is truly a "Founder of Pathologic Anatomy."

TABLE 1.1 Contributions of world leaders in autopsy.

Name	Period	Place and country	Significant contribution
Antonio Benivieni	1443 to 1502	Florentine (Italy)	Correlated clinical symptoms with autopsy findings; Publication of autopsy records in 1507—"The Hidden Causes of Diseases"
Giovanni Battista Morgagni	1682 to 1771	Padua (Italy)	Performed and described 700 autopsies and produced the first exhaustive work on pathology in 1761—"The Seats and Causes of Disease Investigated by Anatomy"; "Founder of Pathologic Anatomy"
Marie Xavier Bichat	1771 to 1802	Paris (France)	Identified 21 types of tissue with the help of physical and chemical tests and without the help of microscope; wrote monograms and books which describe his experiences with tuberculosis, pneumonia, typhoid, and gastroenteritis; "Father of Histology"
Carl von Rokitansky	1804 to 1878	Vienna (Austria)	Performed 30,000 autopsies and supervised 70,000 autopsies; described autopsy technique based on the in situ examination of viscera; Publications: "Handbook of Pathological Anatomy" and "Defects in the septa of the heart; "Father of Modern Autopsy"
Rudolf Ludwig Carl Virchow	1821 to 1902	Berlin (Germany)	Developed simple autopsy technique and published as "Method of Performing Post-Mortem Examinations in the Dead House"; Through the use of microscopic examination and demonstrated that the cellular pathology is the basis of disease; published a book "Cellular Pathology"; first to give names to diseases such as leukemia, embolism, thrombosis, ochronosis, etc. terms named after him: Virchow's node, Virchow–Robin space, Virchow–Seckel syndrome, and Virchow triad; "Father of Modern Pathology"
William Osler	1849 to 1919	Montreal (Canada)	A giant of clinical medicine and pathology; Brought autopsy at the center of medical education; first to note that aneurysm of aorta was a complication of syphilis; on the basis of his autopsy data published in a book "The Principles and Practice of Medicine"

Marie Xavier Bichat (1771–1802), an anatomist and leading physician of Paris, had a great interest in autopsy. In the year he died, he allegedly performed 600 autopsies. He was analytical, and in addition to dissecting the organs he used to carry out physical and chemical tests on the organs. With the help of these tests, he identified 21 types of tissues and this was done without using microscope. He strongly argued that tissues are damaged in diseases. His observations were important milestones in the history of medicine. Bichat wrote monograms and books which describe his experiences with tuberculosis, pneumonia, typhoid, and gastroenteritis.

Carl von Rokitansky (1804–1878) was a great physician of Vienna and is considered as the father of modern autopsy. He was of the opinion that the autopsy will be of great help for physicians. In earlier time when autopsy examination of only diseased organs was performed, Rokitansky described a technique of systematic examination of organs. He not only examined the diseased organ meticulously but also paid attention toward examination of all organs one-by-one systematically. In a span of 45 years of his career, he himself performed 30,000 autopsies and supervised 70,000 autopsies. He had collection of tens of thousands of pathologic specimens. Rokitansky described entities such as acute yellow atrophy of liver to massive hepatic necrosis. His notable contributions are congenital heart disease, bacterial endocarditis, lobar and lobular pneumonia, and pulmonary complications of typhoid. Vienna school of medicine was worldwide recognized because of scientific contributions of Rokitansky; his contribution was published as "Handbook of Pathological Anatomy and Defects in the Septa of the Heart."

Rudolf Ludwig Carl Virchow (1821–1902) was a great pathologist of Berlin (Germany), biologist, prolific writer, an editor, and is known as "The Father of Modern Pathology." When he was appointed as assistant to prosector in the Chariate Hospital, Berlin, he noticed that the working in the autopsy room was disordered. No systematic method for performing autopsy was available. Young untrained surgeons used to perform autopsy and they were not making notes during autopsy. Therefore, for the benefits of beginner in autopsy, Virchow developed simple autopsy technique which was subsequently published in 1876. He studied diseased tissue by microscopic examination and demonstrated that cellular changes are responsible for the development of disease and cellular pathology is the basis of disease. Through microscopy, he made significant contribution for the development of pathology and brought autopsy and pathology to recognizable state. His most important work in the "Cellular Pathology," published in 1858 as a collection of lectures, is regarded as the root of modern pathology. A number of terms are named after him, Virchow's node, Virchow–Robin space, Virchow–Seckel syndrome also known as "bird-headed dwarfism", and Virchow triad. He was first to describe and give names to diseases such as leukemia, embolism, thrombosis, and ochronosis.

Sir William Osler (1849–1919), the giant of clinical medicine, was initially trained for 3 months in Berlin under Virchow and for 5 months in Vienna with Rokitansky. In his era, pathology and autopsy attained the highest position. He performed 800 autopsies, and published papers on autopsy. At McGill University, Montreal, he curated and mounted museum specimens and used this data while writing his textbook "The Principles and Practice of Medicine." He highlighted the importance of pathology for better understanding of medicine. He was among the first to note that aneurysm of aorta was a complication of syphilis. He was among the earliest to show micrococci in the etiology of endocarditis; he also contributed significantly to our understanding of cardiac pathology.

HISTORY OF AUTOPSY IN INDIA

The first medicolegal autopsy in Indian empire was performed on 28th August, 1693, when Mr James Wheeler (Member of Council, Sea Customer and Chief Justice of Choultry) died in Chennai. The progress of pathology in India during British Era began much earlier in preindependence era. The first Bengal medical school was established in 1822 in Calcutta (now renamed as Kolkata) which was converted into a Bengal Medical College (now renamed as Kolkata Medical College) in 1835. In Bengal Medical College, records of creation of the "Pathology Museum" in early 1840 are available. Dr Allen Webb, Professor of Descriptive and Surgical Anatomy, was the main person behind the creation of museum. In those days civilian medical students and medical students of army who passed as graduates, used to perform autopsies and collect specimens of diseased organs. The specimens were collected from the West, the East, from Aden and Singapore, from Moulmein and Lahore, and from the southern confines of the Madras Residency to the Himalayan range. The British Government provided the preservation facility and transportation facility to bring the specimens to Kolkata Medical College to create a pathology museum in 1840. This museum is the central depot of pathological contributions from every part of the British Empire. The descriptions of the specimen are written by Dr Allan Webb, after exposition of parts in the dissecting room, and by the civilian and army doctors. The vast collection of morbid anatomy specimens in the museum, thoroughness of the study and recorded descriptions are simply fascinating. This pathology museum during that time was known to be "one of the finest pathology museums" in the world. Professor Allen Webb subsequently published a book Pathologia Indica: "Anatomy of Indian Diseases" in 1848 (**Fig. 1.1A**). This book contains autopsy notes with short clinical details and treatment prescribed and also has comments on historical and pathophysiological aspects of diseases of different systems of the body.

The review of first edition of the book on the subject of diseased heart and arteries among the native, Parsees, and Hindus, mentions that aneurysm appears to be, if not altogether unknown, a disease of rare occurrence. Hence, remarks as "Are natives of India exempt from aneurysm"? In Southern part of India, Madras Medical College was established in 1835, while in the West, the Grant Medical College was established in Bombay (now renamed as Mumbai) in 1845. The Coroner's act was implemented in Mumbai on January 27, 1871. In the Coroner's system, autopsies were performed 24 hours a day, after obtaining permission from the Coroner's office. The Coroners Act did not apply to the cases in which the death had been caused by cholera or other epidemic diseases. The first clinical postmortem was conducted in the Grant Medical College, Mumbai in January, 1872. Dr Gharpure has published several articles on the autopsy material of GMC and JJH, Mumbai. Dr Gharpure's papers described the incidence of primary carcinoma in India from postmortem records between 1877 and 1926, and also described analysis of postmortem findings of human amebiasis in 426 cases. Currently, The Grant Medical College has preserved autopsy records of 18,578 autopsies from 1884 to 1966. These records are handwritten, contains meticulous descriptions and hand drawings of the pathologic lesions.

Dr MN De, from Kolkata Medical College, studied and published autopsy findings describing pathogenesis of commoner types of splenomegaly met within India" (1938) (**Fig. 1.1B**) and pathologic aspects of "Epidemic Dropsy." In postindependence period (1947–2000), clinical autopsies were performed in all the government run medical colleges and postgraduate institutes. Significant pathological data of nervous system and cardiovascular diseases was published. Recently, Dr Lanjewar et al. described

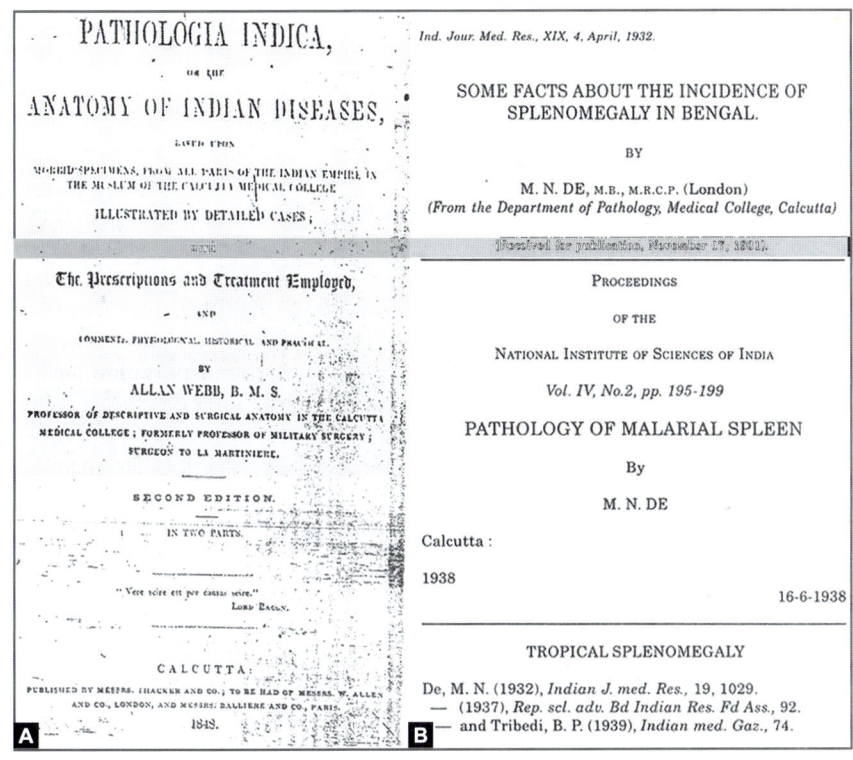

FIGS. 1.1A AND B: (A) Pathologia Indica: Anatomy of Indian Diseases; (B) Publications of Dr MN De.

the largest autopsy report in India from the Department of Pathology, Grant Medical College, and Sir JJ Hospital, Mumbai, wherein autopsy findings of 13,024 adults are described. Currently, 529 medical colleges are providing undergraduate and postgraduate training to several thousand medical students in India. Only 10 out of 529 medical colleges perform clinical autopsies, due to nonperformance of clinical autopsies in many institutes, valuable information is lost; hence, there is a need of reviving clinical autopsy program in India.

FURTHER READING

1. Benivieni A. The Hidden Causes of Disease. Translated by D Singer. Springfield, Ill: Charles C Thomas; 1954.
2. Bichat X. Anatomie generale, appliqué, La physiologie et a la medicine, Vol. 1-4. Paris, Brosson, Gabon, 7 Co; 1801.
3. Bliss M, Osler W. A Life in Medicine. New York: Oxford University Press; 1919. pp. 87.
4. Cary TO. Forensic Hair Comparison: Background Information for Interpretation. Forensic Science Communications. 2009;11(2).
5. Clifton B. Handbook of Death and Dying. California: Sage Publications, Inc.; 2003.
6. Cowles I. Autopsies: Examining the dead to understand the living. [online] Available from https://www.findingdulcinea.com/features/science/milestones/autopsies.html. [Last accessed June, 2020].
7. Crawford DG. A history of Indian Medical service 1600-1913, Vol. II. London: W Thacker & Co. 1914:443-35.

8. Dastur DK, Lalitha VS. The many facets of neurotuberculosis: an epitome of neuropathology. Prog Neuropathol. 1973;2:351-408.
9. De MN, Chatterjee KD. Pathology of epidemic dropsy. Ind Med Gaz. 1935;70:489-93.
10. De MN. Some facts about the incidence of splenomegaly in Bengal. Indian J Med Res. 1932;19:1029.
11. De MN. Trivedi BP. Pathogenesis of the commoner types splenomegaly met within India. Indian Med Gaz Calcutta Med J. 1939;74:9-14.
12. Dodwell H. Records of Fort St. George: Diary and Consultation Book of 1693:128-129. The Superintendent of Government Press; 1921. New York Public Library.
13. Elisabeth SD. "Ancient science and forensics". In: Ayn Embar-Seddon, Allan D Pass (Eds). Forensic Science. Salem, MA: Salem Press; 2008. p. 43.
14. Farber SB. The postmortem examination. Springfield, Ill Charles C Thomas; 1937.
15. GCSE History wiki-Galen. [online] Available from http://gcsehistory.wikispaces.com/galen. [Last accessed June, 2020].
16. Gharpure PV, Saldanha JL. Some observations on human amoebiasis (being an analysis of post-mortem findings in 426 cases). Ind Med Gaz. 1931;66(3):132-5.
17. Gharpure PV. Hundred years of pathology (in the Grant Medical College, Bombay). Antiseptic. 1951;48(5):397-402.
18. Gharpure PV. Incidence of primary carcinoma of the liver and other organs as inferred from autopsy work. 1926–1946. Ind Med Gaz. 1948;83(1):5-6.
19. Gharpure PV. The incidence of primary carcinoma in India as inferred from post-mortem records of fifty years from 1877 to 1926. Ind Med Gaz. 1927;62(6):315-7.
20. Handbuch der pathologischen Anatomie ("Handbook of pathology anatomy", 3 vols; Vienna: Braumullers und Seidel, 1842-1846); English translation by the Sydenham Society, 4 Vols. London.
21. Hill RB, Anderson RE. The recent history of the autopsy. Archives of pathology and laboratory medicine. 1996;120:702-12.
22. Kinare SG. Nonspecific aortitis (Takayasu's disease). Autopsy study of 35 cases. Pathol Microbiol (Basel). 1975;43:134-9.
23. King LS, Meehan MC. A history of the autopsy: a review. Am J Pathol. 1973;73(2):514-44.
24. Lanjewar DN, Sheth NS, Lanjewar SD, Wagholikar UL. Analysis of causes of death as determined at autopsy in a single institute, the Grant Medical College and Sir J. J. Hospital, Mumbai, India, between 1884 and 1966: a retrospective analysis of 13024 autopsies in adults. Arch Pathol Lab Med. 2020;144(5):644-9.
25. Morgagni GB. The Seats and Causes of Diseases, Investigated by Anatomy. Vol 1-3. Alexander B. trans. Mount Kisco, NY: Futura; 1980.
26. Nutton V. [online] Available from https: www.britannica.com//biography/Galen of Pergamum. [Last accessed June, 2020]
27. Osler W. Berlin correspondence. Can Med Surg J. 1874;2:308-15.
28. Osler W. Vienna correspondence. Can Med Surg J. 1874;2:451-6.
29. Porter R. The greatest benefit to mankind: a medical history of humanity from antiquity to the present. London: Fontana Press; 1999.
30. Rodin AE. Osler's autopsies: Their nature and utilization. Med His. 1973;17(1):37-8.
31. Rokitansky. Die Defects der Schidewande des herzen ("Defects in the septa of heart"). Vienna W Braumuller; 1875.
32. Rothenberg K. "The autopsy through history." In: Ayn Embar-Seddon, Allan D Pass (Eds). Forensic Science. Salem, MA: Salem Press; 2008. pp. 100.
33. Talwalkar NG. Men and Memorabilia of Grant Medical College & J. J. group of hospitals. Publisher Research Society, Sir J. J. Group of Hospitals and Grant Medical College, Bombay, 1995.
34. THE CORONERS ACT, 1871. Central Government Act. Chapter III- Duties and Powers of Coroners. Act No. 4 of 1871, 1, 27th January, 1871. [online] Available from https:indiakanoon.org/doc/792853. [Last accessed June, 2020].
35. The Editors of Encyclopaedia Britannica on the topic Autopsy. [online] Available from https:// www.britannica.com/topic/autopsy. [Last accessed June, 2020].

36. The Editors of Wikipedia on the topic Autopsy. [online] Available from https://en.wikipedia.org/wiki/Autopsy. [Last accessed June, 2020].
37. The Egyptians Mummies. [online] Available from https://www.historyonthenet.com/the-egyptians-mummies. [Last accessed June, 2020].
38. Virchow RLK. Description and explanation of the method of Performing Post-mortem Examinations in the Dead House of the Berlin Charite Hospital, with special reference to Medico-Legal Practice. Translated from the 2nd German edition by TP Smith. London: Churchill; 1880.
39. Webb A. Pathologica Indica; or, the Anatomy of Indian Diseases: Based Upon Morbid Specimens, from All Parts of the Indian Empire, in the Museum of the Calcutta Medical Collage. Illustrated by detailed cases, the Prescriptions and Treatment Employed, 2nd edition. London: Messer W Allen and Co. and Paris: Messer Dalliere and Co.; 1848.
40. "Virchow Biography" Berlin Medizinhistorisches Museum der Charite. [online] Available from http://www.biography-center.com/biographies/7415-Virchow-Rudolf. [Last accessed June, 2020].

CHAPTER 2

External Examination at Autopsy

Arvind Valand, Dhaneshwar Lanjewar

INTRODUCTION

Before initiation of postmortem examination, one should thoroughly read clinical history, results of investigations, treatment given, and mode of death. The first step of postmortem procedure is to perform external examination. When patients are hospitalized, findings of general examination are recorded on clinical case papers; during external examination at autopsy, these findings need to be confirmed. When the patient is in the hospital, he/she may show additional signs; these also need to be noted during external examination. Many changes that are noted externally may also mimic antemortem disease hence these should be documented, but interpreted with caution. It often gives significant clues to the pathologists as to which organs of human body are likely to show pathologic lesions and most possible cause of death. External examination should be performed in a well-lighted autopsy room, should be carried out in an orderly fashion, and the findings should be recorded sequentially. Many modern autopsy rooms have voice recorder for recording the findings.

The general points to be noted in the external examination are as below:

- The body built reflects genetic constitution, nourishment, socioeconomic status, and presence of chronic diseases. The corpses can be well built (and at times muscular), averagely built, or poorly built or obese. *Cachexia* is characterized by thin body with loss of muscle mass and fat; it is caused by malnutrition, anorexia nervosa, chronic diseases such as tuberculosis, acquired immunodeficiency syndrome, and malignant tumors particularly those arising from esophagus and stomach. Due to loss of fat and muscle mass, there is hollowness of abdomen, thin camel-like limbs, and dry and sallow skin (**Fig. 2.1A**). In the obese, diseases such as diabetes or other endocrine disorders should be suspected and careful examination of the heart for myocardial infarction and coronaries for atherosclerosis must carried out.

- Height is measured by measuring tape or long ruler; from crown to heel (not up to toes). *Gigantism* can be racial or familial or can be due to endocrine disorders such as pituitary adenoma at a young age, hypogonadism (due to delayed epiphyseal plate fusion). *Acromegaly* is not gigantism; it is characterized by big head, protruding chin, coarse thick skin, and thick lips with large hands, feet, and digits. It is usually produced by increase in growth hormone; and is caused by pituitary adenoma and/or hyperfunctioning of pituitary. *Arachnodactyly* is a hereditary condition, in which long limbs, long fingers, and hyperextensible joints are observed; examination of aorta for dissections or aneurysms in the thoracic segments should be done in arachnodactyly. Short stature is usually constitutional or familial; other causes include endocrine disorders, congenital hypothyroidism, hereditary anemias, renal rickets, cystic fibrosis of pancreas, malabsorption syndromes, and congenital heart diseases. Due to pituitary disorders, the stature is short; the patient has absence of secondary sexual characteristics and small testes, if it is a male. Achondroplasia and osteogenesis imperfecta are responsible for *dwarfism*.
- *Rigor mortis* is muscle rigidity demonstrated by flexing of arms and legs and is first noted in the muscles of the jaw, neck, arms, and feet. It is caused by breakdown of adenosine triphosphate (ATP) to adenosine diphosphate (ADP), which results in contraction of muscle fibers thus producing stiff and rigid muscles. Even after death, this chemical reaction in muscle continues for some time. It begins in 2–4 hours after death and disappears in 24–48 hours and is useful to determine time since death.
- *Changes in the skin*: These can be seen due to underlying diseases as well as postmortem changes. Livor mortis or postmortem lividity (**Fig. 2.1B**) is a bluish black coloration of dependent parts of skin such as back, developing due to gravitational stasis of blood in small superficial vessels; it begins in 30–45 minutes after death. Presence of putrefaction and decomposition should also be noted.

Pallor is pale appearance of not only the skin, but also of the nails and sclerae and is seen in anemias. Cyanosis is blue to black discoloration of the body due to low hemoglobin percentage. Central cyanosis is seen in tongue, tip of nose, skin, nails, tip of fingers, and toes; it indicates presence of cardiac and respiratory diseases. Peripheral cyanosis is indicative of shock. Localized cyanosis is produced due to stagnation of blood in veins. If icterus (yellow discoloration of skin, nails, and sclerae) is present, then examination of liver, biliary system, and pancreas is required. Icterus can also be observed in cases of chronic hemolytic anemias. There is sallow skin in cases of alcoholic cirrhosis, while there may be whitish deposits (uremic frost) in cases of chronic renal failure.

The skin may show hyper- or hypopigmentation. Localized hyperpigmentation is seen in acanthosis nigricans, ochronosis, urticaria pigmentosa, porphyria, Peutz–Jeghers syndrome, heat, irradiation, and neurofibromatosis; distinct and multiple nodularity indicates metastatic melanoma (**Fig. 2.1C**). Generalized hyperpigmentation is seen in Addison's disease, thyrotoxicosis, and hemochromatosis. When hyperpigmentation of skin is identified, it is essential to examine the adrenal glands for causes of their chronic insufficiency. Generalized hypopigmentation is observed in albinism, observed in persons having genetic

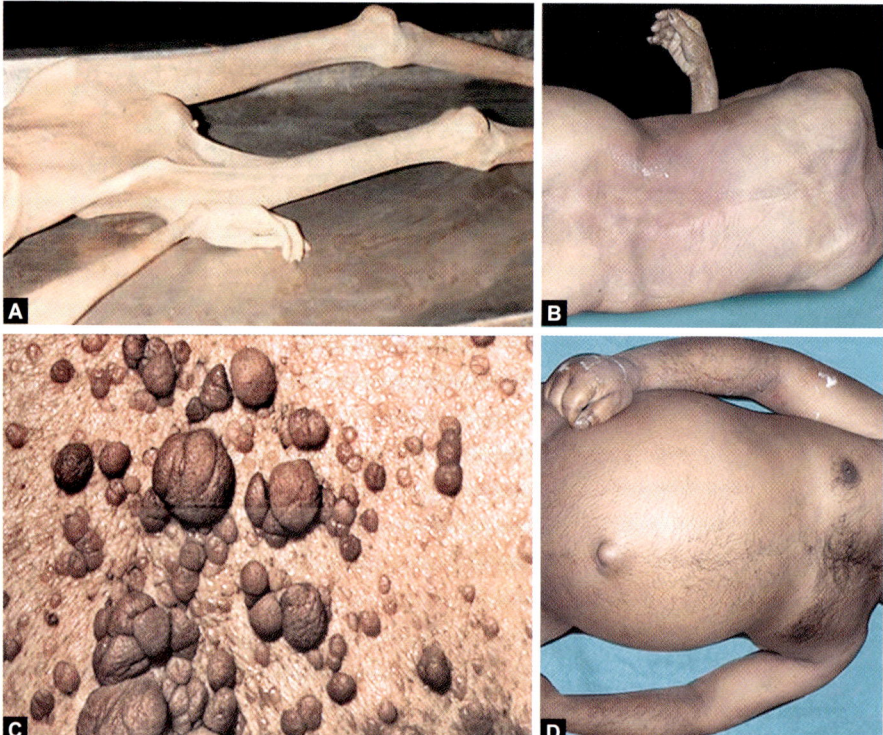

FIGS. 2.1A TO D: (A) Cachexia in an elderly woman due to disseminated cervical cancer. (B) Postmortem lividity on the back. (C) and (D) Gross ascites in a patient with alcoholic liver cirrhosis.
Note: Eversion of the umbilicus and presence of anasarca.
Courtesy: Dr BG Chikhalkar, GGMC, Mumbai.

deficiency of the enzyme tyrosinase. Localized hypopigmentation is seen in the form of vitiligo and leukoderma. It can also be seen in leprosy and fungal diseases; hence, it is important to look for evidence of fungal lesions or leprosy at other places on the skin and in internal organs. Tattooing is decorating body parts by injection of India ink. In ancient times, decorating of body was prevalence in almost all countries. Extensive tattooing is noted in human immunodeficiency virus (HIV)-infected individuals. Diseases such as hepatitis and HIV infection can be transmitted in process of tattooing.
- Injuries, bruises, abrasion, laceration, and skin infections, if present, should be noted. Nowadays, piercings of body parts (apart from ears), are seen at a multiple sites, not only in women but also men. Piercing sites, their numbers, and nature of the jewelry should be noted. Medical intervention and devices such as the presence of tracheostomy, gastrostomy, colostomy, or external pacing wires should be noted in external examination.

  Once general points are noted then examination of corpse should be carried out in a sequential pattern from head to toe.

- Head should be examined for size. A large head is seen in hydrocephalus, while in microcephaly, it is smaller. Examine the head for presence or absence of infections, local tumors, and/or metastatic deposits. The ears should be examined for presence of bleeding; it is suggestive of intracranial bleed. Examination of ear for presence of pus should also be done; it may suggest the presence of pyogenic meningitis. Similarly, examination of mastoid processes for presence of mastoid abscess should be carried out because it may spread to meninges. The eyes are examined for symmetry, exophthalmoses, icterus, Kayser–Fleischer ring, petechial hemorrhages, and tumors. The lips, mouth, teeth, gums, tongue, and nose should be examined for infections, ulcers, and tumors. The face is to be examined for presence of puffiness or presence of any kind of rash. The parotid glands are to be examined for any enlargement or atrophy.
- In the neck, the jugular veins are examined for distention and engorgement (observed in congestive heart failure). The thyroid gland is examined for unilateral or bilateral, diffuse, or nodular enlargement. Even if it is normal, the gland should be removed during dissection for further histopathological study. Similarly, neck should be examined for enlarged cervical and supraclavicular lymph nodes and if found enlarged, then these glands should be removed during dissection. Enlargement of these glands is noted in pyogenic infections, tuberculosis, lymphoma, leukemia, and metastatic deposits. Enlargement of left supraclavicular gland in elderly person indicates the possibility of metastases from a gastric carcinoma. The other sites where examination for enlarged lymph nodes should be carried are the axillary and inguinal regions.
- The upper extremities are examined for unilateral edema, presence of ulcer and tumors. Metastasis of breast carcinoma in axillary lymph nodes can show unilateral edema of hand. In addition, while performing the examination of hands, one must note down congenital abnormalities such as additional digits as it is indicative of anomalies in other organs. The fingers should be examined for presence or absence of gangrene, ulcers, and tumors. Clubbing of fingers shows club-shaped thickening of tip of fingers and toes; it is usually seen in chronic disorders, malignancy, and cyanotic heart diseases. Hence, it is important to look for tuberculosis, bronchiectasis, and malignancy in lungs. Examination of nails should be done for identification of koilonychias, fungal infection, and splinter hemorrhages.
- Thorax should be examined for symmetry and presences of bulges. Asymmetry of chest suggests the possibility of presence of disease process either in lungs and mediastinum. Barrel-shaped chest indicates presence of emphysema. In females, the breasts should be examined and palpated for identification of retracted nipples, ulcers, discharge from the nipple, and presence of firm areas or masses. If tumor is identified, it should be removed from the inside after the skin flaps over the thorax are opened out and subjected to microscopic evaluation. Male breasts should also be examined for gynecomastia, ulcer, and mass lesions. Examination of back of the body is carried out for identifying spinal column deformities and bed sores. Kyphosis is humping of back and is caused by rickets, osteomalacia, and collapse of vertebral bodies due to fracture, tuberculosis, or tumor. Scoliosis a lateral curvature of the spine; it is usually observed in postpoliomyelitis or is

- produced by injury to vertebral bodies. Multiple lipomatosis is observed as nodules and is seen in back and neck in Cushing's disease.
- While performing examination of abdomen, one should note the presence of distension or protuberance. Distensions are due to the presence of fluid (ascites) in peritoneal cavity (**Fig. 2.1D**) or the presence of tumor masses. Distention of abdomen is identified in cirrhosis of liver, bacterial peritonitis, perforation of stomach/intestine, tuberculosis, primary tumors originating in peritoneum or even retroperitoneum, and metastatic tumor deposits. Presence of hernia and dilated veins can also be found in abdominal examination. The genitalia in males and females are examined for presence or absence of sexually transmitted, molluscum contagiosum, tumors, etc. In males, scrotum is examined for hydrocele, gangrene, and size of testis.
- The lower extremities should be examined for unilateral or bilateral edema, ulcers, abscesses, and tumors. Edema can be pitting edema or nonpitting. Pitting edema is mainly seen in cardiac, liver, and kidney disorders while nonpitting edema is seen in filariasis and myxedema. Generalized edema (anasarca) is seen in nephrotic syndrome, anaphylaxis, starvation, liver disorder, and beriberi. Edema of face, arms, and upper limbs suggests the superior vena cava syndrome. Edema of limbs, scrotum, vulva is observed in cardiac diseases, compression of inferior vena cava, and thrombophlebitis. Unilateral edema of feet is noted in filariasis, metastasis in inguinal lymph nodes, and lymphoma of inguinal lymph nodes. The toes should be examined for tropical ulcers, gangrene, and autoamputation.

FURTHER READING

1. Baker RD. Postmortem examination, specific methods and procedures. Philadelphia and London: WB Saunders Company; 1967.
2. Burton JL, Rutty GN (Eds). The Hospital Autopsy. New York: Arnold Publisher; 2001.
3. Camps FE. Establishment of the time of death-a critical assessment. J Forensic Sci. 1959;4:73-82.
4. Gresham GA, Turner AF (Eds). Postmortem procedure (an illustrated textbook). London: Wolf Medical Publication; 1979.
5. Knight B. Medical Jurisprudence and Toxicology. New York: Arnold Publisher; 1990.
6. Knight B. The Post Mortem Technicians Hand Book: A Manual Of Mortuary Practice. London: Blackwell Science Publication; 1984.
7. Lyle HP, Stemmer KL, Cleaveland FP. Determination of time of death. J Forensic Sci. 1959;4:167-75.
8. Rezek PR, Millard M (Eds). Autopsy pathology: A guide for pathologist and clinicians. Springfield, Illinois USA: Charles C Thomas Publication; 1963.
9. Rutty GN (Ed). Essentials in Autopsy practice. London: Springer; 2001.
10. Saphir O. Autopsy Diagnosis and Technique. London: Paul B Hobber Incl.; 1947.
11. Saukko P, Knight B. Knight's Forensic Pathology. London: Arnold Publisher; 2004.

CHAPTER 3

Utility and Techniques of Autopsy

Jaya Deshpande

INTRODUCTION

Western medicine, as we know today, has developed in a large measure due to the insights into connections between patient's clinical symptoms and diseased organs found at death. Though benefits of autopsy to the practice and science of medicine continue to be vast, there has been a steady decline in autopsy rates in the last 50 years. In general, the primary use of autopsy has been the determination or confirmation of the cause and mechanism of death, and this leads to improvement in the practice of medicine through application of autopsy findings to clinical practice.

In the modern era, autopsy has played a critical role in understanding newly diagnosed diseases, such as acquired immunodeficiency syndrome (AIDS), Ebola virus infections, severe acute respiratory syndrome (SARS), and Lyme disease, by allowing investigators to correlate tissue changes with epidemiologic and clinical data. Specialties such as neurology sciences and cardiovascular disorders have progressed and made giant strides due to contributions from autopsy services. The autopsy continues to provide new insights into diseases such as Alzheimer. Research in Alzheimer and dementia is progressing due to establishment of National Repository, which provides biological material and data for studies in such fields. This is done by establishing brain banks—human brain tissue repository (HBTR) worldwide to promote research in neurobiology using human nervous tissues. Newer developing specialties such as transplants and fetal autopsies are emerging areas of new dimensions in autopsy services with additional tools like molecular studies. There has been an increase in the rates of terminations of pregnancy for fetal anomaly. When a prenatal diagnosis is based on the results of scan only, the additional information from an autopsy by a pediatric pathologist can be important. In published data (Boyd et al. 2004), autopsy findings changed the estimated risk of recurrence in 27% cases and in 8% this was to higher risk strata. Shankar and Phadke (2008) in their study of fetal autopsy confirmed the utility of such procedure particularly with regards to genetic counseling of the affected couple. Also, the ever-expanding horizon of transplant surgery also needs the services of a good autopsy service with experienced pathologists and clinician participating in the autopsy program.

Today molecular studies can be done using paraffin-embedded tissue samples. Even archival material can be utilized for molecular analysis. In cases of sudden unexpected deaths, genetic analysis may be of use to identify inherited genetic causes, so that counseling of the family may prevent further such casualties. With use of gene therapy and genetic modulation, autopsy material will help in understanding disease patterns and the changes brought about by gene therapy.

Furthermore, the medical field ensures the quality of their services in part by continuously backing up clinical diagnoses with a pathological diagnosis. In studies spanning many decades, authors have found that autopsy has added value in 11–21% cases with serious undiagnosed findings, which could affect clinical outcome and management. Roulson et al. (2005) also carried out a meta-analysis to identify the value of autopsy histology and discrepancies between clinical and autopsy diagnosis. In a College of American Pathologists (CAP) survey of 248 institutions in US, in 40% autopsies, there was at least one unexpected finding that contributed to the patient's death. In the Indian scenario, a few recent studies have shown that discrepancy rates between antemortem and postmortem findings ranged from 23 to 45%. These data in a simple way are a form of audit and a measurement of quality assurance of medical diagnostics and service. It also re-emphasizes the importance of autopsy as an essential part of medical services.

It is often felt that Hi-tech diagnostic tools make autopsy superfluous and redundant. However, the impact of imaging/ancillary tests still remains unproven. Many studies have highlighted that discrepancies in diagnosis were due to misleading diagnostic test results. Today the potential use of autopsies goes beyond a simple audit and teaching aid. There is also a definite use in postgraduate teaching programs. The benefits of autopsy, therefore, are manifold such as:

- Quality assurance of medical diagnostics and service.
- Reservoir of tissue for research and education both for physicians and for the public.
- To develop accurate mortality statistics.
- Early identification of environmental infections and occupational hazards to health.
- Evaluation of new forms of therapy and diagnostics modalities.
- Information documentation for future legal, financial, and medical evaluation.

In spite of such apparent benefits of autopsy, today the autopsy rates continue to be dismal with a falling trend. The decline has been ongoing for the last 50 years, with <15% cases being subjected to autopsy in the US. The Joint Commission for hospital accreditation has eliminated autopsy as a requirement.

Various publications from 1988 to 2013 have noted discrepancy in diagnosis ranging from 11 to 45%. This wide range of figures is due to the different modalities of study. The hospital administration facing financial constraints does not often support such nonremunerative procedures. Moreover, most clinicopathological meetings are poorly attended; autopsies are performed by the junior most staff with inordinate delays in completing autopsy studies. Lack of investigative autopsy tools results in many unanswered questions. An in-depth audit of autopsy may help to reduce this trend and improve quality of autopsy services, making it once more an essential part of any hospital service.

PRELIMINARY SKIN INCISIONS

Before commencement of the autopsy, the general examination of the body (Chapter 2) should be carried out as meticulously as one would perform the general examination of a patient before systemic examination. Even in the absence of detailed clinical history, a lot of information can be made available by a thorough external examination that will provide clues about ongoing and pre-existing diseases. The preliminary body incision depends on local institutional customs and needs. The incision should provide maximum exposure, permit adequate reconstruction at the end of the procedure, and the incision should be safe for the prosectors.

In complete autopsy, the incisions for opening the thoracic and abdominal cavities are essentially I, T, Y, or I with a U-shape on the top part of the incision (**Figs. 3.1A to D**). The most common type of incision generally followed is a straight

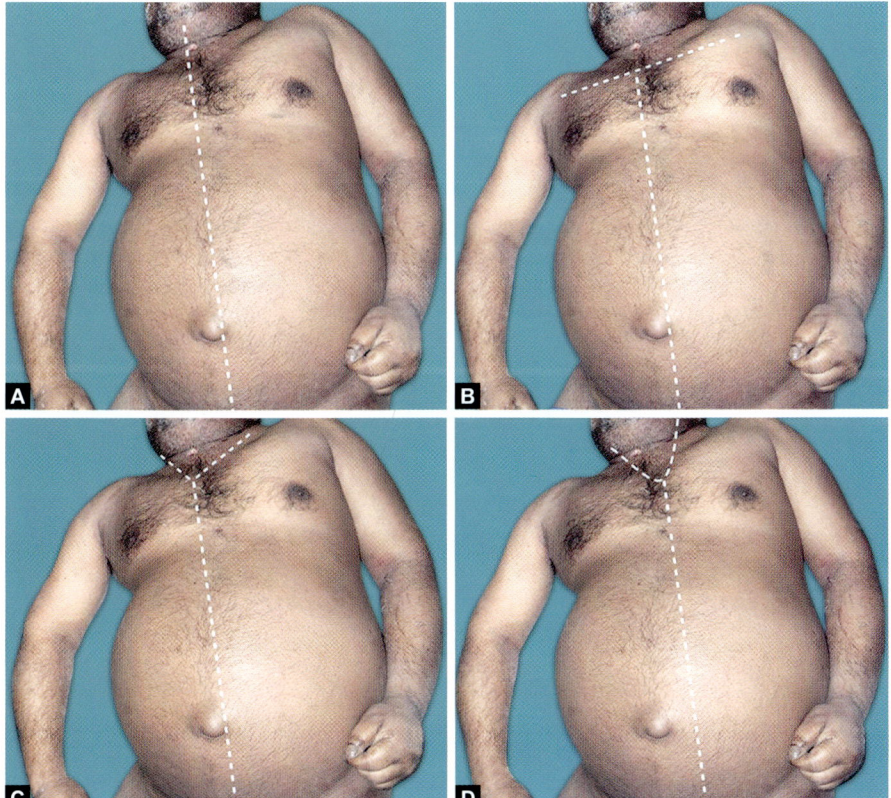

FIGS. 3.1A TO D: The incisions for opening the thoracic and abdominal cavities. (A) I-shaped; (B) T-shape; (C) Y-shape; and (D) I-shape with a U-shaped on the top part of the incision.

line incision from the chin to symphysis pubis, going around the umbilicus on the left. A T-shaped incision begins at the shoulders, meets at the level of sternum, and is extended incision up to the symphysis pubis. A Y/U-shaped incision starts 1 cm behind external auditory meatus, along the lateral aspect of neck, crosses the clavicle to meet the opposite side incision at the sternal angle. The incision is then followed downward along the midline to the symphysis pubis. Whatever may be the type of incision, the body is placed supine with a block under the shoulders to extend the neck. The preliminary incision is made after positioning the body thus.

A complete autopsy is the best method, but limited autopsy can be offered as a substitute to overcome resistance on the part of relations or where there are hazards of infections. Limited autopsy may focus on an organ or body cavity, which is primarily suspected. Where only a limited autopsy is permitted, the autopsy may be restricted to the abdomen, chest, or skull. For opening only the abdomen, a midline incision extends from xiphisternum to symphysis pubis, with a T-shaped subcostal incision. The skin flaps so produced allow safe and wide access to the abdominal and pelvic cavity. If the diaphragm is cut and separated, one may gain access to thoracic organs also. If the autopsy is limited to the chest, the incision extends from the suprasternal notch to the xiphisternum. The rib cage is cut in the usual manner and thoracic cavity is exposed. The diaphragm can be cut to provide access to the abdominal organs. For opening of the skull cavity (refer to Chapter 5).

OPENING OF THE THORACIC AND ABDOMINAL CAVITIES

The skin and muscles are dissected from the chest wall taking care not to disrupt the intercostal muscles. Presence of pneumothorax can be tested at this point. If indicated, breast examination is to be carried out when it is freed from the ribcage. One can palpate the breast internally for lumps and cysts. If necessary, the breast can be sliced internally at 1 cm intervals and followed up to the axillary tail. Care is to be taken that the skin is not incised.

Before opening the chest cavity, the abdominal cavity should be laid open (**Fig. 3.2**). The abdominal skin and fat are reflected to display the abdominal organs. If the abdominal skin is thick, the fat needs to be cut to gain access to the organs (particularly in obese individuals). Any fluid within the abdominal cavity should be noted and quantity and quality of fluid should be observed. Some fluid can be collected for detailed biochemical and cytological examination. For opening the chest cavity, the sternoclavicular joints are first disarticulated with a long blade or bone shears. The rib cage can be separated by cutting through the costochondral cartilages. This can be done with a bread knife or bone shears. The ribs are separated up to the 1st rib, which is initially left intact. The chest contents are inspected. Any fluid collection in the pleural cavity is collected, measured for quantity and collected for biochemical and cytological examination. Another method for opening the chest cavity is the use of a lateral incision from the sternocleidomastoid along the anterior axillary line. Rib shears are used to cut the ribs. This provides a wider window with fewer shape edges. The anterior rib cage is detached and reflected, care being taken not to damage underlying structures. The cut ends of the ribs are covered by the skin flaps or with cloth to prevent sharp injuries to the prosector.

Utility and Techniques of Autopsy

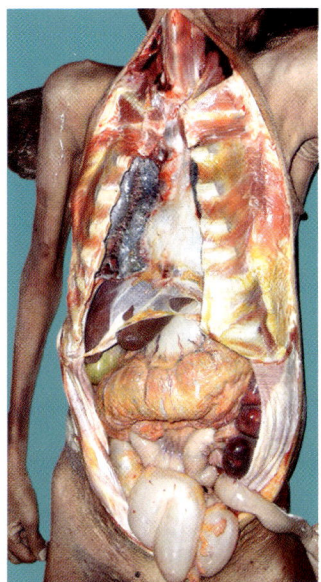

FIG. 3.2: Thoracic and abdominal viscera seen after the I-shaped incision and further dissection.

The intercostal muscles are cut so that underlying adhesions can be cut and lungs pushed away from parietal pleura. The cuts should be superficial and gentle. Loose adhesions are easily separated by blunt dissections while more dense adhesion may be difficult, and one needs to find a plane of cleavage for blunt dissections. Dense adhesions are often seen in healed tuberculosis, chronic lung diseases, or tumors. While disarticulating the sternum from the clavicle considerable force may be used and care should be taken so that underlying important vascular structures are not damaged.

TECHNIQUES OF EVISCERATION

En Masse

This was originally described by Letulle. This involves removal of all organs from neck downward in one swoop. Start the dissection from under the chin, getting a plane along the mandible ridge. One can then pull the tongue out along with nasopharynx and detach the aerodigestive tract along the vertebral column by a scalpel or blade. As you go down, separate the diaphragm from its attachment to the ribs. Retract the thoracic organs and detach the abdominal organs as a block up to the pelvis. Reach down into the pelvis and tie the rectum with a stout thread before cutting it. Likewise the bladder neck is also cut. The entire block of thoracic organs and abdominal organs is thus made available. It provides a bulky mass of organs, which can subsequently be dissected out. It is a rapid technique, but requires practice. It keeps the relationships between various organs intact. Pathologies occurring on both sides of the diaphragm can be best demonstrated by this method. It is followed in perinatal autopsies, as the block of organs is smaller. An inexperienced prosector may find the entire block removal and subsequent dissection a daunting task. There are several ways of separating the organs. In Ghon's method, organ blocks are separated for further detailed examination. Sometimes, the site of interest/main lesion is first dissected out. In the Saphir's method, the retroperitoneal vessels (descending aorta and inferior vena cava) are first dissected, followed by removal of adrenal glands, urogenital tract, and then esophagus and finally thoracic and abdominal organs are dissected out. Whichever way is followed, it is advisable to separate the intestinal loops before further separation is attempted.

Virchow's Method

It is to remove each organ individually one-by-one and then subsequent carry out dissection. This method is quick, but difficult to study relationships of various organs and lesions.

Rokitansky Method

This involves in situ dissection. The method is not very satisfactory, but can be used, if highly transmissible disease is suspected.

Other Autopsy Techniques

Since consent for autopsy by dissection is often difficult to obtain immediately after death, few institutions advocate imaging as a method of noninvasive autopsy. Few studies are in progress evaluating the effectiveness of magnetic resonance imaging (MRI) and computed tomography (CT) in adult death, especially in the backdrop of cultural and religious objections. However, both are expensive tools and it remains an incomplete modality of autopsy since no microbiological culture studies are possible, no histological studies can be done and spatial resolution is not possible. However, it can be best used as an option in special circumstances. Few studies have proposed endoscopic/laparoscopic/thoracoscopic collection of tissue samples. It is believed to be of value in trauma-related death, but less sensitive in nontraumatic causes of death. Needle biopsies of various organs can offer some information as to the cause of death. Huston (1996) has observed that needle autopsy could provide a diagnosis in 67% cases. The advantage is that tissue samples are fresh and samples for microbiology can also be collected.

FURTHER READING

1. Boyd PA, Tondi F, Hicks NR, Chamberlain PF. Autopsy after termination of pregnancy for fetal anomaly: retrospective cohort study. BMJ. 2004;328(7432):137.
2. Huston BM, Malouf NN, Azar HA. Percutaneous needle autopsy sampling. Modern Pathol. 1996;9(12):1101-7.
3. Landefeld CS, Chren MM, Myers A, Geller R, Robbins S, Goldman L. Diagnostic yield of the autopsy in a university hospital and a community hospital. N Engl J Med. 1988;318(19):1249-54.
4. Medscape. (2019). Autopsy quality metrics. [online] Available from https://emedicine.medscape.com/article/1701295-overview [Last accessed June, 2020].

5. Roberts IS, Benamore RE, Benbow EW, Lee SH, Harris JN, Jackson A, et al. Post-mortem imaging as an alternative to autopsy in the diagnosis of adult deaths: a validation study. Lancet. 2012;379(9811):136-42.
6. Roulson J, Benbow EW, Hasleton PS. Discrepancies between clinical and autopsy diagnosis and the value of post mortem histology: a meta-analysis and review. Histopathology. 2005;47(6):551-9.
7. Sankar VH, Phadke SR. Clinical utility of fetal autopsy and comparison with prenatal ultrasound findings. J Perinatol. 2006;26(4);224-9.
8. Sarode VR, Datta BN, Banerjee AK, Banerjee CK, Joshi K, Bhusnurmath B, et al. Autopsy findings and clinical diagnoses: a review of 1,000 cases. Hum Pathol. 1993;24(2):194-8.
9. Sebire NJ, Weber MA, Thayyil S, Mushtaq I, Taylor A, Chitty LS. Minimally invasive perinatal autopsies using magnetic resonance imaging and endoscopic postmortem examination ("keyhole autopsy"): feasibility and initial experience. J Matern Fetal Neonatal Med. 2012;25(5):513-8.
10. Shanks JH, McCluggage G, Anderson NH, Toner PG. Value of the necropsy in perioperative deaths. J Clin Pathol. 1990;43(3):193-5.

CHAPTER 4

In situ Examination

Dhaneshwar Lanjewar

INTRODUCTION

In situ examination is the process of the examination of surfaces and coverings of the organs and the organs itself when they are in their normal anatomical position. A careful in situ examination gives clues to the pathologists of appropriate dissection to find out pathology in various organs and to know the cause of death. During in situ examination, all the body cavities are examined.

EXAMINATION OF CRANIAL CAVITY

After cutting through skull bone, the skull cap is removed; the cranial cavity and dura are visible. Examine inner surface of the skull and external surface of dura mater for the presence of metastatic tumors. Metastasis in skull and dura is commonly observed in carcinomas of breast, prostate, lung and thyroid, and head and neck cancer. Also, examine dura for presence or absence of hemorrhages on its surface (extradural/epidural hemorrhage). An extradural hemorrhage is bleeding between the inside of the skull and the outer covering of the brain. The confirmation of extradural hemorrhage can be done by scraping hemorrhagic area with the blunt end of scalpel. If blood clots come out with the scraping, it is extradural hemorrhage. It is most frequently associated with head injury, vascular malformations, and in patients with hemorrhagic diathesis. Remove the dura and palpate the superior sagittal sinus. Normally, the superior sagittal sinus is collapsed as blood in it is fluid; however, if it feels cord-like, it indicates presence of thrombosis. Thrombi are commonly observed in deaths occurring during pregnancy, puerperium, polycythemia, meningitis, middle ear infection, mastoiditis, sickle cell anemia, thyrotoxicosis, homocystinuria, dehydration, etc. Such thrombi can lead to hemorrhagic venous infarcts. After removal of the dura, surface of the brain is examined for presence of subdural hemorrhages. Presence of subdural hemorrhage can be also confirmed by scraping the hemorrhage with knife; if scraping shows blood clot, then it is subdural hemorrhages and if scraping does not show blood clot, it is subarachnoid hemorrhage. Subarachnoid hemorrhage, which occurs between arachnoid and pia, is most commonly seen in hypertensives, head injuries, arteriovenous malformations, berry aneurysms, bleeding disorders, use of blood thinners, etc. Normally leptomeninges are thin, shiny, and clear. Superior surface of brain is examined for flattening of gyri and narrowing of sulci; if these are noted, it indicates presence of brain edema. Yellowish green exudates on the superior surface of the brain along with congested meningeal vessels indicate presence of pyogenic meningitis. Once pyogenic meningitis is identified, it is necessary to search for primary source of infection reaching to meninges such as skin infection/abscess, otitis media, pneumonia, and infective endocarditis. Plastic membrane like exudates and presence of tubercles along the course of blood vessels indicates tuberculous meningitis. The meninges in cryptococcal meningitis appear hazy and glistening and when fingers are gently moved over meninges, a slippery feel is felt. Intense gray appearance of the brain indicates cerebral malaria. Localized swelling of cerebral hemisphere results in asymmetry and suggests space-occupying lesion, which can be inflammatory or neoplastic. Noninflammatory lesions of brain such as infarcts are soft to feel while brain tumor is firm to feel. The inferior surface of the brain is examined for atherosclerosis, thrombosis, and aneurysm of circle of Willis, plastic membrane such as exudates in tuberculous meningitis, and herniation of unci, cingulate gyri, and cerebellar tonsils.

PERICARDIAL CAVITY

One should look for position of the heart. Note down the size of the heart and examine the layers of the pericardium. Cut the parietal pericardium and examine the pericardial fluid. Normal pericardial fluid is 5–50 mL in quantity; it is clear or pale yellow. Note down excessive fluid, which may be transudate (as in pericardial effusion, **Fig. 4.1A**), exudate, or even frank blood (hemopericardium). When purulent pericarditis is identified (**Figs. 4.1B** and **C**), then there is a need to carry out microbiological study of the pus in the pericardial sac. If hemopericardium is identified, it is usually occurs as a result of rupture of the myocardium or intrapericardial great arteries (particularly the ascending aorta). Note the position of apex and size of the heart. Palpate the pulmonary artery; a cord-like feel indicates the presence of pulmonary embolism. Give a Y-shaped incision in the pulmonary trunk, if embolus is present, it can be seen clearly. If embolus is not identified, through Y incision, insert little finger into right and left branches of pulmonary artery and if firm feeling is felt to the tip of finger, then it confirms the presence of embolus. Petechial hemorrhages on heart are seen in thrombocytopenia, sudden hypoxia, blunt trauma on chest, leukemia, and septicemia. Examine the heart for metastatic deposits; usually in such cases, primary sites of tumor are melanoma, mediastinal tumor, and cancer of colon, prostate, urothelial carcinoma, and lymphoma. Aneurysm of ascending aorta can also be identified at in situ examination of thoracic cavity.

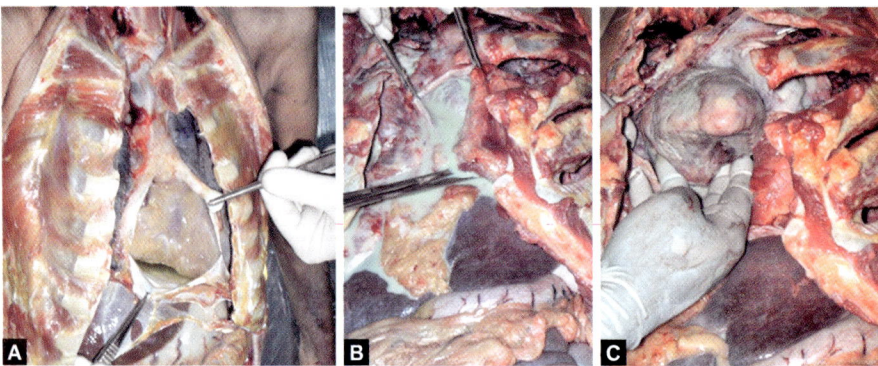

FIGS. 4.1A TO C: (A) Amber-colored slightly hazy fluid in a case of pericardial effusion. (B) Incision of the parietal pericardium has resulted in an outpouring of pus that was present in the pericardial cavity. (C) The visceral pericardium showing yellowish white shaggy purulent exudates: A case of pyogenic/suppurative pericarditis or pyopericardium.

PLEURAL CAVITY AND LUNGS

In varied pathologic conditions, transudates/exudates accumulate in the pleural cavities. Transudate is clear watery fluid and its accumulation is noted in congestive cardiac failure, hypoproteinemia, cirrhosis, end-stage renal disease, nephrotic syndrome, etc. The character of exudates is fibrinous, serofibrinous, and purulent and may be caused by bacterial, viral, fungal, and protozoal infections, but is also seen in acute rheumatic fever and collagen vascular diseases. In empyema thoracis, collection of pus is observed in pleural cavity. Pre-existing pleural effusion is required for the development of empyema. Hemorrhagic effusion is noted in primary pleural or lung cancers and also in metastatic disease. In situ examination of lungs is done for identification of collapse of lung, pleuritis, bronchopneumonia, lobar pneumonia, miliary tubercles, pulmonary infarcts, and hemorrhages and for the presence of pleural mesothelioma and metastatic deposits. The diaphragm should be examined for congenital defects through which contents of abdominal cavity (stomach, intestines, **Fig. 4.2A**) enter into the thoracic cavity. Inspect the inner part of the thoracic cage for any pathology (**Fig. 4.2B**).

ABDOMINAL CAVITY

With the first postmortem incision, the presence of excess fluid (ascites) in the peritoneal cavity is noted. Normally, 50 mL of clear pale yellow fluid is present in the peritoneal cavity. The collected fluid can be transudate or exudate. Transudate is usually seen in cirrhosis of liver. Some variation in the fluid may be encountered.

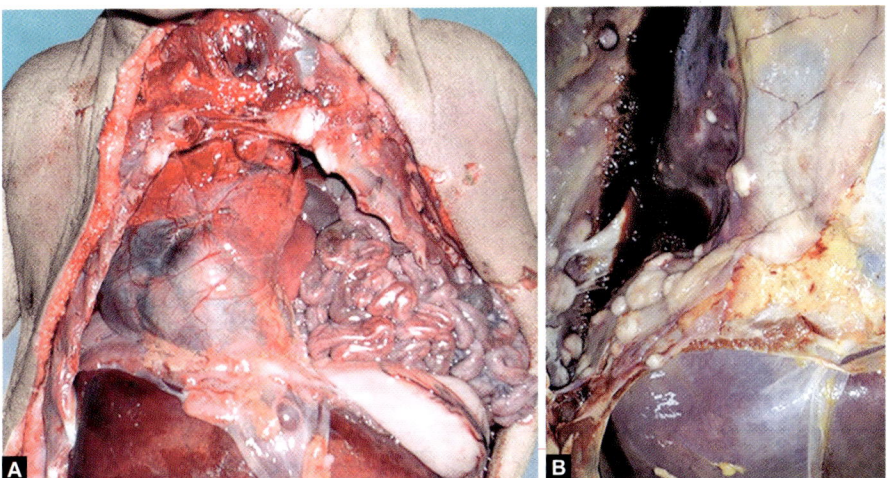

FIGS. 4.2A AND B: (A) Congenital diaphragmatic hernia with coils of small intestine within the left thoracic cavity. This has displaced the left lung and heart. (B) The right lung has been pulled toward the left side of the thoracic cage to show the hemorrhagic effusion and multiple metastatic nodules present on the inner surface of the chest wall.

The fluid will be yellow or green when jaundice is present and is generally blood tinged when caused by tuberculosis or malignancy of the peritoneum. The volume of ascites can reach up to 20 L giving abdomen the appearance of term pregnancy with the diaphragm pushed up high. In such cases, the superficial veins of the abdominal wall are prominent and the umbilicus is everted. In acute peritonitis, the abdomen is distended due to the presence of purulent exudate and it can be seen with infections, with or without perforations of the intestines.

Bleeding into peritoneum can be observed in bleeding disorders and due to ruptures of large retroperitoneal hematomas. A massive pelvic hematoma may occur before or during pregnancy or after delivery. Gangrene of the intestine can also be identified during in situ examination. For peritoneal nodules, differential diagnosis of peritoneal nodules metastasis of carcinoma, tuberculosis, and fat necrosis must be considered. Metastases (from stomach, colon, gall bladder, ovary, and pancreas) and tuberculosis produce rigid greater omentum, which spreads out in a flat thick cake-pattern, and dense adherence of loops of intestines (**Fig. 4.3A**). There is also associated mesenteric lymphadenopathy. With mucin-producing tumors, there may be accumulation of abundant mucin in the peritoneal cavity (pseudomyxoma peritonei). The liver and spleen can be seen in the *in situ* examination only in cases of moderate to marked enlargement (**Fig. 4.3B**). After removal of the coils of the intestines, the retroperitoneal structures, such as the kidneys, pancreas, and vertebral column are palpated for any pathology.

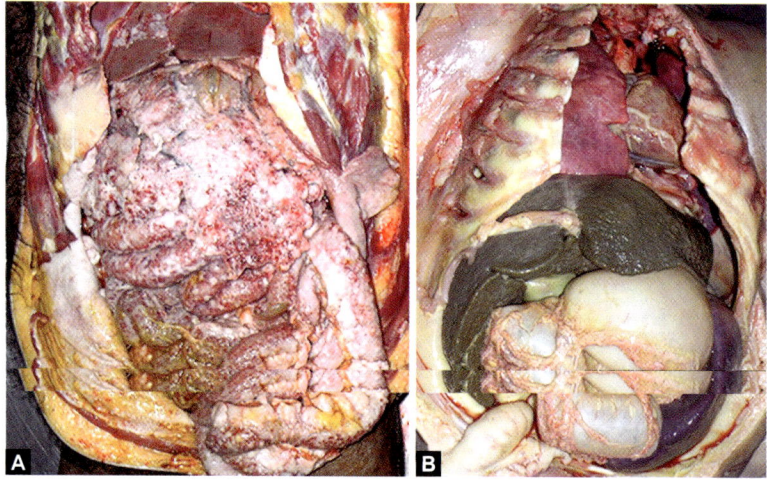

FIGS. 4.3A AND B: (A) An icing of gray-white tissue has produced complete plastering of the greater omentum with associated adherence of intestinal loops. These cannot be separated by blunt dissection. (B) An enlarged green, obviously cirrhotic liver along with enlarged spleen is seen as an in situ finding.

FURTHER READING

1. Baker RD. Postmortem examination, specific method and procedure. Philadelphia and London: WB Saunders Company; 1967.
2. Burton JL, Rutty GN. The Hospital autopsy, 2nd edition. New York: Arnold Publisher; 2001.
3. Chiari H. Pathologisch-anatomische Sektionsteehnik. Berlin: H Kornfeld; 1894.
4. Farber SB. The Postmortem Examination. USA, Springfield, Ill: Charles C Thomas; 1937.
5. Finkbeiner WE, Ursell PC, Davis RL. Autopsy Pathology: A Manual and Atlas. Philadelphia: Churchill Livingstone; 2004.
6. Gresham GA, Turner AF. Postmortem procedure (an illustrated textbook). London: Wolf Medical Publication; 1979.
7. Knight B. Medical Jurisprudence and Toxicology. New York: Arnold Publisher; 1990.
8. Knight B. The Postmortem Technicians Hand Book: A Manual Of Mortuary Practice. London: Blackwell Science Publication; 1984.
9. Letulle ME. La pratique des autopsies. Paris; C Naud; 1903.
10. Rezek PR, Millard M. Autopsy Pathology: A Guide for Pathologist and Clinicians. Springfield: Charles C Thomas Publication; 1963.
11. Saphir O. Autopsy Diagnosis and Technique. London: Paul B. Hobber Incl.; 1947.
12. Saukko P, Knight B. Knight's Forensic Pathology. London: Arnold Publisher; 2004.
13. Virchow RL. Description and Explanation of the Method of Performing post-mortem Examinations in the Dead House of the Berlin Charite Hospital, with special Reference to medico legal practice. Translated from 2nd edition by TP Smith. London: Churchill, 1880.

5

CHAPTER

Systemic Examination

Bishan Radotra, Pradeep Vaideeswar, Gayathri Amonkar, Anjali D Amarapurkar, Ashim Das, Vinaya Shah, Daksha Prabhat, Shubhangi Agale, Subhash Yadav

5A: Central Nervous System

Bishan Radotra

INTRODUCTION

In clinical practice, autopsy is carried out to confirm clinical diagnosis and bring out pathology not known to clinicians during life. The importance of central nervous system (CNS) autopsy cannot be underestimated. The precise aim of performing a CNS autopsy remains by and large the same as for a general medical autopsy, i.e., to confirm clinical neurological diagnosis, to find out the immediate cause of death, the underlying basic disease, complications of the disease, and its treatment. It is important to remember that a pathologist, at the end of CNS autopsy, should be able to answer the queries of the neurologists or neurosurgeons and also be able to demonstrate a good correlation with clinical and radiological findings. Postmortem examination of the CNS should ideally include examination of the brain, spinal cord (SC), orbital cavities including the eyeballs, paranasal sinuses, the auditory apparatus, other structures at the base of the skull, and samples of peripheral nerves and muscles. However in most places, routinely, only brain is examined and other structures are examined only when a specific request and consent are given.

Before doing an autopsy on CNS, a proper plan should be made. The prosector should go through the clinical notes, imaging, etc., and prepare a list of what all is required to be preserved at the end of autopsy and which areas require a close observation. It is essential to keep the following ready just as in any autopsy procedure: Glass slides for touch imprints, syringes and needles, containers for biochemical investigations, culture bottles for microbes, glutaraldehyde for electron microscopy, media for immunofluorescence and genetic studies, containers for fresh tissue for polymerase chain reaction (PCR), and pencil, pen and other materials for labeling.

BRAIN REMOVAL PROCEDURE

The brain removal is performed on a body placed in a supine position. A 6–8 inch high wooden block, with a groove in the center, is placed under the nape of neck (**Fig. 5.1A**). The hair are parted on either side of an assumed incision line which joins the two mastoids in the coronal plane. A deep incision is made through the whole thickness of the scalp so as to reach the level of bone without removing too much hair (**Fig. 5.1B**). In females, it is better to tie the hair in anterior and posterior half of scalp preferably after combing (**Fig. 5.1C**). The skin and subcutaneous tissue is peeled off by blunt dissection to the level of the eyebrows as anterior flap over the face. Similarly, a posterior flap is made up to the occipital protuberance and folded under the neck. Using a scalpel, the temporalis muscles on either side are cut along the periphery and reflected on the sides.

The skull removal is one of the difficult steps in brain autopsy, although in experienced hands, it does not take much time and effort. It is cut along a line which joins from one temporal fossa to the other, passing anteriorly about two fingers above the orbital ridges. The posterior cut in the skull is made in such a way that forms an angle of about 120° or so with anterior cut and passes above the inion. This would eventually ensure a proper realignment of skull cap after postmortem. The skull can be cut by using a handsaw. In most places, a vibrating bone saw also referred to as "Stryker saw" is used for cutting skull. The vibrating saw should preferably be attached with a bone dust vacuum collector (**Fig. 5.2A**), which prevents bone dust, tissues, and secretions from aerosolizing. Placing a wet towel on skull can be helpful tip to prevent aerosols but it obstructs the full view of working area. The prosector should be more careful while cutting skull and the skin flap in subjects who have had craniotomies and in patients with head trauma, etc. While using the vibrating saw, it is important to gently tilt it from side to side rather than cutting deep at one place. If saw is kept at one place, it tends to penetrate suddenly and damages the brain. It is generally advisable not to cut the inner table of the skull with vibrating saw, which can be achieved with the help of a hammer and chisel (**Fig. 5.2B**). The temporal bones can be cut by tilting the head to the opposite side. Since the dura is usually firmly attached to inner table of the skull, it should be gently separated using either a dura mater elevator or scalpel handle. A gentle pressure with a hook can be applied to lift the skull cap but only after

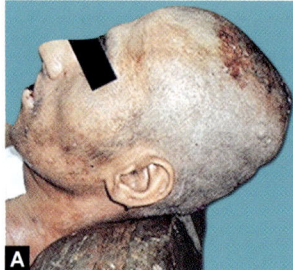 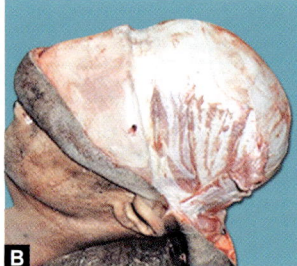 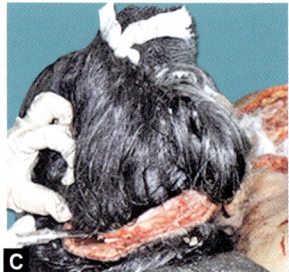

FIGS. 5.1A TO C: (A) A wooden block is placed beneath neck of the deceased; (B) Removal of temporalis muscle by scalpel after reflecting anterior and posterior flaps of scalp; and (C) In females, the parted hair lock can be tied with gauze piece for ease of dissection.

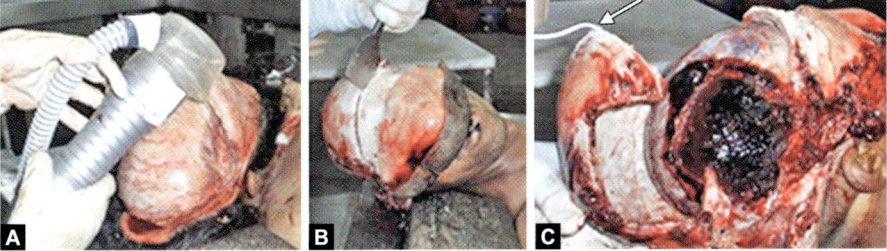

FIGS. 5.2A TO C: (A) The skull cap is being cut with a vibrating saw attached to a vacuum collector; (B) The inner table of the skull is cut with a hammer and chisel to avoid damaging the dura and underlying brain by vibrating saw; and (C) The skull can be gently pulled out antero-posteriorly with a hook (arrow) after separating the dura in order to avoid any damage to underlying brain.

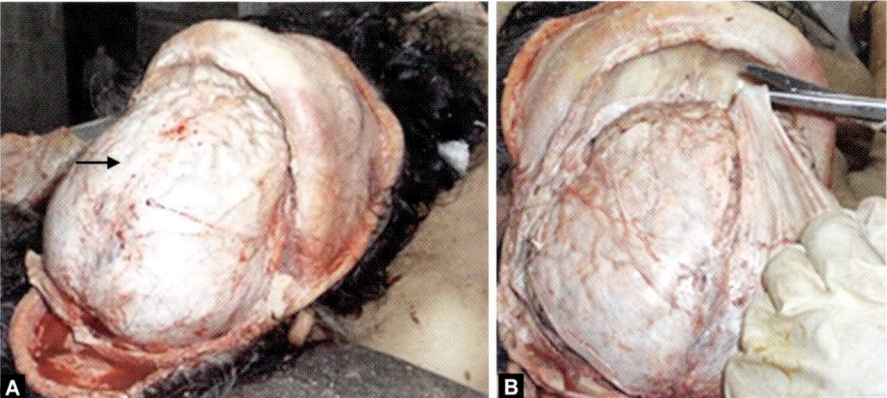

FIGS. 5.3A AND B: (A) The skull cap is removed and the dura is exposed. The superior sagittal sinus runs in the middle of dural covering (arrow); (B) The dura mater is cut with a pair of sharp scissors along parallel to cut edges of the skull.

separating the anterior part of the dura (**Fig. 5.2C**). Forceful pulling the skull from the dura and underlying brain may result in damage.

Removal of the skull cap exposes the dura (**Fig. 5.3A**) where superior sagittal (longitudinal) sinus (SSS) can be palpated for any thrombosis. Any other pathology such as extradural pathology as hematoma, abscess, or tumor deposits is noted. The skull cap is examined at this stage for any pathology as fractures. The superior longitudinal sinus is best left to be opened later after removing dura. Using a pair of scissors, the dura is incised along cut edges of the skull bone except at its anterior (**Fig. 5.3B**) and posterior attachments. Then anterior attachment of the falx to the crista galli is then cut under vision by retracting two frontal lobes posteriorly. The dura can now be pulled back along with falx cerebri and any attachment in the midline such as superficial cortical veins entering SSS are severed with scalpel. It is allowed to hang freely near its posterior attachment. Damage to leptomeninges must be avoided during all preceding maneuvers while cutting dura. It cannot be overemphasized that even though the leptomeninges are thin structures, they hold the brain parenchyma very well. An edematous brain or a softer brain resulting from various acute pathological processes is very likely to pour out through damaged leptomeninges.

After removal of dura, the brain is removed by using minimum number of instruments. The frontal lobes are lifted from the anterior cranial fossa using left hand fingers which expose the optic nerves. These are cut by a scalpel at its exit into the cranium (**Fig. 5.4A**). The infundibulum of pituitary is then cut. Subsequently, the internal carotid arteries, the third, fourth, and fifth cranial nerves are cut where they enter the skull. The next step is to separate the temporal lobes from middle cranial fossa which is done by inserting fingers beneath them. The tentorium cerebelli on either side is now cut under direct vision either by a long-handed scissors or scalpel. It is preferable to start from the hiatus and proceed posteriorly as close as possible to the petrous ridge of temporal bone (**Fig. 5.4B**). During this procedure, due care should be taken not to pull the brain too much so as to avoid damage to midbrain. The rest of the cranial nerves are then cut close to their exit points. The vertebral arteries and cervical SC are cut as low as possible below the level of the foramen magnum (**Fig. 5.4C**). If all

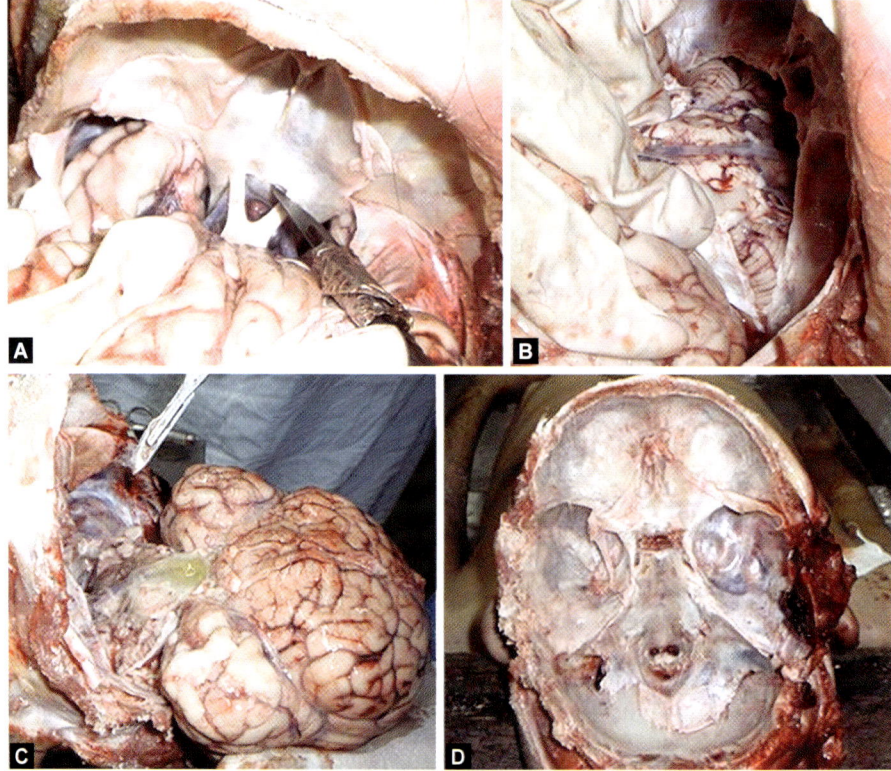

FIGS. 5.4A TO D: (A) The lifting of frontal lobes exposes optic nerves which should be cut close to its exit in the skull; (B) The tentorium cerebella are being used to expose the posterior fossa; (C) The lower cranial nerves and medulla or cervical cord should be cut under vision; and (D) Examination of base of skull after stripping the basal dura.

the structures at the base are cut, the brain can be delivered now in the left hand; tilting the head backward and a few jolts at the chin may be required. If brain does not come out, look for any remaining attachments which should be cut. Lastly, the posterior dural attachment is severed. The weight of the unfixed brain is recorded.

The base of skull (**Fig. 5.4D**) is examined after stripping the basal dura using a bone forceps. The base of skull is inspected for any fractures in cases of head trauma, infective pathology, venous thrombosis, tumors and status of the pituitary fossa and the parasellar regions, the internal auditory meatuses, the cribriform plates, the orbits, the openings of the cranial nerves, and the internal carotid arteries. Using a saw and chisel, the pathological structures are cut along with some normal bone. The skull fractures can be easily missed, if dura is not peeled off. The pituitary is removed at this stage by breaking the dorsum sella by a hammer and a chisel along its upper anterior surface. It will expose the diaphragm of the sella turcica which is held by a toothed forceps and cut along its margins with a pair of scissors. Pulling the diaphragm raises the pituitary gland, which can then be taken out by scooping it out by sharp dissection. In cases of pituitary pathology, e.g., tumors, the sellar fossa with adjacent structures can be cut out using a saw.

EXAMINATION OF THE BRAIN BEFORE FIXATION

Many a times, the prosector is in a hurry to immerse the brain in formalin for fixation. This is out of apprehension and lack of plan for brain autopsy. It is important to take a quick look at the unfixed brain and record baseline findings (**Fig. 5.5A**). At this stage, samples for investigation are taken depending upon the clinical diagnosis and gross appearance of the brain at autopsy. Cerebrospinal fluid (CSF) from the lateral ventricle can be obtained at this stage by passing a long needle through frontal lobes convexity. This can be used for determining antigen and antibody levels in the fluid. In cases of meningitis and subdural empyema, microbiological examination from visible exudates should be sent for culture. One should take tiny fresh tissue rather than swabs from the exudates; however, care should be taken not to damage the brain in anyway. The frontal lobes can be chosen for biochemical estimations which require larger tissues. Samples of brain tissue should be taken for RNA/DNA extraction for further molecular and genetic studies. Small fresh pieces of brain tissues from hippocampus/cerebellum should be sent immediately to virology department in cases suspected of viral encephalitis and rabies. For electron microscopy (EM) in viral encephalitis, few millimeters of tissue in glutaraldehyde including gray as well as white matter could be taken at this stage. Larger chunks should be avoided for EM because they may not fix adequately and tissue preservation is compromised. In cases of subarachnoid hemorrhage and cerebral arterial aneurysms, examination of circle of Willis and proximal parts of the main arteries should be done in fresh state because it is easier to wash off the blood with a gentle stream of water. The aneurysmal walls are usually fragile and a planned and deliberate dissection is required. After formalin-fixation, the blood clots become too hard which are difficult to do dissect. The demonstration of deeper aneurysms and their relationship to the hemorrhage, if any, is best avoided at this stage and better confirmed by serial slicing after fixation.

FIXATION OF THE BRAIN

The brain is fixed by suspending it in a bucket containing large volume of 20% formalin for about 10–15 days. A strong thread is passed under the basilar artery. Immerse the brain in a bucket containing fixative and tie the thread to both sides of bucket handle (**Fig. 5.5B**). Do not use cotton or gauze-piece to wrap the brain; rather put enough formalin to cover the brain surface so as to avoid drying artifacts. The brain should not touch the bottom or sides of the bucket otherwise it distorts its shape during fixation (**Fig. 5.5C**). The dura should not be left attached to the brain while fixation.

REMOVAL OF THE SPINAL CORD

The SC can be removed either by anterior approach or by a posterior approach. The latter is time consuming and painstaking and necessitates cutting of spinal muscles and vertebral bodies. However, many prefer this approach, as it allows removal of entire cord under direct vision. The anterior approach exposes the spinal canal by cutting vertebral column anteriorly after the removal of thoracic and abdominal organs. This is relatively easy but exposure of spinal canal is not optimal.

For posterior approach the body is placed in prone position. The vertebral column needs to be fully flexed and, therefore, wooden blocks are placed under the abdomen and the anterior surface of the neck. A sharp midline incision is given from the level of foramen magnum to the tip of coccyx and skin is reflected on either side. The paraspinal muscles are cut to expose spinal processes. A preliminary cut is made all along the laminae on either side using vibrating saw. The direction of the cutting has to be changed according to the angles of the laminae. A bone forceps should be used for cutting individual vertebral laminae. The sacral canal is better exposed with the help of a hand saw. Trauma to the cord is avoided at all stages and, therefore, one has to be patient. The SC is removed with intact dural sac.

After opening the spinal canal and exposing the cord, the anterior as well as posterior nerve roots are cut from above downward. A few posterior nerve roots are traced up to the dorsal root ganglia and those roots are cut beyond the ganglia.

Now, gradually the cord is lifted by holding the dura with a toothed forceps and cut all epidural attachments. At cauda equina level, cut the bunch of nerves, take

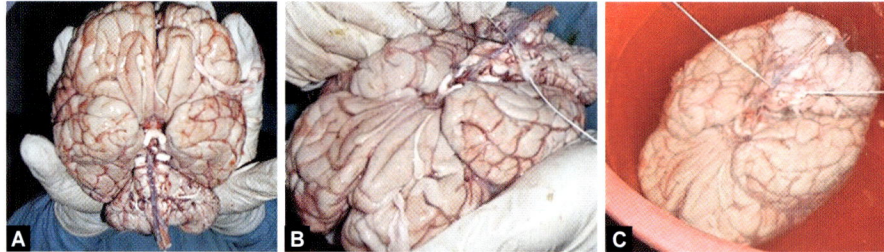

FIGS. 5.5A TO C: (A) The brain is examined for its external anatomy and obvious lesions such as exudates, hemorrhages, etc.; (B) A thread is passed under basilar artery which is then tied to the handle of the bucket; and (C) The brain is suspended in the bucket with sufficient formalin and is not allowed to touch the sides or bottom of the bucket.

out the cord, and lay it on a flat surface. Now the anterior and the posterior aspects of dural sac are opened in the midline before fixation. It prevents any artifacts and distortion of SC during fixation.

Collect material for examinations requiring unfixed tissue. The cord can be fixed either by just dropping in the brain bucket or suspending vertically in a cylinder containing fixative by passing a thread through the dura at the cervical end and tying the ends of the thread around the cylinder. The spinal canal is examined for any pathology, e.g., tumors, granulation tissue, disc material, etc.

After removal of brain and SC, the body needs to be sutured. The skull is placed back in its position in such a way that it stays in position. The two portions of reflected scalp are aligned and sutured with thread. Since the original incision did not cut much hair, the sutured scalp is not visible. It is better to comb the hair. Similarly, the back muscles are kept back in position. The back skin is neatly sutured. A final cleaning should be done to remove any blood stains and body is handed over.

EXAMINATION OF BRAIN AFTER FIXATION

The examination of the brain is done after washing the brain overnight or at least for 2 hours in running tap water. It ensures minimum eye irritation by formalin vapors. Ideally, a separate set of sharp instruments should be reserved for brain cutting or at least a knife with a long sharp blade should be kept separately for brain cutting. There is no fixed method of sectioning of the brain for internal examination. The whole idea is to find out the pathology in relation to the various anatomical structures of the brain. The most frequently used method is coronal sectioning because most people are familiar with anatomy of coronal slices. Additionally, most anatomy atlases have photographs showing coronal slices for ready reference. If computed tomography (CT) scans are available for comparison, it may be preferable to slice the brain horizontally. In conditions where brain is diffusely involved such as neurodegenerative diseases and demyelinating diseases, one-half the brain can be cut sagittally and the other half can be preserved for research purposes. The whole aim is to identify lesions and describe them in such a way that they are easily recalled later on and understood by other pathologists as well. The weight of the brain is recorded after fixation. Extradural pathology such as hemorrhage (**Fig. 5.6A**) is noted and dural sinuses are explored for any venous thrombosis. A thorough external examination carried out for herniations (**Fig. 5.6B**), leptomeningeal exudates (**Figs. 5.6C** and **D**), swelling, atrophy, or asymmetry. Examination of the arterial circle of Willis for atherosclerosis, occlusions, aneurysms, and anatomical variations is done at this stage.

The cerebellar hemispheres are gently lifted posteriorly with fingers and the leptomeninges close to superior cerebellar vermis are cleared. The brain stem and cerebellum are separated from the cerebral hemispheres by a sharp axial cut at about 45° angle passing through the midbrain just inferior to the exit of the third cranial nerves.

Traditionally, the cerebral hemispheres are divided into two halves by a coronal cut at the level of mammillary bodies which ensures that both hemispheres are symmetrically cut for proper orientation. It is preferable to use a wooden board to obtain serial coronal slices of 1 cm thickness, which are laid on a tray (**Fig. 5.7**).

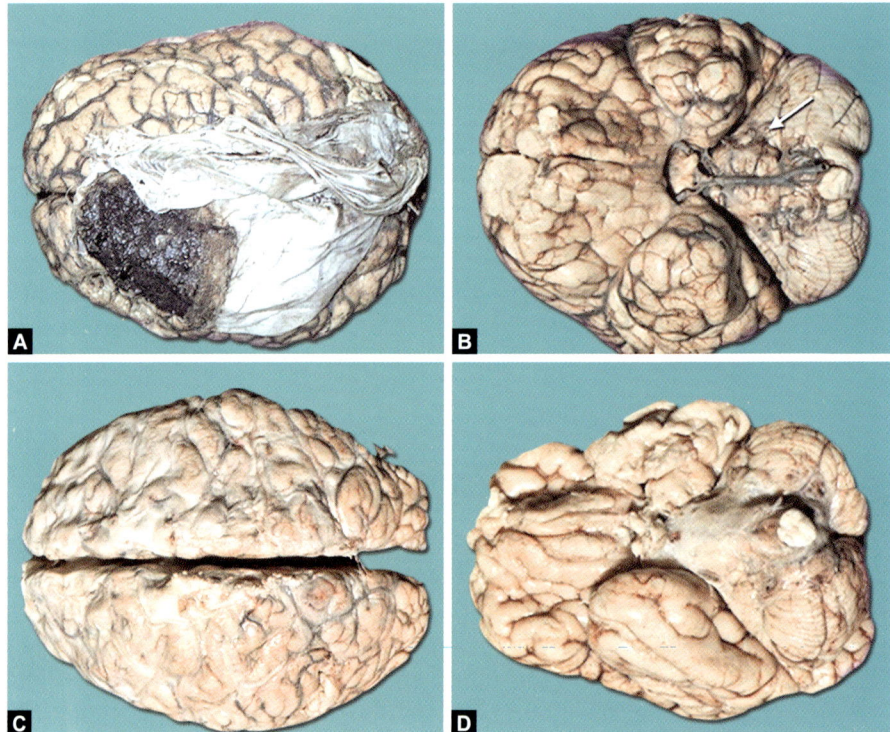

FIGS. 5.6A TO D: (A) Extradural hematoma over left frontal lobe following removal of a meningioma; (B) Cerebellar tonsillar herniation compressing medulla due to left cerebellar infarct caused by basilar artery thrombosis; (C) Diffuse purulent leptomeningeal exudates on the convexities in a case of pyogenic meningitis; and (D) Thick gray–white basal exudates covering interpeduncular fossa and ventral surface of the brainstem.

The wooden boards can be locally manufactured. For neurodegenerative diseases, 5-mm thick slices are preferred to demonstrate neuroanatomical landmarks. Various devices can be used to get 1-cm or 5-mm thick slices.

The brain stem and cerebellum are examined together by axial cuts or they are divided in two halves by cutting through the midline. Alternatively, the brainstem can be separated from cerebellum by incising superior, middle, and inferior cerebellar peduncles and then examined by axial 5-mm cuts. The cerebellum can be examined by 5-mm parallel cuts from medial to lateral surface. It is not necessary that all the slices must be of same thickness. If brain is soft due to any reason or if there is a large hematoma which is difficult to cut, then slices are cut according to pathologist's convenience. It is more important that the cuts should be straight so that one is able to compare the structures on two sides. Thick cuts can also be used if there are large lesions, which need to be preserved for demonstration purpose or for museum. It is necessary to use a sharp knife so that meninges are cut cleanly otherwise a blunt blade carries meninges with it and causes crushing artifact of the parenchyma. Sawing effect should be avoided as such slices cannot be used for photography. The description is recorded in such a way that other pathologists are able to comprehend and localize the lesions later on and the dissector also remembers the description. The cut slices

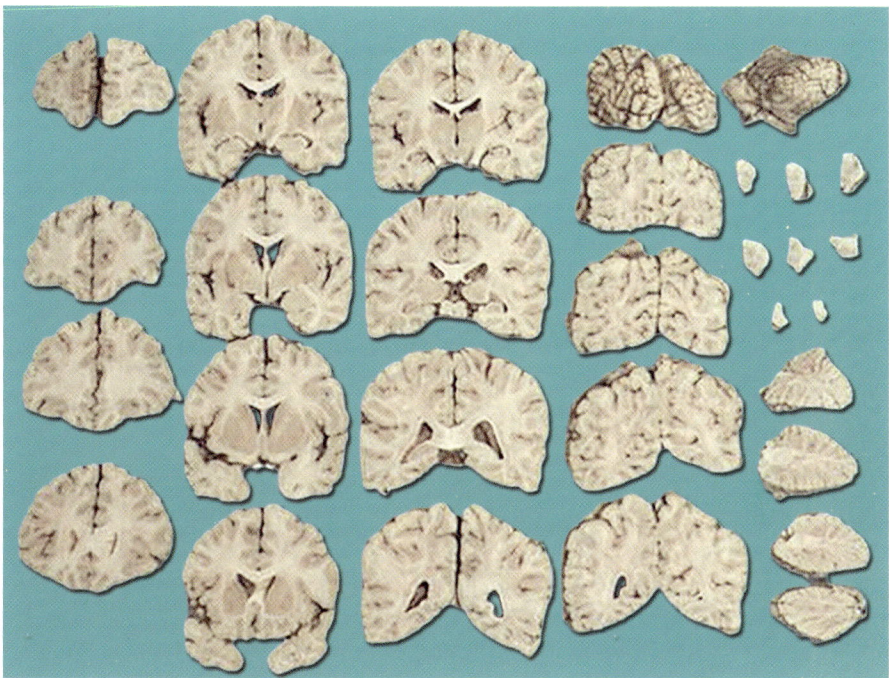

FIG. 5.7: Slices of brain laid down for gross examination.

are examined for any pathology (**Figs. 5.8A** to **D**). Ventricular size is noted since it is a reliable indicator of either atrophy or swelling according to whether these are wider or narrow respectively (**Figs. 5.9A** to **E**). Ventriculitis or choroid plexitis is noted in cases of meningitis. Photography should be done of external pathology and after slicing of brain.

SAMPLING FOR HISTOLOGY

There is nothing fixed about sampling and it depends upon the resources of the concerned laboratory and interest of the neuropathologist. Blocks are taken according to the following broad situations:
- In grossly visible lesions, take samples to represent the lesion adequately along with part of normal brain. Tissue samples should be taken from areas where lesion is expected according to neurological findings or clinical diagnosis. The number and extent of sampling in such situations would depend upon the experience of the pathologist.
- Standard protocols are used for neurodegenerative diseases and these are universally available for different diseases (average 20–25 blocks). Extensive histology is advised in such cases to compare data with other centers.
- When no grossly visible lesions are identified, standard sampling is carried out. It is advisable to use large cassettes for processing brain blocks so that anatomical relationship in sections is easily identifiable. Five-to-six standard samples from the following sites should be fairly representative of the entire brain:

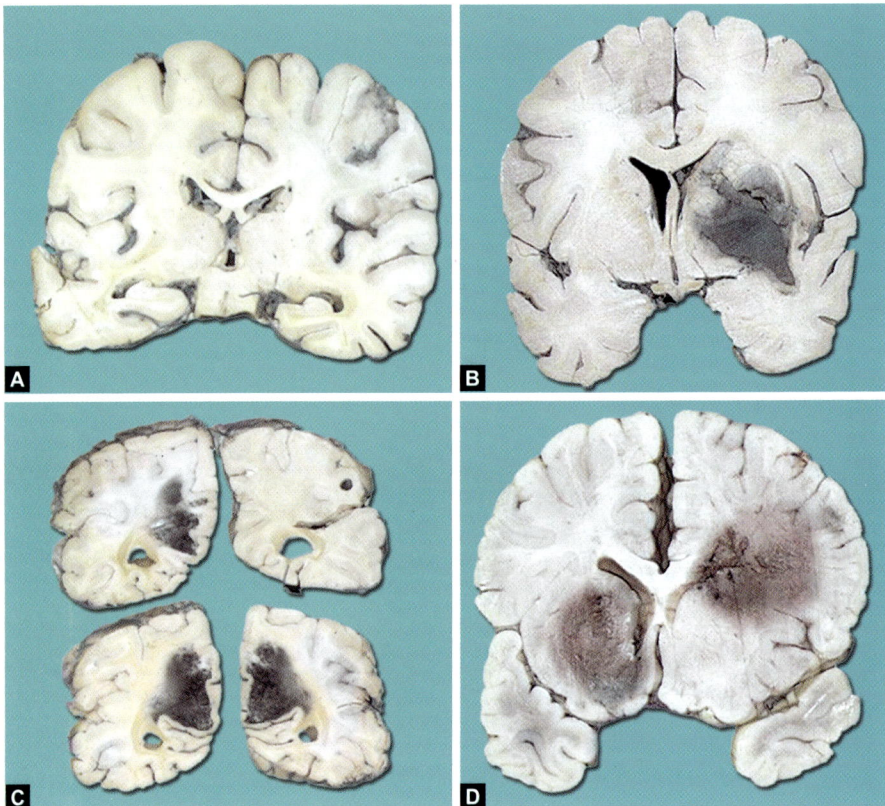

FIGS. 5.8A TO D: (A) Fresh infarct in middle cerebral arterial territory affecting right frontal lobe; (B) A case of hypertension causing right lenticular hemorrhage with edema; (C) Multifocal hemorrhages due to leukemic infiltration in a case of acute myeloid leukemia; and (D) Multifocal hemorrhagic necrosis in a case of disseminated aspergillosis.

- Parietal/frontal cortex with white matter; about 3 cm away from the midline and including a sulcus;
- Basal ganglia (BG)—Ependyma of lateral ventricle to insula, which would include the caudate nucleus, lentiform nucleus, and part of thalamus;
- Hippocampus—Ammon's horn;
- Midbrain and pons;
- Cerebellum including cortex, white matter, and dentate nucleus
- When there is no history of neurological illness and brain examination (including microscopy) does not demonstrate any lesions, it can be safely presumed that there is no pathology in brain.

SPINAL CORD EXAMINATION AND SAMPLING

The SC should be laid on a flat surface and is best examined by slicing at 5 mm intervals in the transverse plane. Grossly visible lesions such as infarcts, softening,

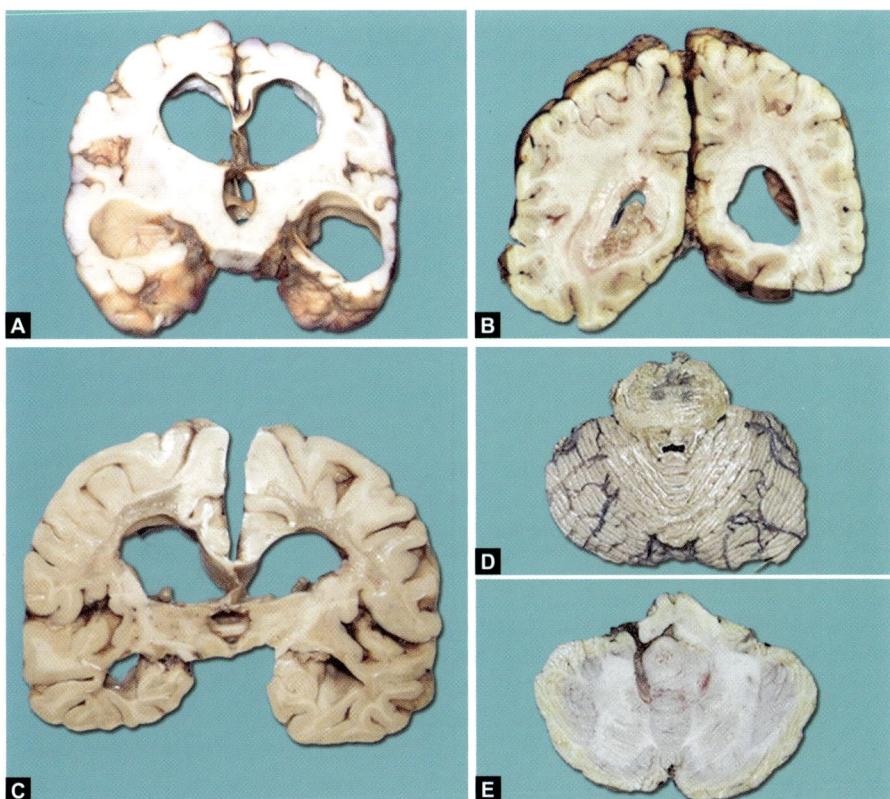

FIGS. 5.9A TO E: (A) Marked hydrocephalus with dilatation of both lateral and third ventricles; (B) Choroid plexitis and ventriculitis in a case of pyogenic meningitis; (C) Periventricular demyelinating plaques in a case of multiple sclerosis; (D) Pontine infarction due to atherosclerosis of basilar artery; and (E) Medulloblastoma occupying the fourth ventricle.

hemorrhages, demyelination, atrophy, etc., are recorded. Samples for microscopic examination should include segments from the level of lesion as well as from above and below the level. If there is no obvious lesions, at least four blocks (cervical, upper dorsal, lower dorsal, and lumbar segments) should be examined. A dorsal root ganglion is usually sampled. Knowledge as to how individual segments are identified is important for the pathologist. It is always better to ink the cutting surface so that right and left could be identified later. Keep the nerve roots attached to the cord while taking blocks.

FURTHER READING

1. Banejee AK. Postmortem examination of the nervous system. Neurol India. 1997;45:120-5.
2. Connolly AJ, Finkbeiner WE, Ursell PC, Davis RL. Autopsy Pathology: A Manual and Atlas, 3rd Edition, Elsevier, Philadelphia, 2016.

5B: CARDIOVASCULAR SYSTEM

Pradeep Vaideeswar

INTRODUCTION

Cardiovascular diseases are the leading causes of death due to noncommunicable diseases the world over, and they are fast becoming the number one killer in developing countries. In India, we continue to grapple with our twin problems of ischemic and valvular heart diseases. The high burden of ischemic heart disease in India is as a result of an increasing incidence of diabetes mellitus coupled with an "intrinsic" dyslipidemia and rising prevalence of obesity. Similarly, rheumatic heart disease continues to be major health problem largely due to socioeconomic issues such as poverty, overcrowding, poor sanitation, and availability of healthcare facilities. Both diseases, along with a variety of other cardiovascular disorders are also important causes of sudden death and hence one confronts cardiovascular diseases in forensic pathology practice as well.

There has been tremendous progress in the diagnostic and therapeutic modalities in the specialties of radiology, cardiology, and cardiac surgery. Hence, it follows that the pathologist too must understand the functional changes to arrive at a good functional-morphological correlation in every case. But, it is a fact that cardiac pathology the world over is largely autopsy-based and autopsy methodology by itself has changed very little. But it must be remembered to this day that examination of the heart has played a pivotal role in understanding several cardiovascular diseases. In all such cases, the mantra to be followed is "inspect, probe, photograph, dissect, and cut". The limits of traditional morphology (where offending organisms and structural defects tend to escape even ultrastructural imaging) can be bypassed when new tools like PCR or gene sequencing can be incorporated in the armamentarium of postmortem investigations.

SEPARATION AND FIXATION OF THE HEART

The heart and lungs are received as a block with the trachea-bronchial tree (**Fig. 5.10A**). The pericardium and its cavity are kept intact in the beginning. The outer layer is the parietal layer, which is translucent or opaque and variably infiltrated by adipose tissue (often age-dependent). If an infective pericardial pathology is suspected, then the pericardial surface is seared with a heated spatula and then incised with sterile scalpel blade so that necessary material for culture is collected with a swab; alternatively, the material is collected by sterile needle/syringe. Preferably, this procedure is usually performed near the cardiac apex. Furthermore, since the opening is small, the rims can be held with blunt forceps so that excess amounts of fluid can be sucked out for measurement of its volume. If there is no significant pathology, the parietal pericardium is excised, and all major arteries and veins are carefully dissected (**Fig. 5.10B**). Normally, it is not easy to flip the heart upward due to normal pulmonary arterial and venous connections to the lungs.

Systemic Examination

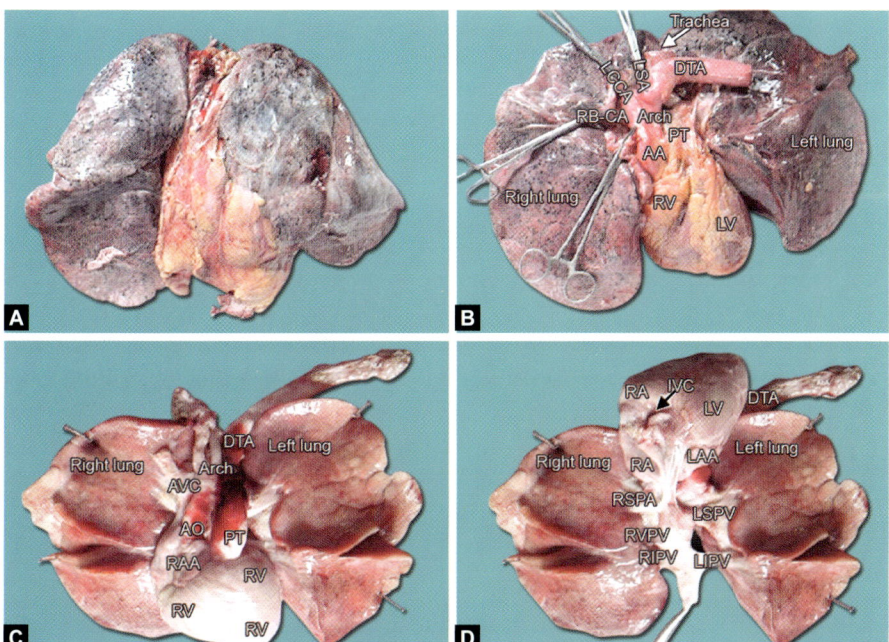

(AA: ascending aorta; Ao: aorta; DTA: descending thoracic aorta; LAA: left atrial appendage; LCCA: left common carotid artery; LIPV: left inferior pulmonary vein; LSA: left subclavian artery; LSPV: left superior pulmonary vein; LV: left ventricle; RBCA: right brachiocephalic artery; PT: pulmonary trunk; RAA: right atrial appendage; RIPV: right inferior pulmonary vein; RSPV: right superior pulmonary vein; RV: right ventricle)

FIGS. 5.10A TO D: (A) The heart and lung block received after separating and reflecting the descending aorta and esophagus. The esophagus is further dissected with the gastrointestinal tract. If kidneys are diseased, then part of the abdominal aorta is usually kept with the kidney block. (B) The parietal pericardium has been excised and the systemic veins and great arteries/branches have been dissected. (C) The heart and lung block in an infant. Please note that the left ventricle is hardly seen from the anterior aspect. (D) The heart is easily reflected backward because the anchorage provided by the pulmonary veins is lost due to their congenital anomalous infradiaphragmatic connection, which was missed and inadvertently cut.

This flipping is an important step to be performed in all pediatric autopsies, as it may point to a supracardiac or infracardiac (**Figs. 5.10C** and **D**) total anomalous pulmonary venous connection. In such cases, the heart and lungs should be ideally kept with upper aerodigestive tract, stomach, "C" of the duodenum, pancreas, liver, and spleen. The pulmonary trunk may also be incised to rule out a massive embolism (a cause of sudden death) due to "saddle embolus" (see Chapter 5C).

The heart is then separated from the lungs (**Figs. 5.11A** to **D**). It is best to commence the separation from the left side. The left pulmonary veins and left pulmonary artery are incised with a sharp scalpel blade as close to the lung hilum as possible. These structures are separated by blunt dissection from the left main bronchus and trachea, by pulling the heart to the right. Similar cuts are made on the right side by lifting the heart, where along with pulmonary vasculature, the superior caval vein is also separated from right bronchus.

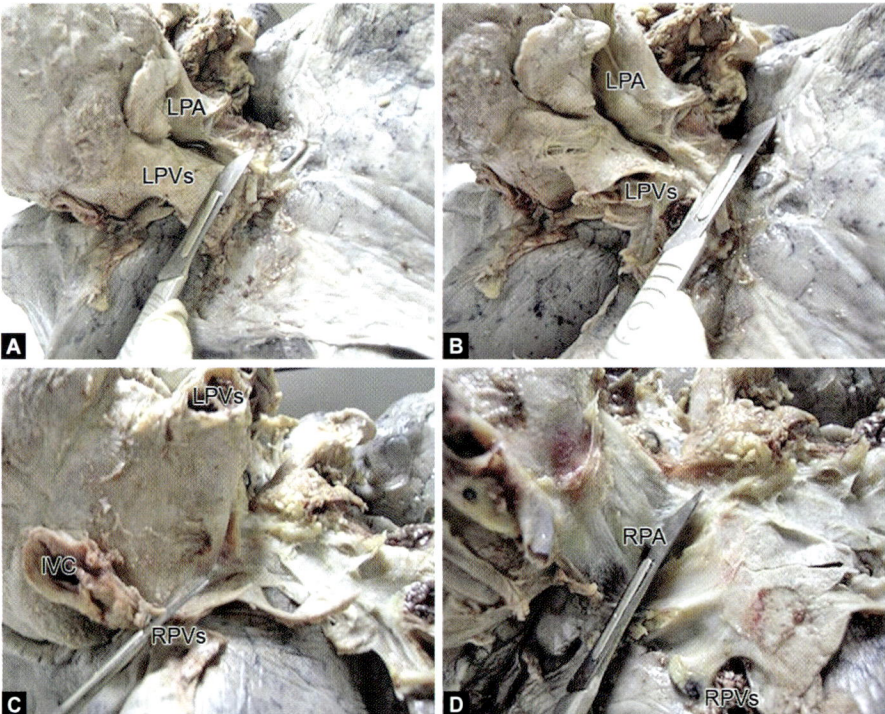

(IVC: inferior vena cava; LPA: left pulmonary artery; LPV: left pulmonary vein; RPA: right pulmonary artery; RPV: right pulmonary vein)

FIGS. 5.11A TO D: Once the prosector is convinced that there are no anomalies in the pulmonary arteries and veins, the heart is separated from the lungs, preferably commencing from (A and B) the left side and then (C and D) from right side.

The heart may then be dissected in the fresh state or after overnight fixation with buffered formalin. If overnight fixation is adopted, then care should be taken to flush out all the blood clots otherwise the endocardial and intimal surfaces will appear blood-stained. In cases of coronary artery disease and in all patients above the age of 40 years, we routinely practice the process of coronary arterial perfusion (**Figs. 5.12A and B**). The arch arteries are clamped after checking that there are no pathological lesions within them. An adequately sized cannula is inserted into the thoracic aorta or through one of the arch arteries and passed into the ascending aorta in such a way that it lies well above the coronary arterial ostia. Buffered formalin is allowed to run into the cannula from a height of 30 cm for at least 10 minutes. With the formalin running, the cannula is gently eased out and the aorta is clamped. This retains the formalin at adequate pressure within the arteries to preserve their circular contours. This may be performed in the autopsy room as sufficient time elapses during other organ dissections. It is preferable to photograph the heart in the fresh state as fixation alters the natural colors. The photography of any specimen including that of the heart may be easy due to digital cameras and mobile phones, but care should be taken to take esthetically pleasing image and avoid distracting backgrounds.

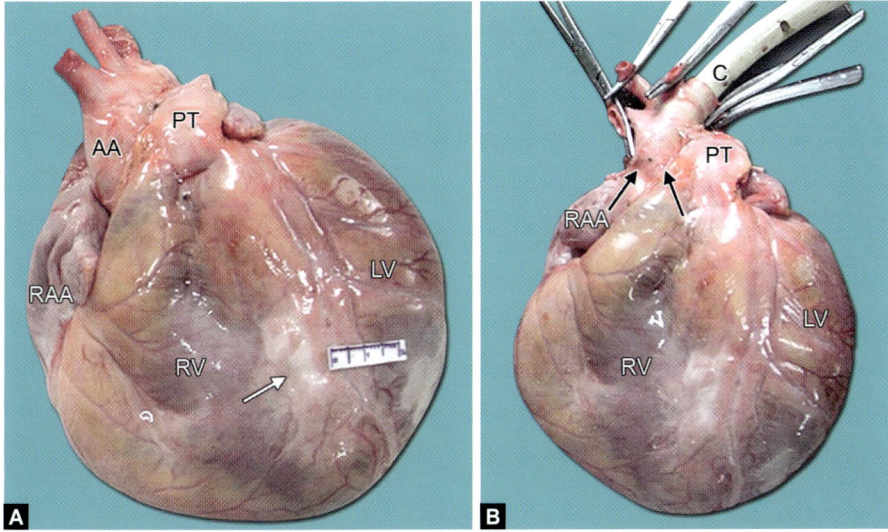

(LV: left ventricle; PT: pulmonary trunk; RAA: right atrial appendage)

FIGS. 5.12A AND B: (A) The heart from a patient with a history of ischemic heart disease has been separated from the lungs and oriented in a normal anatomic position. The arrow shows a milk patch over anterior surface of right ventricle (RV). (B) For coronary arterial perfusion, the cannula (C) has been passed into the ascending aorta (AA) till it lies at least a centimeter above (arrows) the coronary arterial origins.

EXTERNAL EXAMINATION OF THE HEART

Before opening the heart, it is important to spend time over the external anatomy, which may provide clues to the inner pathology and may also alter pattern of further dissection. The features to be noted are: Orientation, appearance of epicardial surface, the cardiac surfaces, atrial appendageal morphology, great arterial relations/sizes, and coronary arterial anatomy/dissection and cardiac size.

- *Orientation:* The heart has to be oriented in the normal anatomic position whereby the axis of the ventricles is oriented laterally to the left from base to the apex, extending anteriorly and slightly inferiorly. The apex of the heart is pointed to the left and is usually formed by the left ventricle; this is levocardia.
- *Appearance of epicardial surface* (**Figs. 5.13A to D**)*:* The epicardial surface, which is normally smooth, shiny, and transparent, is inspected for presence of thickening, increase in adipose tissue, tortuosity of epicardial vasculature and presence of increased fluid and exudates, and also even for the presence of any deficiency. These abnormalities may be localized or generalized. If the exudate is minimal, it usually collects over the right atrial aspect. If the visceral pericardium is normal, color of the underlying myocardium also has to be noted.
- *The cardiac surfaces:* The anterior surface of the heart (**Fig. 5.14A**) shows the atrial appendages, superior vena cava, and great arteries toward the base, and most of the right ventricle and small part of left ventricle toward the apical aspect. The posterior surface of the heart (**Fig. 5.14B**) shows the atria proper, inferior

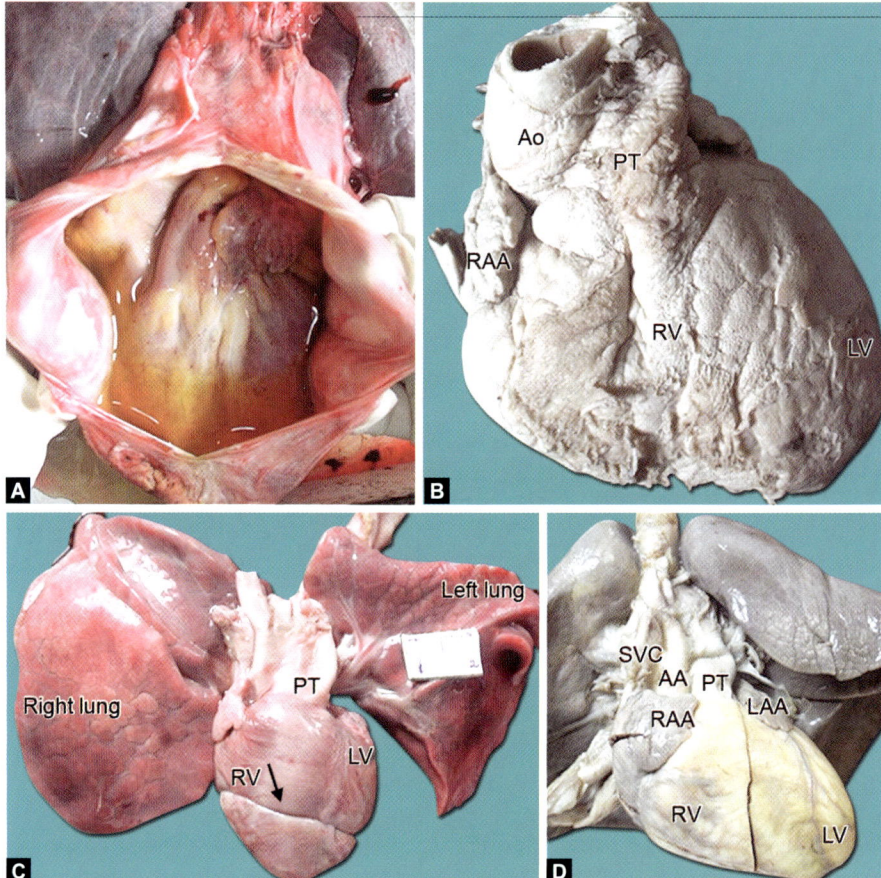

(AA: ascending aorta; Ao: aorta; LAA: left atrial appendage; LV: left ventricle; PT: pulmonary trunk; RAA: right atrial appendage; RV: right ventricle; SVC: superior vena cava)

FIGS. 5.13A TO D: (A) The parietal pericardium is incised to show the amber colored slightly hazy pericardial fluid in a case of moderate pericardial effusion. (B) The anterior surface of the heart is covered by a layer of grayish white, granular fibrinous exudate. (C) Neonatal heart showing partial deficiency of the pericardium, which has produced a ring of constriction in the mid-portion (arrow). (D) Neonate with perinatal asphyxia. The myocardium has a distinct yellow hue due to myocardial fatty change.

vena cava, longitudinally placed coronary sinus, pulmonary veins, larger portion of left ventricle, and small part of right ventricle. All chambers appear to meet at a common point, the crux of the heart. On the basal aspect, the superior wall of left atrium is related to pulmonary arterial bifurcation, while ascending aorta is wedged between pulmonary trunk and right atrium.
- *Morphology of atrial appendages:* In the external anatomy, the most characteristic feature of the atria is their appendage. The right atrial appendage (**Fig. 5.15A**) is large, triangular with a broad base and is characteristically pectinated. It is to be noted that the entire anterior wall of right atrium is formed by its appendage. The

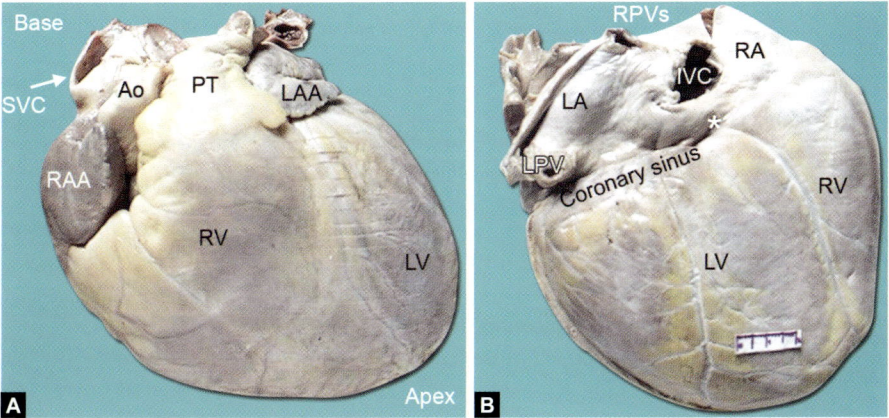

(Ao: aorta; IVC: inferior vena cava; LAA: left atrial appendage; LPV: left pulmonary veins; LV: left ventricle; PT: pulmonary trunk; RAA: right atrial appendage; RPV: right pulmonary veins; RV: right ventricle; SVC: superior vena cava)

FIGS. 5.14A AND B: (A) Anterior and (B) posterior, surfaces. Please note that all chambers meet at a common point, the crux (*) of the heart.

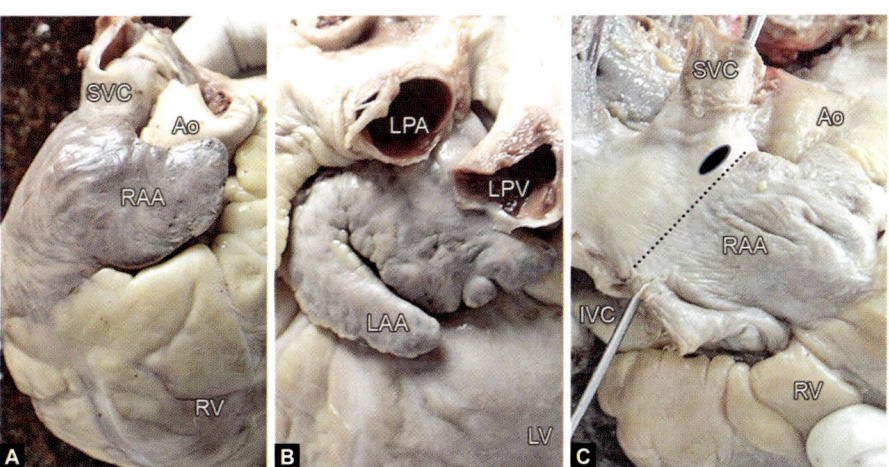

(Ao: aorta; IVC: inferior vena cava; LAA: left atrial appendage; LPA: left pulmonary artery; LPV: left pulmonary vein; LV: left ventricle; RAA: right atrial appendage; RV: right ventricle; SVC: superior vena cava)

FIGS. 5.15A TO C: Characteristic morphology of (A) the right atrial appendage and (B) the left atrial appendage. (C) The sinoatrial node (black ellipse) occupies a lateral position at superior cavoatrial junction.

left atrial appendage (**Fig. 5.15B**), on the other hand, resembles a crenellated, crooked little finger, which has a distinctive narrow junction with main chamber. The superior and inferior caval veins enter the right atrium nearly in alignment. Demarcating the pectinated appendage from the smooth-walled venous component of the atrium is the sulcus terminalis. Important in this area is the location of sinoatrial node, which occupies a lateral position at superior cavoatrial junction

(**Fig. 5.15C**). For examining the sinus node, the entire block of tissue should be taken and serially sectioned.

- *Great arterial relations:* The pulmonary trunk or main pulmonary artery is situated anterior and to the left of the ascending aorta, which constitutes the normal great arterial relationship. The arch of aorta is left-sided and gives off three branches—right brachiocephalic, left common carotid, and left subclavian, arteries (see **Fig. 5.1B**).
- *Coronary arterial anatomy and dissection:* The right coronary artery (**Fig. 5.16A**) arises from the root of the ascending aorta and passes into the right atrioventricular groove. The left main coronary artery also arises from the aortic root and is seen behind pulmonary trunk. Without much ado, it breaks into two branches (**Fig. 5.16A**), the left anterior descending artery that courses over the anterior interventricular groove, and the left circumflex artery that enters left anterior atrioventricular groove. In right coronary dominant hearts (**Fig. 5.16B**), the right coronary artery terminates as the posterior descending artery that supplies the posterior wall of the left ventricle and posterior one-third of interventricular septum.
- Coronary arterial dissection is best achieved by serial cross-sections with a sharp scalpel blade at an interval of 0.5 cm (**Fig. 5.17A**). Degree of stenosis is traditionally classified into three categories (**Fig. 5.17B**): less than 50%, more than 50% to less than 75% and greater than 75%; the latter is considered as critical stenosis. Perception of color and texture plays an important role in identification of the type of atheroma (major cause of stenosis), which may be fibrous, fibrofatty, or fatty (**Figs. 5.17C to E**) and its complications in the form of calcification, thrombosis, plaque rupture, or intraplaque hemorrhage (**Figs. 5.17F to H**). If the arteries are

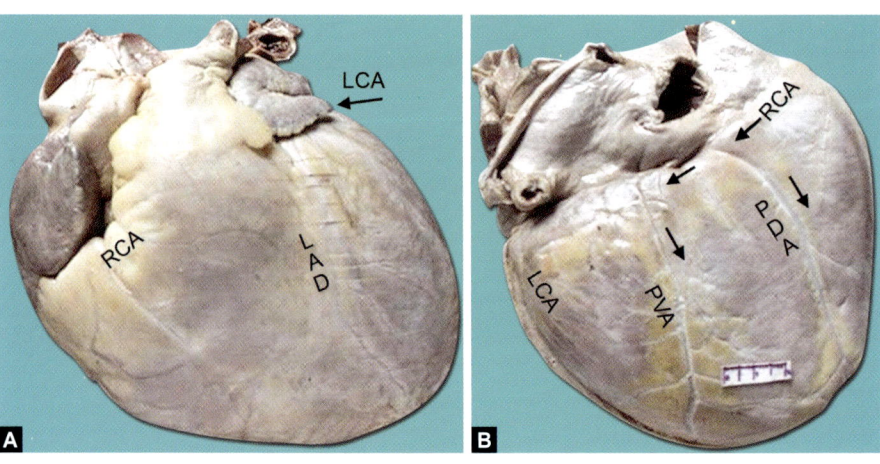

(LCA: left coronary artery)

FIGS. 5.16A AND B: (A) The right coronary artery (RCA) courses in the right anterior atrioventricular groove and is usually embedded within the epicardial fat. The left anterior descending (LAD) artery lies over the anterior interventricular groove. The origins of the left main artery and left circumflex artery (LCA) is not seen on the anterior aspect. (B) The dominant RCA in this heart has given rise to the posterior descending artery (PDA) as well as posterior ventricular artery (PVA).

Systemic Examination

extremely calcified, they are dissected out of their beds, excised, decalcified and then serially sectioned. X-rays, especially after infusion of radio-opaque dyes may also be advocated for this purpose, as it shows the entire arterial tree and points to the position of stents if any.

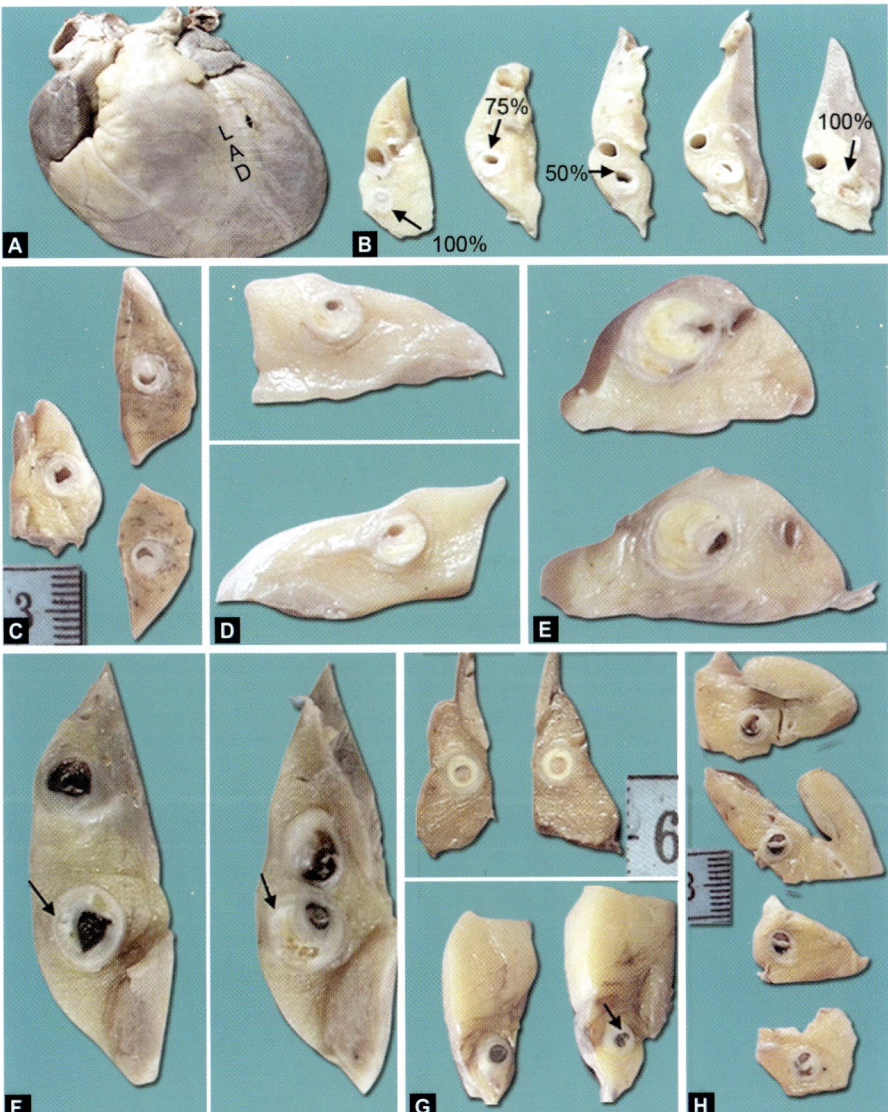

FIGS. 5.17A TO H: (A) The left anterior descending (LAD) artery has been cut at an interval of cm (arrow). (B) The same artery showing various degrees of stenosis that ranges from 50% to complete occlusion. The atheromatous plaques may be (C) fibrous, (D) fibro-fatty, or (E) fatty. The complications noted in these plaques may be (F) calcification (arrows) seen as whitish gritty lesions surrounding the grumous material, (G) occlusive fresh red-brown thrombus and plaque rupture. The arrows indicate region of rupture, or (H) intraplaque hemorrhage.

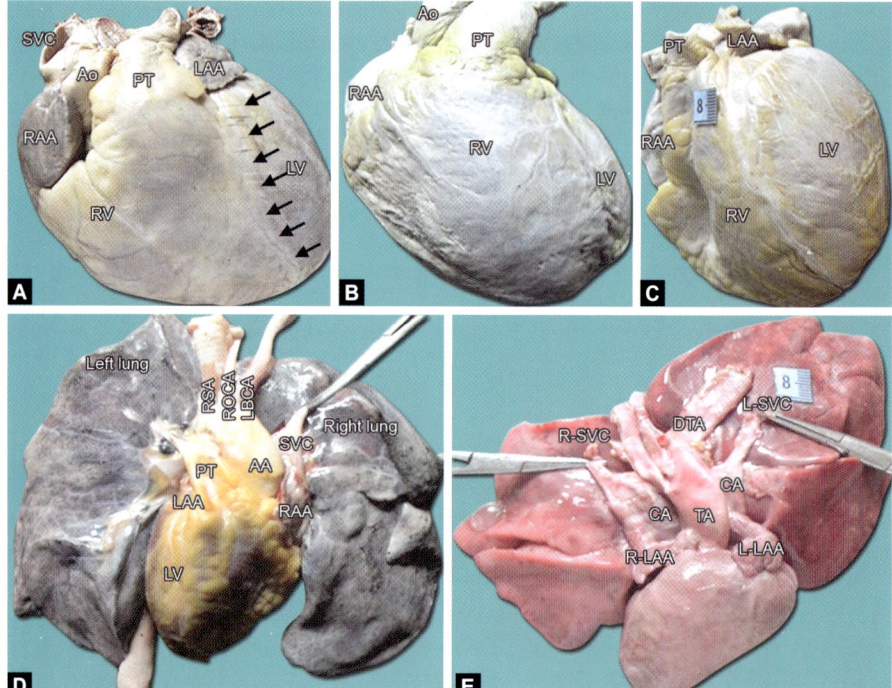

(AA: ascending aorta; Ao: aorta; DTA: descending thoracic aorta; LAA: left atrial appendage; LBCA: left brachiocephalic artery; LCCA: left common carotid artery; LIPV: left inferior pulmonary vein; LSA: left subclavian artery; LSPV: left superior pulmonary vein; LSVC: left superior vena cava; LV: left ventricle; PT: pulmonary trunk; RAA: right atrial appendage; RBCA: right brachiocephalic artery; RCCA: right common carotid artery; RIPV: right inferior pulmonary vein; RSA: right subclavian artery; RSPV: right superior pulmonary vein; RSVC: right superior vena cava; RV: right ventricle; SVC: superior vena cava)

FIGS. 5.18A TO E: (A) The left anterior descending (LAD) artery offers a natural delineation (arrows) for the position of the interventricular septum. The apex is pointing to the left (levocardia) and formed by left ventricle. (B) Moderate cardiomegaly has resulted from marked enlargement of RV. The apex in this instance is formed by the RV and is slightly rounded. (C) This heart shows marked hypertrophy of the LV so that there is a right-ward shift of the LAD. (D) Situs inversus seen as an incidental finding at autopsy. Note that all the relations are reversed but veno-atrio-ventriculoarterial connections are normal. (E) A case of situs ambiguus with left isomerism, associated with complex congenital heart disease - common atrium (CA) and single ventricle (cor biloculare), and single arterial trunk - truncus arteriosus (TA). Note the dextrocardia and bilateral superior vena cavae.

- *Cardiac size:* The heart may be normal, small, or enlarged in size and these alterations may be subjectively graded as mild, moderate, or marked. More importantly, we have to assess the chamber/s, which are responsible for this change. The surface anatomy of the LAD offers an excellent guide to the position of the interventricular septum (**Figs. 5.18A** to **C**).

At this point, a mention must be made of the importance of correlating the morphology of the atrial appendages and corresponding bronchi (the broncho-atrial situs) with the arrangement of the abdominal viscera (the abdominal situs). This gives rise to three arrangements of situs solitus (normal arrangement, **Fig. 5.1B**), situs inversus (mirror-image arrangement, **Fig. 5.18D**), and situs ambiguus (intermediate arrangement, **Fig. 5.18E**). The latter is usually associated with near identical morphology of the atrial appendages and bronchi, i.e., right isomerism with asplenia or left isomerism with polysplenia. In such situations, the apex may point to the right (dextrocardia) or left or may even be in the center (mesocardia).

OPENING THE HEART AND HEART WEIGHT

The heart is usually cut as per the flow of blood (Virchow's or inflow/outflow method). Three cuts each are taken on the right and left sides of the heart. The first cut is made in the mid-portion of the right atrium, extending it into its appendage (**Fig. 5.19A**). Alternatively, the chamber is cut along a probe, which is passed from the inferior caval vein into the superior caval vein. This has to be done only after careful inspection of the veins. After opening, the tricuspid valve is inspected for any pathology. The orifice usually admits three fingers, which is a rough estimate. The second incision (**Fig. 5.19A**) is then taken a little behind right border of the heart from the right atrium into the right ventricle through tricuspid valve orifice (cutting the posterior tricuspid leaflet). The third cut (**Fig. 5.19A**) is taken along the right ventricular outflow tract into the main pulmonary artery and its branches via the pulmonary valve.

On the left side, the first incision is through the two superior pulmonary veins (**Fig. 5.19B**). Again the mitral valve is inspected, and its orifice usually admits two fingers (rough estimate). The second (**Fig. 5.19A**) is a little behind the left border of the heart (cutting the posterior mitral leaflet), reaching the apical aspect of the left ventricle. The third cut (**Fig. 5.19C**) is usually taken through the anterior mitral leaflet and wall of the left atrium to open into ascending aorta.

In all the second and third incisions, care should be taken not to cut through the commissures of the valves. Often the sinuses of the pulmonary valve are faintly visible on the external aspect. With the above pattern, the mitral valve has been cut twice. Whenever there is a mitral valvular pathology, a valve sparing cut is employed where an incision parallel to the left anterior descending artery is taken to enter the ascending aorta (**Fig. 5.19D**). After opening the heart, the blood clots are removed and the arch of aorta is separated from the ascending portion. The heart is then weighed. The weight is approximately 0.45% of the body weight. For the average Indian male and female, it is usually 300 g and 250 g, respectively. The aorta is opened longitudinally along its posterior aspect through the bifurcation and into both common iliac arteries (**Fig. 5.20A**). The vessel is usually described from within outwards, i.e., appearance of the intima, the appearance and thickness of the wall and appearance of the adventitia. It is important to check the size and appearance of the para-aortic lymph nodes, present in the periadventitial tissue. Serial sections of the aorta may be resorted to in cases of aneurysmal disease (**Fig. 5.20B**).

If a myocardial pathology is suspected (or even otherwise), it is better to take a transverse section through mid-portions of the ventricles, from the posterior aspect before taking the third incisions on both sides. I usually prefer to do this before opening the heart so that the myocardium is seen in its entirety. Further, the transverse slicing should not be through and through. The reason for this step is that if there is

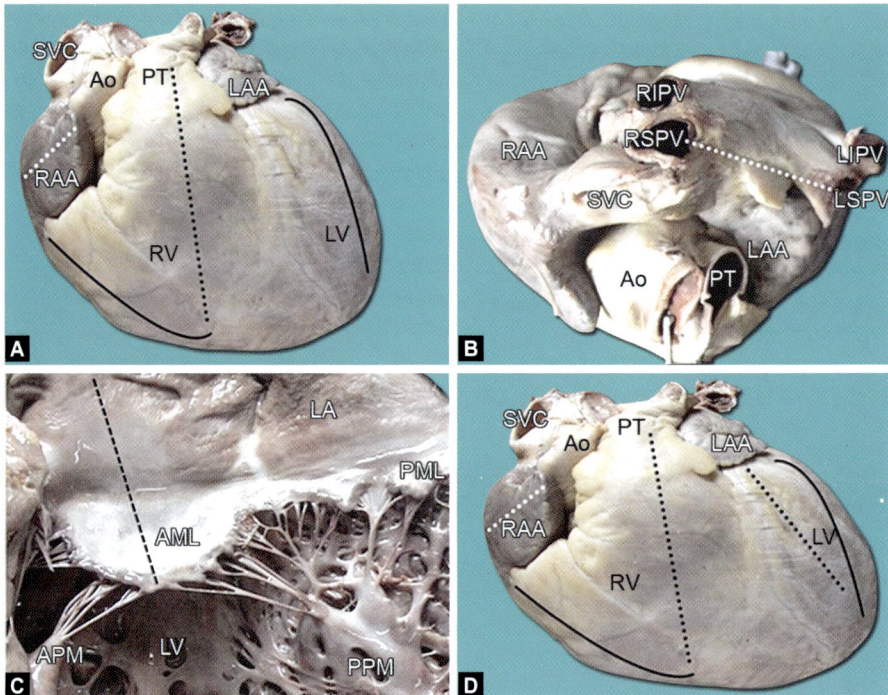

(AML: anterior mitral leaflet; Ao: aorta; LA: left atrium; LAA: left atrial appendage; LIPV: left inferior pulmonary vein; LSPV: left superior pulmonary vein; LV: left ventricle; PML: posterior mitral leaflet; PT: pulmonary trunk; RAA: right atrial appendage; RIPV: right inferior pulmonary vein; RSPV: right superior pulmonary vein; RV: right ventricle; SVC: superior vena cava)

FIGS. 5.19A TO D: (A to C) Shows pattern of cardiac dissection following the flow-of-blood method. (D) In this mitral valve-sparing technique, a cut parallel to the interventricular septum is taken and extended into the ascending aorta.

an incidental finding in the heart, the anterior surface of the specimen can still be photographed with minimal distortion. If there is a myocardial pathology, the heart may be bread-loafed. The myocardium should be inspected for its color, consistency, and thickness, which may change depending on the type of pathology. Most often, it is the left ventricular myocardium that is involved in cardiac diseases. The pathology may be regional or circumferential (uncommon) restricted to one or more walls, i.e., anterior, lateral, posterior, and/or septal (**Figs. 5.21A to C**). This cross-sectioning is also useful for detecting presence of mural thrombi within intertrabecular spaces (**Fig. 5.21D**), which can easily be missed.

INTERNAL EXAMINATION OF THE HEART

Both right- and left-sided chambers are described as their inflow (**Figs. 5.22A and B**) and outflow (**Figs. 5.23A and B**) tracts. It is important to remember right-

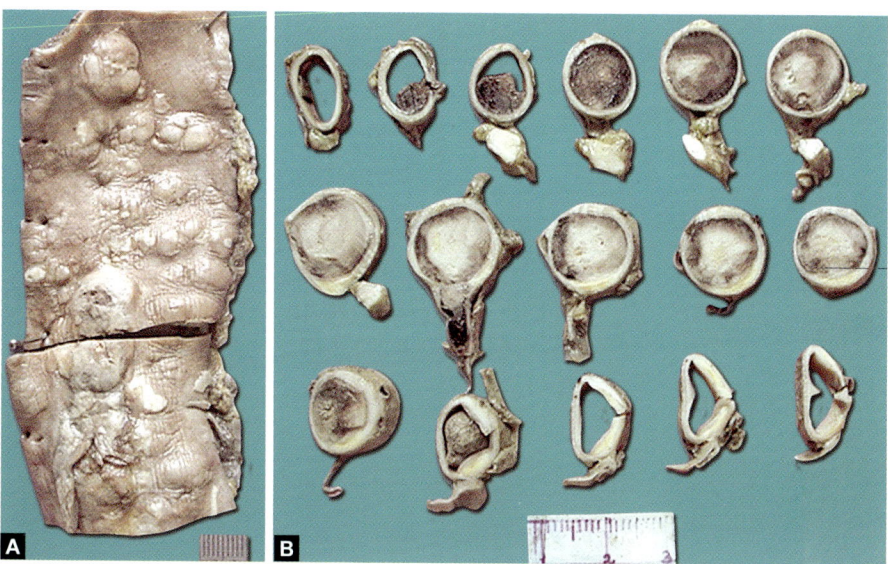

FIGS. 5.20A AND B: (A) Opened out descending thoracic aorta showing the presence of atheromatous plaques. Some of them show focal ulceration; (B) Serial cross-sections of the thoracoabdominal aorta showing luminal occlusion by fresh thrombus.

or left-sidedness to the cardiac chambers and valves are assigned not because of their location, but because of their morphology. The right atrium has two important landmarks. The true extent of the interatrial septum is limited to the fossa ovalis with its muscular anteroinferior rim, the limbus fossa ovalis. Three veins enter the atrium, superior, and inferior caval veins, and coronary sinus. At times, the inferior vena cava and coronary sinus openings are guarded by Eustachian and Thebesian valves, respectively. The smooth-surfaced venous component or the sinus venarum is separated from the pectinated or rough portion of the atrium by the second landmark, the crista terminalis, or terminal crest. In contrast to right atrium, the topography of the left atrium is almost featureless. The pectinate muscles are confined to the appendage. The endocardium is naturally thick and opaque. The septal aspect is marked by shallow irregular pits.

The tricuspid valve has three leaflets, the anterior, septal, and posterior and hence three commissures, the anteroseptal, posteroseptal, and anteroposterior. The leaflets are anchored to the ventricle via the tendinous chords to constantly well-developed anterior, usually developed posterior and occasionally developed medial, papillary muscles. The mitral valve has two leaflets, anterior and posterior and two commissures, anterolateral, and posteromedial. The anterior leaflet has a greater width and appears a little tongue-shaped. The subvalvular apparatus is represented by chords anchored to fairly constant anterior and posterior papillary muscles.

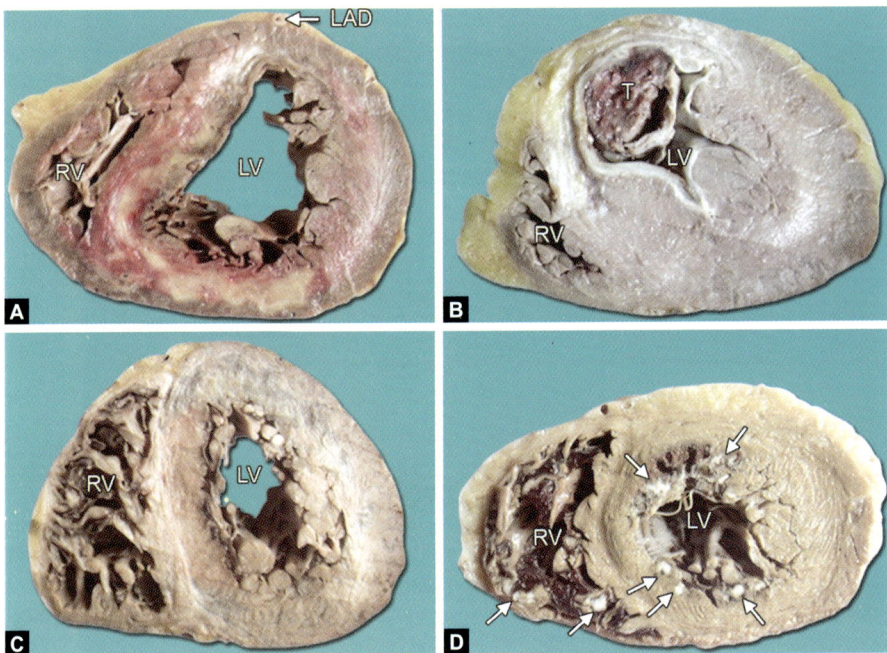

(LAD: left anterior descending artery; LV: left ventricle; RV: right ventricle; T: thrombus)

FIGS. 5.21A TO D: All images are transverse sections taken at the mid-portion of the heart. (A) Acute transmural myocardial infarction affecting the posterior wall and posterior half of the interventricular septum. The right coronary artery had been dominant. The infarct is distinctly yellow with an irregular rimming by zones of hyperemia. (B) Hypertensive heart disease (note concentric left ventricular hypertrophy) complicated by transmural healed infarction and mural fresh thrombus. The small ventricular cavity is obliterated by the thrombus. (C) Sudden cardiac death in a young woman caused by acute myocarditis. The myocardium shows foci of congestion all around. (D) Gray-white fresh thrombi that have obliterated the intertrabecular spaces in both ventricles. The patient was a diabetic with lower limb cellulitis.

The morphology of the right atrium and tricuspid valve provides the landmarks of the Koch's triangle (**Fig. 5.22A**), an established guide to the location of atrioventricular node. The base is formed by the opening of the coronary sinus. The sides are formed by the hinge-line of septal tricuspid leaflet and the Eustachian ridge, which contains the tendon of Todaro. At the apex lies the central fibrous body, which is pierced by the bundle of His. For pathology at this site, the entire block containing the "triangle" is taken. It is divided into upper (containing atrioventricular node and bundle of His) and lower (containing proximal bundle branches) blocks, each of which is longitudinally sliced and processed for histology.

The right ventricle is coarsely trabeculated with a thin compact portion that measures 0.5–0.7 cm. In addition, its outflow tract is also trabeculated due to prominent muscle bands. On the other hand, the left ventricle is finely trabeculated with a thicker compact portion measuring about a 1 cm. The left ventricular outflow tract is relatively smooth with white endocardium over the basal, subaortic aspect of the interventricular septum. The thickness of the ventricular walls is measured

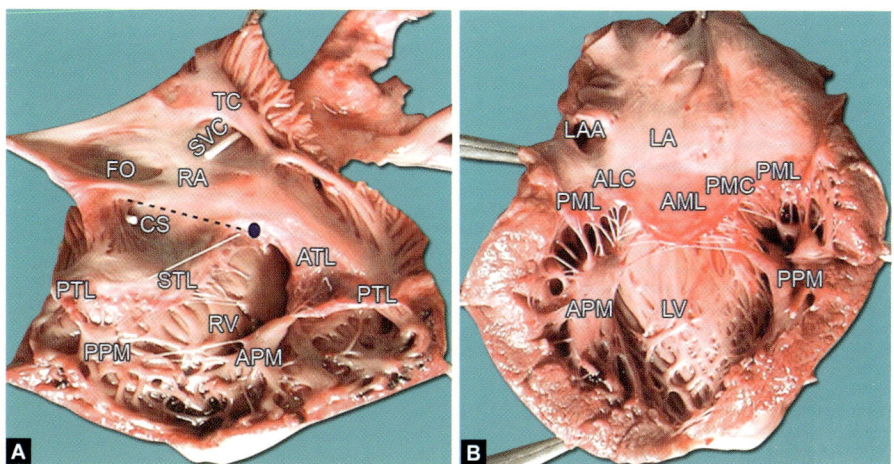

(ALC: anterolateral commissure; AML: anterior mitral leaflet; APM: anterior papillary muscle; ATL: anterior tricuspid leaflet; CS: coronary sinus; FO: fossa ovalis; LA: left atrium; LAA: left atrial appendage; LV: left ventricle; PMC: posteromedial commissure; PML: posterior mitral leaflet; PPM: posterior papillary muscle; PTL: posterior tricuspid leaflet; RA: right atrium; RV: right ventricle; TC: terminal crista; STL: septal tricuspid leaflet; SVC: superior vena cava)

FIGS. 5.22A AND B: The right (A) and left (B) inflow tracts of the heart are displayed to show the various landmarks that especially characterize the right-sided chambers. The black ellipse indicates the location of the central fibrous body at the apex of the triangle of Koch.

at a point 1 cm below the atrioventricular valves or arterial valves. The epicardial fat and the trabeculae are not included. It is to be noted that right ventricular thickness has a slight variation in the inflow and outflow portions. A more sensitive method is a ratio of the weights of the left and right ventricles. The excess fat and atria with atrioventricular valves are separated from the ventricles. The septum is weighed with the left ventricle. The process is tedious and is best done after complete cardiac assessment. The procedure is particularly useful in cases of cor pulmonale.

The morphology of right ventricle leads to subdivisions into three components. The inlet extends from tricuspid annulus to attachment of the chords. The trabecular portion lies between chordal attachments and apex, while the outlet portion lies beyond the septal band. The septal band or trabeculo septomarginalis is an important landmark. Another muscular band, the moderator band, connects it to the base of anterior papillary muscle, but this may not always be prominent. The left ventricle is divided into basal (from mitral annulus to tips of the papillary muscles), middle (tips to the bases of the papillary muscles), and apical thirds (beyond the site of attachment of papillary muscles).

The right ventricle leads to the pulmonary trunk via the pulmonary valve. The outflow tract (**Fig. 5.23A**) is also trabeculated with an additional muscular band, designated as the crista supraventricularis. This connects the free wall of the right ventricle to the interventricular septum, where it is seen inserted between the anterior and posterior limbs of the septal band. The pulmonary valve has three cusps, one anterior and two posterior. They are semilunar and translucent. The left ventricular outflow tract (**Fig. 5.23B**) is smooth and shows thickened endocardium below the

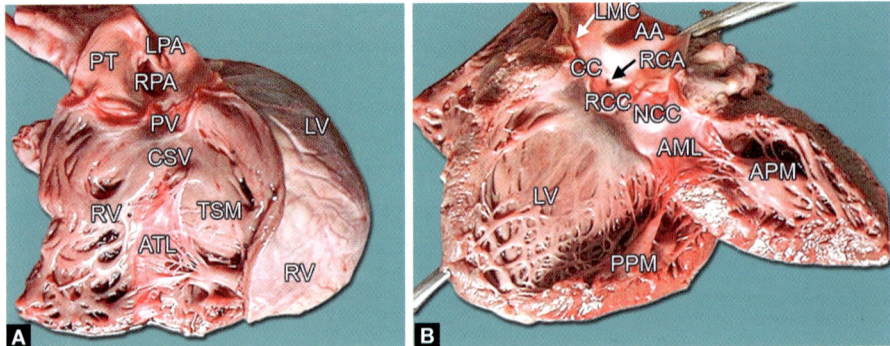

(AA: ascending aorta; AML: anterior mitral leaflet; APM: anterior papillary muscle; ATL: anterior tricuspid leaflet; CSV: crista supraventricularis; LCC: left coronary cusp; LMC: left main coronary artery; LPA: left pulmonary artery; LV: left ventricle; NCC: noncoronary cusp; PPM: posterior papillary muscle; PT: pulmonary trunk; PV: pulmonary valve; RCA: right coronary artery; RCC: right coronary cusp; RPA: right pulmonary artery; RV: right ventricle; TSM: trabeculo septomarginalis)

FIGS. 5.23A AND B: Opened out (A) right and (B) left ventricular outflow tracts, showing their characteristic morphology.

aortic valve. The cusps of the aortic valve are two anterior and one posterior. The space between the cusps and proximal aorta (including those in the pulmonary trunk) is called as sinuses-of-Valsalva. Most often, the sinuses are separated from the ascending aorta by a discontinuous ridge transverse ridge, the sinutubular junction. The right and left coronary arterial ostia are seen below it within the sinuses-of-Valsalva. Hence the cusps are designated as right coronary, left coronary, and noncoronary cusps. Importantly please also note that the anterior mitral leaflet has a fibrous continuity with left coronary cusp. Thus the mitral valve has only a true posterior annulus. It is to be noted that there are variations in the number of aortic valve cusps (bicuspid aortic valve is the most common congenital anomaly) and origin of the coronary arterial ostia. Sometimes, the conal branch of the right coronary artery arises directly from the ascending aorta. Some diseases also produce narrowing of the ostia.

The interventricular septum has two components, muscular and membranous. The muscular component has a sigmoid contour and can also be subdivided into inlet, trabecular, or sinus and outlet portions. Similar divisions can be applied to the sigmoid muscular interventricular septum. The roof of the membranous portion on the right side is formed by the attachment of anteroseptal commissure of tricuspid valve and on the left side; its roof is formed by adjoining halves of right and noncoronary cusps.

In general, the chambers are described with respect to the size, texture of the endocardium, and thickness of their walls. The endocardium may show thickening which at times can be rugose. Presence of localized plaques, jet lesions, and mural thrombi should be noted. The valve circumferences should be measured with a length of string. The circumferences of the valves are as follows: Tricuspid valve: 3.8–4.0 cm, pulmonary valve: 2.3–2.5 cm, mitral valve: 2.8–3.0 cm, and aortic valve: 2.2–2.5 cm. Valvular deformities produce changes in all parts of the valves, to a lesser or greater extent (**Fig. 5.24**). The atrioventricular valves are described in reference to the annuli, commissures, leaflets, chordae and papillary muscles, and the arterial valves as annuli,

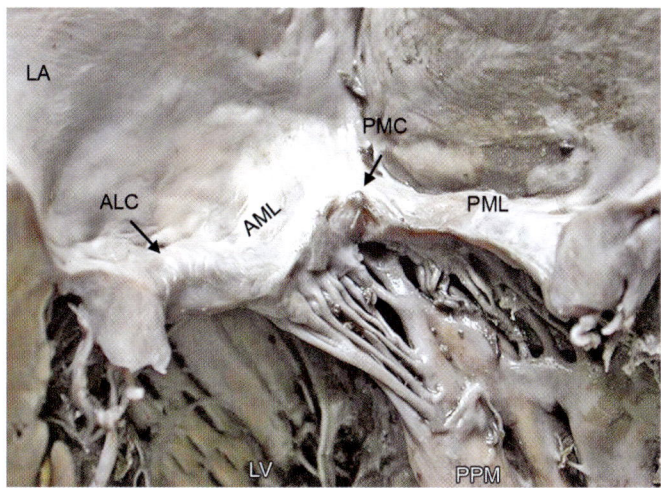

(ALC: anterolateral commissure; AML: anterior mitral leaflet; LA: left atrium; LV: left ventricle; PMC: posteromedial commissure; PML: posterior mitral leaflet; PPM: posterior papillary muscle)

FIG. 5.24: Rheumatic mitral stenosis showing involvement of all components of the valve. There is fusion of the commissures (arrows), thickening of the leaflets with chordal thickening, shortening, and fusion.

commissures, cusps, and their number. The valvular annuli may be normal, small, or dilated. The commissures may be normal, fused, or widened, while leaflets may be myxomatous, dysplastic, fibrotic, and/or calcified. Presence of vegetations and their characteristics (number, site, size, appearance, color, and friability) should be noted. The chordae may appear thick/thin, discrete/fused, long/short, and intact/ruptured. The number, position, and appearance of the papillary muscles should also be noted.

ALTERATIONS IN DISSECTION

The Virchow's method is useful as a teaching specimen, but it may not be possible to apply this method in certain cardiovascular diseases. This is especially true when there is extensive pericardial disease, where the heart may have to be longitudinally sectioned (**Fig. 5.25**). Furthermore, this four-chamber view is also useful in some myocardial diseases like dilated cardiomyopathy. Also alterations may be applied in postoperative cases as well as in congenital heart diseases.

SAMPLING FOR HISTOPATHOLOGY

Most often, the sampling depends upon the resources of the histopathology. By and large, if the heart appears normal, then a section each of the atria, ventricles, valves, and great arteries are taken along with the three coronary arteries. In diseases of the myocardium, relevant sections are taken from all the walls of the ventricles, along with additional sections from the atria, while in valvular deformities, samples are taken

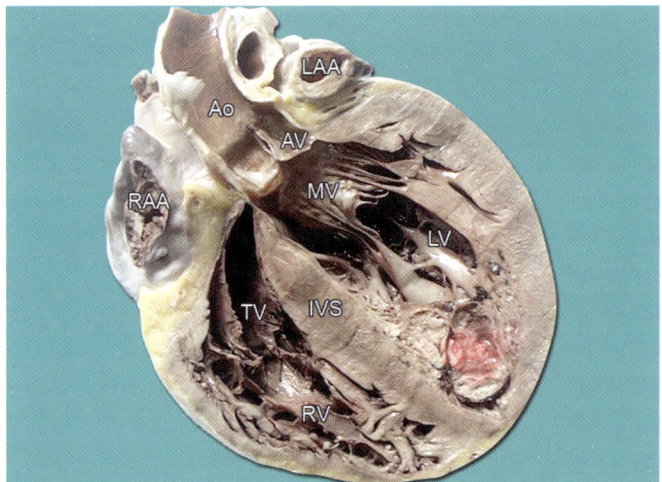

(Ao: aorta; AV: aortic valve; IVS: interventricular septum; LAA: left atrial appendage; LV: left ventricle; MV: mitral valve; RV: right ventricle; TV: tricuspid valve; RAA: right atrial appendage)

FIG. 5.25: The heart has been longitudinally bisected in a case of dilated cardiomyopathy to demonstrate biventricular dilatation and mural thrombus at the left ventricular apex.

from the diseased as well as normal looking valves as well. For coronary artery disease, the area of maximum narrowing or occlusion is always taken along with proximal and distal parts of the artery (where it is near normal or normal). All these segments, which already been serially sliced, are completely "blocked." Circumferential sections of the great arteries or their branches are taken. Accompanying elastic van Gieson (for the arteries) and additional connective tissue stain (for the myocardium, Masson's trichrome) is always preferred.

FURTHER READING

1. Alwan A, Maclean DR, Riley LM, d'Espaignet ET, Mathers CD, Stevens GA, Bettcher D. Monitoring and surveillance of chronic non-communicable diseases: progress and capacity in high-burden countries. Lancet. 2010;376:1861-8.
2. Edwards WD. Photography of medical specimens: Experiences from teaching cardiovascular pathology. Mayo Clin Proc. 1988;63:42-57.
3. Kim AS, Johnston C. Global variation in the relative burden of stroke and ischemic heart disease. Circulation. 2011;124:314-23.
4. Kumar RK, Tandon R. Rheumatic fever & rheumatic heart disease: The last 50 years. Indian J Med Res. 2013;137:643-58.
5. Virmani R, Ursell PC, Fenoglio JJ. Examination of the heart. Hum Pathol. 1987;18:432-40.

5C: Examination of the Respiratory System

Gayathri Amonkar

INTRODUCTION

Respiratory disorders are one of the leading causes of deaths worldwide. They account for around 16% of deaths in India, especially related to acute respiratory infections, tuberculosis, and chronic obstructive pulmonary diseases. In all cases of respiratory diseases, it is extremely important to note details pertaining to occupation, smoking, allergies, and concomitant cardiovascular disorders.

IMPORTANCE OF EXTERNAL AND IN SITU

EXAMINATION (SEE CHAPTER 2 AND 4 FOR DETAILS)

The respiratory system extends from the nares down to the alveoli. The autopsy procedure starts with the external inspection of the thoracic cage, particularly for chest wall deformities, curvature of the vertebral column, and the presence of swelling, fractures, or crepitus. Before opening the rib cage, presence of pneumothorax has to be ruled out. Pneumothorax can be tested by the following ways (**Figs. 5.26A to C**):
- A syringe filled with water may be inserted in the intercostal space before or after skin reflection; care should be taken not to insert it too deeply and puncture the lungs. Air bubbles entering the water in the syringe following aspiration are diagnostic of pneumothorax, or

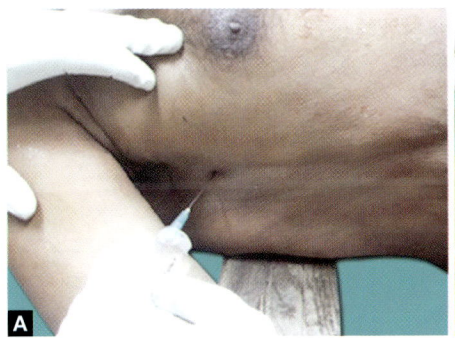
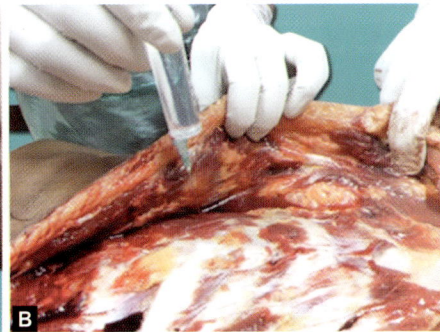
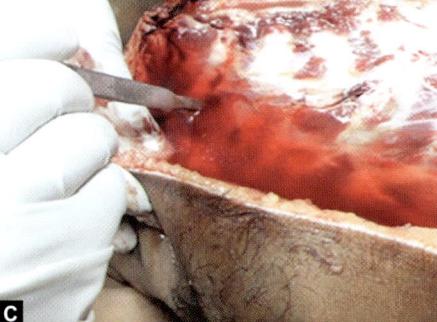

FIGS. 5.26A TO C: Methods for the demonstration of pneumothorax.

- The skin flap can be reflected and once the intercostal muscles are exposed, water is poured into the chest cavity. The chest is opened under water and escape of air is diagnostic of pneumothorax. In cases of pediatric autopsy, the entire body may be submerged under water and the procedure can be carried out.

Normally, the lungs are voluminous and cover the entire surface of the heart. During in situ examination, the pleural cavities are examined for morphological alterations, adhesions, and presence of exudates. Chronic diseases, particularly tuberculosis, often produce dense adhesions between the parietal and visceral layers of the pleura. The visceral pleura, which normally is smooth, shiny, and transparent, is inspected for the presence of rib markings, intense anthracotic pigment deposition, thickening, puckering, and presence of exudates, tubercles, plaques, or nodules (**Figs. 5.27A** and **B**). Exudates in the pleural cavity may be serous, fibrinous, suppurative, or hemorrhagic in nature. It is collected and examined microscopically and sent for microbiology studies.

The pulmonary arteries are examined for pulmonary thromboembolism. The main pulmonary artery must be felt and palpated first; emboli if present often feel cord-like. After palpation, a nick is made in the pulmonary artery. They appear friable greyish brown in color. Saddle-shaped thromboemboli occlude the pulmonary artery and its branches causing sudden death (see later). Air embolism can be seen in fatal cases of pneumothorax, pneumoperitoneum, operative procedures, postpartum cases, intravenous procedures, and in cases of injuries. For demonstration of air emboli, an incision of the skin is taken up to the sternal notch. The skin, subcutaneous tissue, and muscles are reflected and the sternum with the anterior ribs are dissected and carefully removed. The aorta is ligated and the pericardial sac is cut open. One should examine the heart carefully for any bulging which is seen in an embolism due to the distension by the entrapped air.

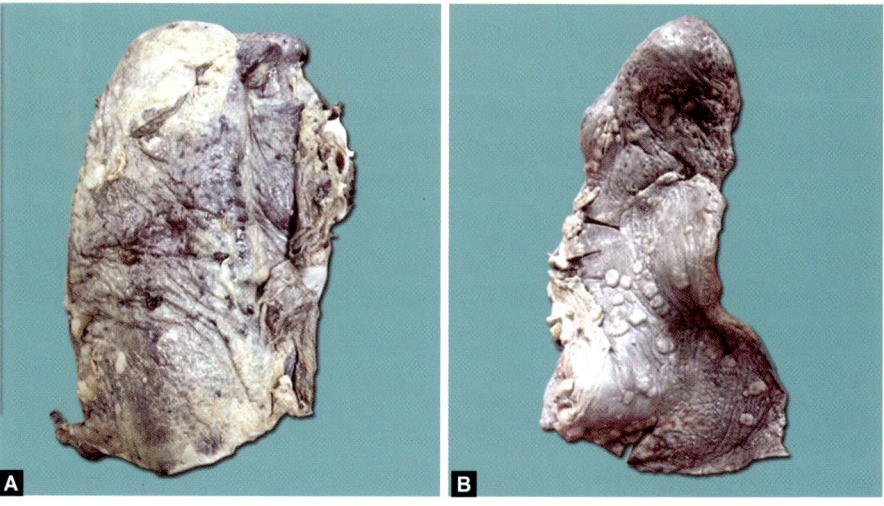

FIGS. 5.27A AND B: (A) Granular to flaky pale yellow purulent exudate over the visceral pleural surface; (B) Multiple small gray-white to pale yellow metastatic nodules and plaques over the pleura. Some of them even appear umbilicated.

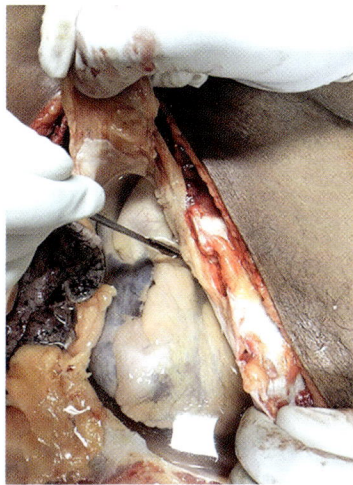

FIG. 5.28: Method for the demonstration of air embolism.

Water is poured in the pericardial cavity covering the heart completely (**Fig. 5.28**). When right-sided chambers or the pulmonary artery are incised with the scalpel, air bubbles will be seen coming out in the water in the pericardial cavity. When massive, bubbles will be seen even after cuts in the left-sided chambers or the coronary arteries.

LUNG DISSECTION, FIXATION AND CUTTING

The block (after separation of the heart) is placed with the posterior surface uppermost. The larynx, trachea, and the main bronchi are cut along their posterior aspect. The left bronchus is long, horizontal, and hyparterial, while the right bronchus is short, oblique, and eparterial; the left bronchus is also narrower than the right (**Fig. 5.29**). One should look for the presence of mucus, pus, blood, aspirated material (**Fig. 5.30A**), or tumor. The pulmonary arteries should always to be inspected for the presence of thromboemboli (**Fig. 5.30B**); the appearance of the hilar lymph nodes should also be noted (**Fig. 5.30C**).

The lungs are separated by cutting the bronchial stems as close to their hila as possible. The lungs should be weighed before their dissection; they weigh 250–400 g each in adults. The normal lungs are often difficult to cut in the fresh state. Some advocate fixation and lung inflation by formalin perfusion (**Figs. 5.31A** and **B**). This can be performed even with the heart and lung block. Formalin is passed through a cannula into the trachea or the individual bronchus from formalin container that is placed at a height (at least 30 cm). This ensures that formalin is perfusing the lungs at a pressure of 25–30 cm of water. The cannulated trachea or the bronchus is secured firmly by thread. Care should be taken to ensure the pleural surface is intact so that the fixative is preserved within the lungs. The perfusion should continue till the pleural surface is smooth (usually 10 minutes or less). The lungs are placed in formalin and the lungs then can be dissected 24 hours later. After perfusion fixation, morphology of

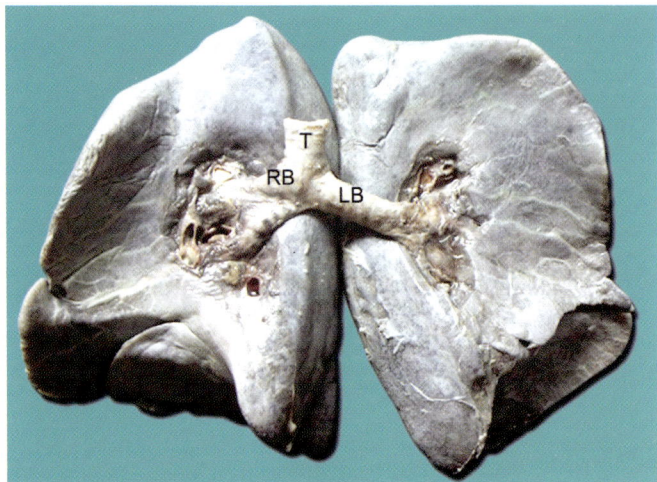

(T: trachea; RB: right bronchus; LB: left bronchus)

FIG. 5.29: Hilar aspects of the lungs to show the characteristic bronchial morphology.

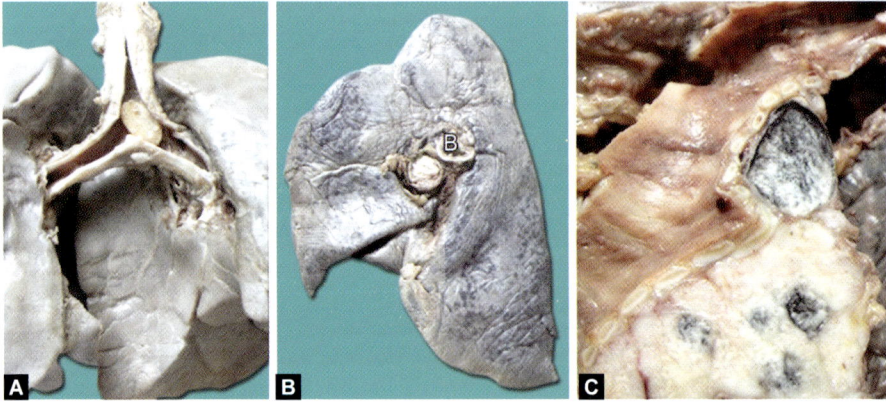

FIGS. 5.30A TO C: (A) A 6-month child choked to death. Note a groundnut astride the tracheal bifurcation. (B) Fatal pulmonary thromboembolism. The left pulmonary artery is occluded by a pale-red brown granular fresh thromboembolus. (C) The hilar lymph nodes are enlarged in size and almost completely replaced by metastatic tumor.

the lungs is better preserved and it is also easier to cut the lungs. A sharp, long-bladed knife is used to cut the lungs. It is important to palpate the lungs before cutting as some lesions are better felt than seen. There are different ways of cutting the lung, the next common being plain slicing of the lungs (parallel to the hilar surface) from the apex to the base aspect with the hilum facing downwards (**Figs. 5.31C** and **D**). Some authors advice dissecting the airways or the pulmonary arteries using probes from the hilum towards the pleural surfaces for predominant bronchial or pulmonary arterial

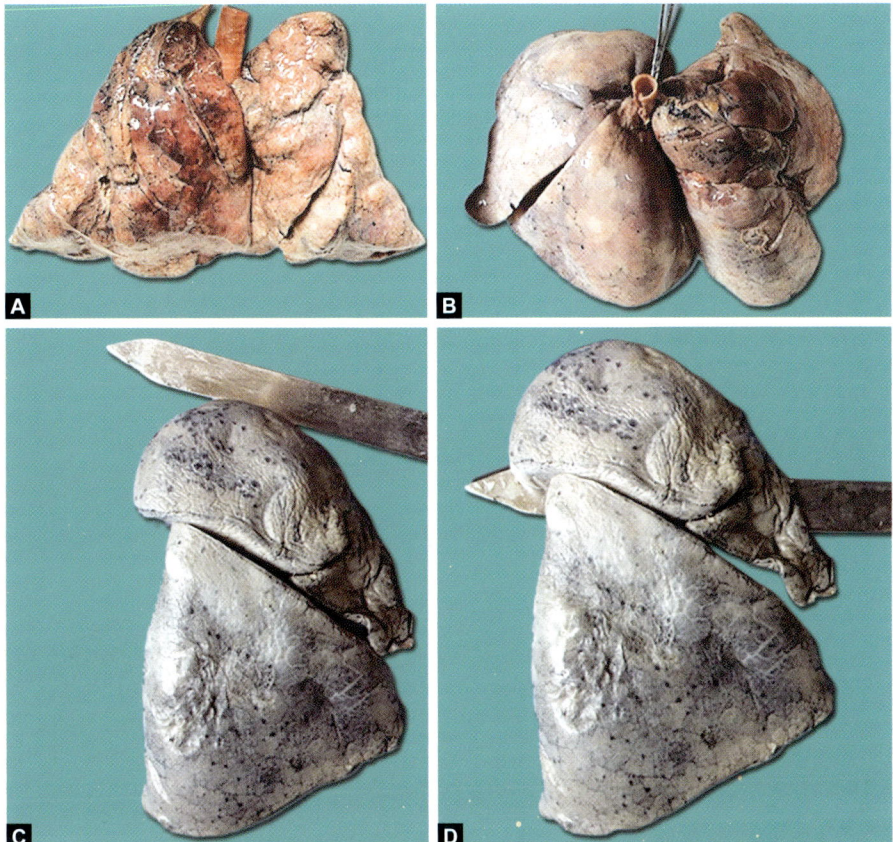

FIGS. 5.31A TO D: (A) Lungs in the fresh state; (B) Lungs immediately after perfusion with formalin; and (C and D) pattern of bisection the lung.

diseases, respectively. McCulloch et al. have described a modified technique where the upper lobe vessels are dissected from the hilum and the middle and right from the pleural surface. This preserves better anatomy of the lung for further examination. Transverse sectioning of the lungs has been recommended for correlation with CT and magnetic resonance imaging (MRI) scans. Gough Wentworth slices were whole lung slices used to study chronic obstructive diseases like emphysema, particularly in the pre-CT era, through a very laborious process; this is now no longer needed.

EXAMINATION OF THE LUNGS

The various gross pathologies of the lungs can be classified into localized and diffuse lung diseases. There may be instances of overlapping of some conditions being localized at times and diffuse in some other cases. The pathologies need to be correlated with radiological findings whenever available. The normal lung parenchyma is subcrepitant. In cases of edema, the lungs are heavy, wet, and frothy fluid

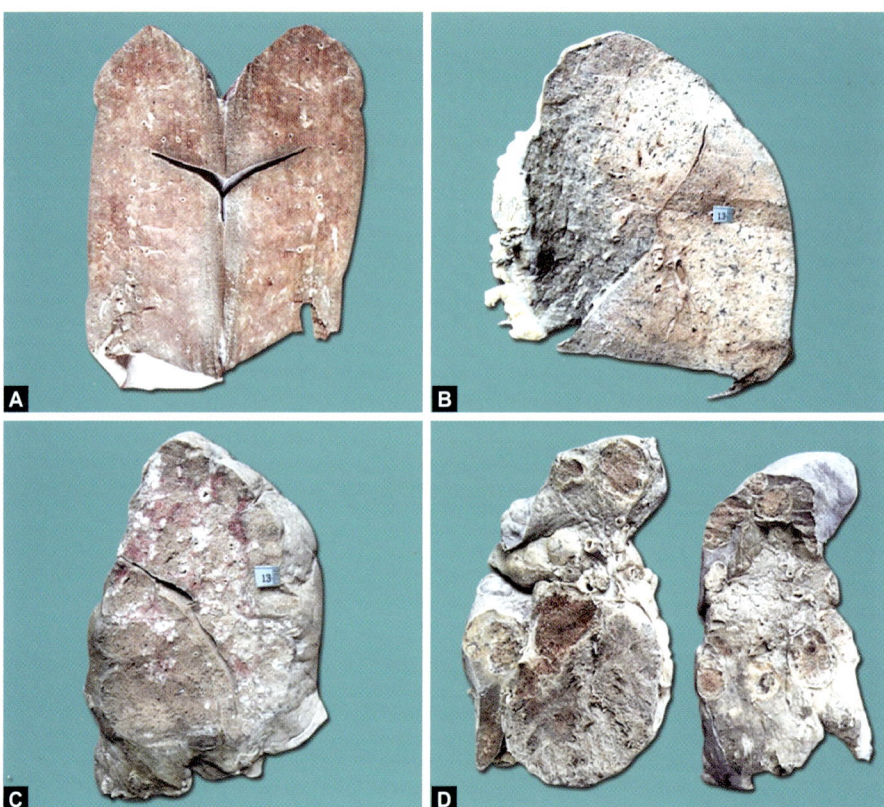

FIGS. 5.32A TO D: (A) Bisected left lung showing a diffuse uniform reddish discoloration due to diffuse alveolar damage; (B) The entire left lower lobe and parts of the upper lobe of the left lung show a uniform reddish consolidation—case of lobar pneumonia. Note accompanying fibrinous pleuritis; (C) The cut surface of the right lung shows scattered large and small areas of caseation necroses; the surrounding congested parenchyma showed hyaline membranes on histology; and (D) Serial slices of the right lung show well-circumscribed yellowish to hemorrhage metastases due to choriocarcinoma present in malignant testicular germ cell tumor.

oozes out on cutting the lungs. The lungs feel rubbery, firm, or solid in some localized or diffuse lungs diseases (**Figs. 5.32A** and **B**). The sinking test can be performed where a small piece of lung parenchyma is placed in a container of water; the piece sinks in cases of consolidation. Their locations and distinct colorations often enable one to make a tentative gross diagnosis. Some diseases are characterized by the presence of small or large, localized (solitary), or diffuse nodules; commonly these include tuberculosis and tumors (**Figs. 5.32C** and **D**).

Another common pathology seen in the lungs is cavitary, cystic, or bullous lesions. Cavities are sharply demarcated, usually air-filled spaces with regular or irregular walls, which have a thickness of >0.1 cm; the surrounding parenchyma

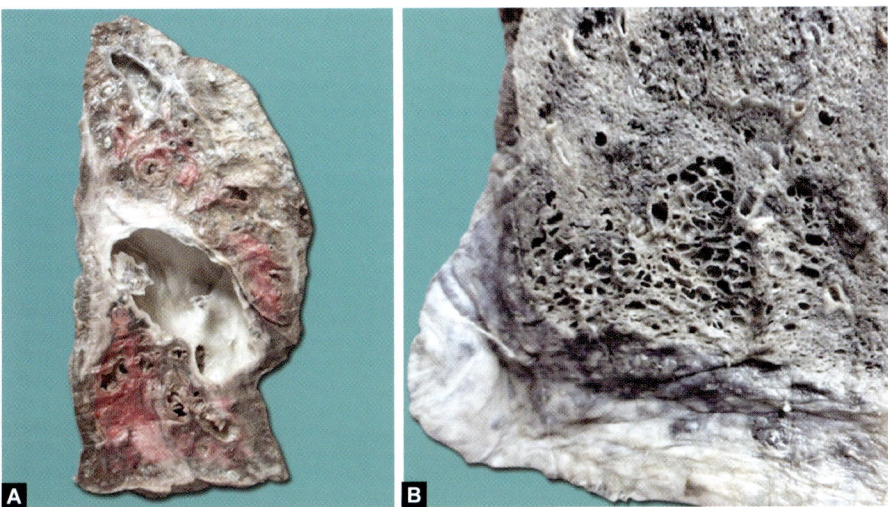

FIGS. 5.33A AND B: (A) Bronchiectasis of the left lung with formation of a large cavity; (B) Classic honey combing in a case of usual interstitial pneumonitis.

is usually diseased. Cavities occur in the lung occur due to the diseases involving the airways and/or the parenchyma. One should document the site, location, wall thickness, contents, inner lining, and the surrounding parenchyma (**Fig. 5.33A**). In cases of malignancies, the wall thickness of the cavitary lesion may be >1 cm. Cysts are thin walled and filled with air or liquid lined by respiratory epithelium. Bullae usually measure 1 cm or more, are sharply demarcated and are subpleural in location. They can get infected or may lead to pneumothorax. A predominant diffusely fibrotic gross pattern on lung is seen in a number of conditions, included under the umbrella of interstitial lung diseases. Their distribution serves as an important clue, e.g., in usual interstitial pneumonitis, the basal regions of the lungs that are involved, whereas in cases of silicosis the upper lobe is affected. In end-stage lung disease, the lungs are stony hard in consistency and show honeycombing (**Fig. 5.33B**), which externally resembles cirrhosis.

FURTHER READING

1. Baker RD. Postmortem examination: Special methods and procedures. Philadelphia: WB Saunders; 1967.
2. Ludwig J. Handbook of Autopsy Practice, 3rd edition, Totowa: Humana Press; 2002.
3. McCulloch TA, Rutty GN. Postmortem examination of the lungs: a preservation technique for opening the bronchi and pulmonary arteries individually without transsection problems. J Clin Pathol. 1998;51:163-4.
4. Nair S, Abraham A, Ramachandran R, Mohan D, Kutty RV. Pattern and determinants of respiratory mortality in Kerala, South India. Int J Med Public Health. 2014;4:467-71.
5. Shaeff, Michael T, Hopster, Deborah J. Post Mortem Technique Handbook, 2nd edition. Verlag London: Springer; 2005.

5D: Gastrointestinal Tract at Autopsy

Anjali D Amarapurkar

INTRODUCTION

The gastrointestinal tract (GIT) is a long tubular system that starts with mouth and ends at anal canal. It is capable of digesting/absorbing food as well as expelling the undigested material. The entire system is under hormonal control. After food is mixed with saliva, it is swallowed and passes down in esophagus. With the help of esophageal musculature, it is propelled into the stomach. Stomach is J-shaped organ with two openings, one is at distal esophagus and other is at proximal duodenum. Stomach helps in preliminary digestion of food. It produces acid and has antibacterial action. Small bowel is site where chemical and mechanical digestions are carried out with absorption of major nutrients. Large bowel absorbs water and passes semisolid feces into rectum to be expelled out through anus.

Common gastrointestinal symptoms are abdominal pain (acute or chronic), dysphagia, dyspepsia, nausea, vomiting, and diarrhea. This symptomatology is primarily related to gastrointestinal disorder. Acute abdominal pain <24 hours can be due to acute appendicitis, cholecystitis, acute pancreatitis, diverticular disease, perforated duodenal ulcer, small bowel obstruction, or ischemia. In majority of them, diagnosis is arrived with clinical, endoscopic, and radiological findings. However, in occasional cases diagnosis remains obscure despite investigations. However, it is important to note that there are many extraintestinal conditions, which can present with similar symptoms. Extraintestinal causes for acute abdominal pain are cardiac (myocardial ischemia), pneumonitis, uremia, infections, hypersensitivity reactions, or neurological cause. Hence, while performing autopsy not only gastrointestinal but other systems should be examined carefully. Chronic abdominal pain is multi-dimensional and its diagnosis is challenging due to varied etiology. Some patients have functional causes. At times, diagnostic tests also fail to find the cause of chronic abdominal pain.

Dysphagia, regurgitation, or reflux is common symptoms pointing towards esophageal diseases such as esophagitis, gastroesophageal reflux disease, neuromuscular causes, or carcinoma esophagus. Dyspepsia affects >20% of general population. It is caused by peptic ulcer disease, esophageal infections, malignancy, and food intolerance. Nongastrointestinal causes are medications, pancreatobiliary disorders (chronic pancreatitis, cholelithiasis, biliary obstruction, and pancreatic neoplasms) or systemic diseases such as diabetes mellitus or thyroid diseases. Almost 30% of patients with chronic dyspepsia do not have significant focal or structural lesions. They are labeled as functional dyspepsia.

Nausea and vomiting are very common symptoms. Mechanical gastric outlet obstruction, small bowel obstruction, peptic ulcer disease, infections, drugs, acute appendicitis, cholecystitis, pancreatic disease, and ischemia are various causes, which should be looked for while performing dissection. Extraintestinal causes include mainly CNS disorders such as infections, migraine, increased intracranial pressure, and neoplasms.

Diarrhea is another common symptom and not a disease. It can occur in many conditions. Diarrhea frequently represents protective response to variety of intestinal insults. Common causes of diarrhea are bacterial infection, parasite, food poisoning, or allergy. Chronic diarrhea is seen in inflammatory bowel disease, vasculitis, or neoplasms. Since extraintestinal diseases also present with gastrointestinal complaints, meticulous examination of organs other than GIT is essential. At least 2% of autopsies reveal causes other than suspected clinically.

IN SITU EXAMINATION

Once abdominal cavity is opened, one sees the stomach with greater omentum, coils of small intestine, and the transverse colon. Normally, the liver is usually not seen, but if there is an enlargement, then the liver is seen below the right subcostal margin to a variable extent. Examine the omentum carefully for blood vessels and lymph nodes, and then displace the omentum and transverse colon superiorly. While removing intestinal loops, observe for any surgical anastomosis, if present examine anastomotic site for sutures, gaping wound, inflammation, or ischemic change at that site. Shift coils of small intestine to one side, exposing the duodenojejunal junction. The duodenum is identified by its fixity to underlying retroperitoneal structures. It is shortest and widest part of the small intestine measuring about 25 cm in length. Clamp, ligate, and cut the small intestine at the duodenojejunal junction.

Start removing small bowel loops by cutting mesentery close to the serosa (**Fig. 5.34A**). Pull the bowel loops toward the prosector, which makes removal of the bowel easy. The mesentery should be thoroughly checked for presence of lymph nodes and status of blood vessels, which is best achieved by spreading out of mesentery. Identify ileocecal junction and appendix, lift it up, and remove adherent fibroadipose tissue. At hepatic flexure, return the omentum and transverse colon back to their anatomical position. Cut through transverse mesocolon and continue along with the descending colon till the rectosigmoid junction is reached. Put ligature at rectosigmoid junction and transect the bowel. Rectosigmoid junction is indicated by the lower end of the sigmoid mesocolon. Then the rectum follows concavity of the sacrum and coccyx. The rectum ends by becoming continuous with the anal canal at the anorectal junction which is 2-3 cm in front of the tip of coccyx. In males, it corresponds to the apex of prostate. The esophagus, stomach, and duodenum with liver, pancreas, spleen, and kidneys are as thoracoabdominal block and further dissected depending on the case history of the deceased.

SYSTEMIC EXAMINATION

The small intestine is about 6 meters long, which includes the duodenum, jejunum and ileum. The large intestine is 1.5 meters long divided into cecum, appendix, ascending, transverse, descending, sigmoid colon, rectum, and anal canal. As compared to small intestine, the large intestine is wide in caliber with presence of taenia coli and appendices epiploicae. Opening of the intestinal loops is done with an instrument called enterotome (**Fig. 5.34B**). It is nothing but a larger scissor with one blunt end that lies in the lumen of the intestine. Then intestinal loops are cut along

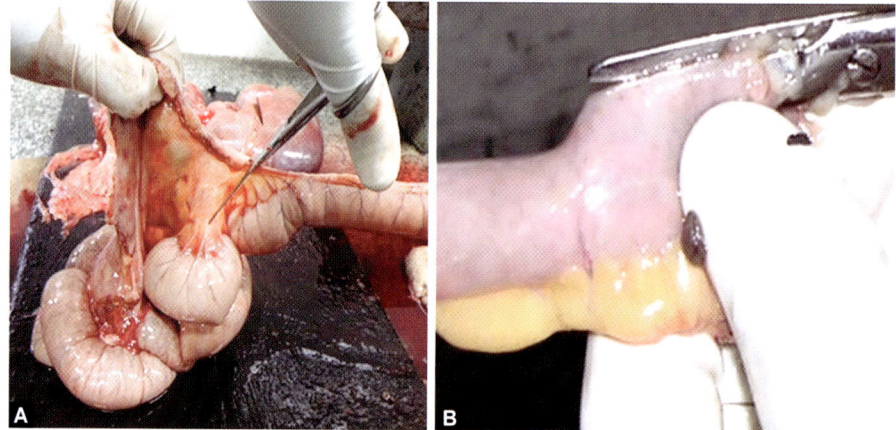

FIGS. 5.34A AND B: (A) Separating mesentery from bowel wall; (B) The small intestine is cut through the antemesenteric border with an enterotome.

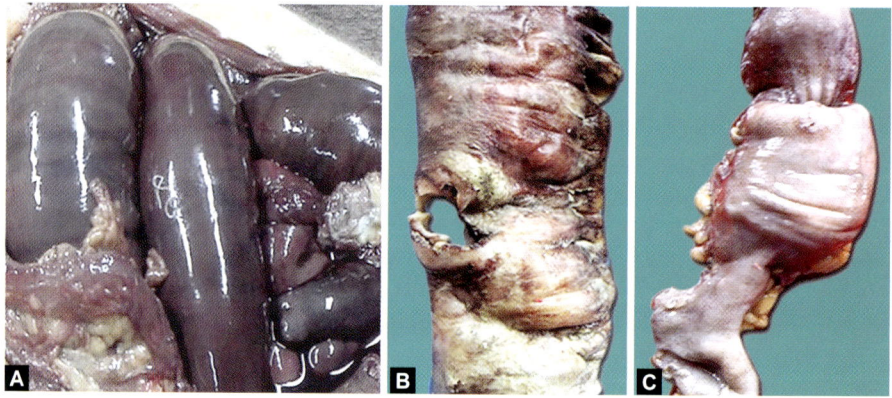

FIGS. 5.35A TO C: (A) Dilated extremely congested gangrenous small intestinal loops; (B) Perforated small bowel with exudate on serosa; and (C) Ileoileal intussusception.

its long axis, through the antimesenteric border, under running tap water. Observe serosal surfaces for exudates, gangrene (**Fig. 5.35A**), perforation (**Fig. 5.35B**), stricture, intussusceptions (**Fig. 5.35C**), or tumor deposits. In intussusception, a part of bowel slides into adjacent bowel loop. It is common in pediatric age group. In adults, it may be due to underlying tumor. It can be associated with complications such as infection, bowel perforation, or ischemia. Hence, every intussusception should be opened to check for tumor or its complications. Expose the mucosa and look for ulceration, mucosal irregularities, polyps, or tumor. Patients with severe infective colitis on antibiotic therapy can show presence of pseudomembranes (**Fig. 5.36A**). The large bowel can show ischemic ulcers, which are superficial but with hemorrhagic borders (**Fig. 5.36B**). Tumors are usually diagnosed antemortem. However, one can get incidental tumor at autopsy. Intestinal loops should be handled as little as possible.

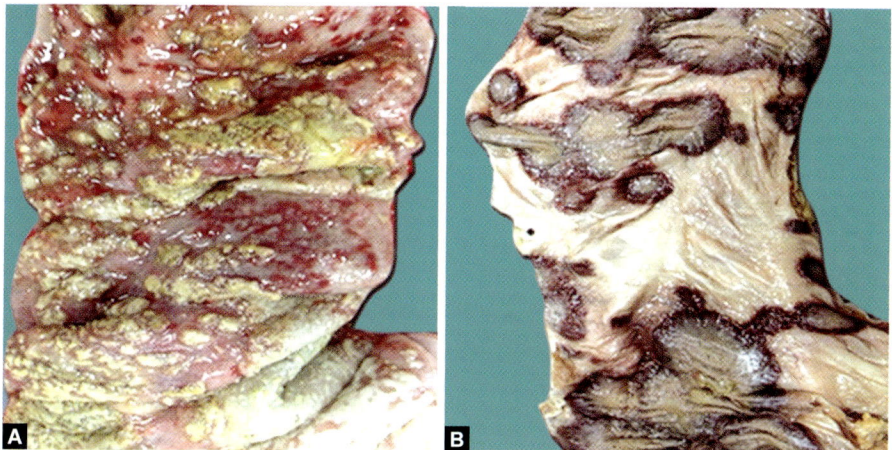

FIGS. 5.36A AND B: (A) Pseudomembranous colitis, in which mucosa is extensively ulcerated and covered with a pseudomembrane; (B) Multiple superficial ulcers with hyperemic borders suggestive of ischemic ulcers.

They should be kept in formalin (10%) at least for 24 hours to get good fixation. Satisfactory results are obtained, if the fixation begins within 6 hours after death. If there is any lesion, it is advisable to pin the representative bowel loop on paraffin tray covered with cotton and soaked in formalin. This method exposes the lesion well so that photography and section taking becomes easy. If tumor or any pathology is suspected in duodenum, periampullary region, or head of pancreas, then duodenum should be opened in situ. Specimen can be suspended in formalin bath. Locate pathological lesion and take representative sections as that of surgical specimen.

Remove omental fat from greater curvature of stomach. The esophagus is opened along its length and examined for mucosal lesions or tumors. The esophageal mucosa is white as compared to gastric mucosa, which can be well appreciated at gastroesophageal junction. Various types of ulcers (superficial or deep) can be seen in esophagus, majority of these have infective etiology. Representative sections are taken from those ulcers. Esophageal carcinoma is rare finding at autopsy, since it is diagnosed early on clinical and radiological grounds. However, occasional carcinomas grow outward and develop fistula with adjacent organs. When tracheoesophageal fistula or infiltrating cancer is suspected, esophagus should be left attached to the mediastinal organs. Tracheoesophageal fistula can be demonstrated by opening the esophagus along its posterior wall and opening the trachea anteriorly. Note down the connection between two.

Fix specimen well and take representative sections. Tracheoesophageal fistula in adults is found in cases of esophageal perforation, tuberculosis, or infiltrating malignancy. A different method is followed for demonstrating esophageal varices. In such cases, esophagus should be left attached to the stomach, which should be opened along the greater curvature. Remove the contents of the stomach. A string is tied at the upper end of the unopened esophagus and then pulled through the lumen to evert the esophagus (**Fig. 5.37A**). With this method, varices are well visualized at

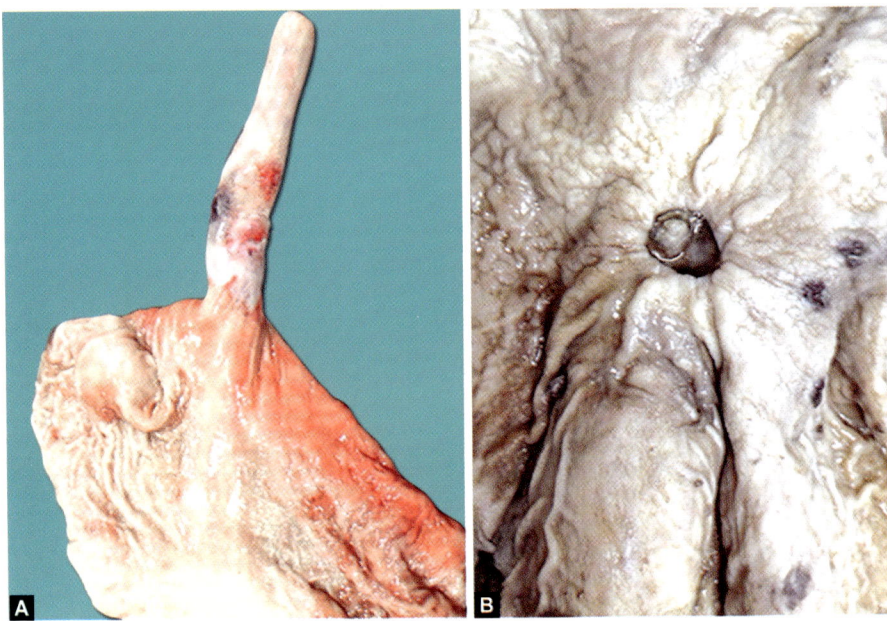

FIGS. 5.37A AND B: (A) The esophagus has been everted to show varices, which are tied up with bands; (B) Benign gastric ulcer showing clean base and radiating mucosal folds.

gastroesophageal junction and become more prominent with the formalin fixation. Esophageal varices can be enhanced by injecting varices by barium sulfate-gelatin.

The stomach is opened along its greater curvature. Observe gastric mucosa for the mucosal folds, ulceration, erosions, vascular malformations, or tumor. Benign gastric ulcer (peptic ulcer) was a common finding few years back. However, due to effective treatment for acid peptic disease, it is not very common to get such ulcerations at autopsy (**Fig. 5.37B**). In cases of penetrating ulcers or infiltrating tumors, it is advisable to keep the stomach with adjacent organs, or whatever the infiltrating organ might be. Then give representative sections and note infiltrative nature of the lesion. Due to early autolytic changes, microscopic examination of gastric mucosa is unsatisfactory especially to determine intestinal metaplasia or *Helicobacter pylori*. Collection of stomach content is useful in some of the medicolegal cases. The stomach and small bowel contents are collected in properly labeled jar with saturated solution of sodium chloride for analysis of poisons, drugs, or toxins in suspected cases. Entire stomach and segment of duodenum can be sent to reference toxicology laboratory. Mesenteric angiography is performed in cases where gastrointestinal vasculature needs to be studied; the celiac axis, superior, and inferior mesenteric arteries can be injected with barium sulfate-gelatin mixture either in situ or after removal of the block.

Special Situations

Following are common situations where autopsy procedure can be modified.

Peritoneal Adhesions

Adhesions are most common cause of bowel obstruction. It is also very common situation after abdominal surgery. When multiple adhesions are seen, dissection is done layer by layer. One may have to do blunt dissection using fingers. Avoid damage to adjacent viscera while dissecting. When numerous adhesions are present due to metastasis or because of peritonitis, leave intestines attached to other abdominal organs. Some bowel loops can be kept unopened to maintain anatomical relations. Careful sections are taken from adjacent organs.

Peritonitis

Inflammation of peritoneum or peritoneal cavity caused by localized or generalized infection by bacteria, virus, or fungi without GI perforation is labeled as primary peritonitis; while in the presence of GI perforation, it is secondary peritonitis. In peritonitis, exudates are seen over bowel loops or within peritoneal cavity. Exudate is usually well appreciated as soon as abdominal skin flap is opened. Note down color of exudates. It can be collected in culture tube for microbiological examination. In presence of peritonitis dissection of bowel loops is done carefully. While doing so, rule out perforation of any part of GIT. When numerous adhesions are present, it is advisable to leave the intestinal loops attached to adjacent abdominal organs.

Gastrointestinal Perforation

Perforation of any part of GIT is very frequent finding at autopsy. Most common site of perforation is duodenum and pyloric perforation by peptic ulcer disease. Small bowel and colonic perforations are not uncommon. Various common causes for GI perforation are stress ulcers in stomach, *H. pylori* infection, nonsteroidal anti-inflammatory drug (NSAID) use, alcohol, smoking, typhoid/paratyphoid infection, *Yersinia*, diverticulitis, Crohn's disease, tuberculosis, and iatrogenic or noniatrogenic trauma. Peforations can also occur with appendicitis or cholecystitis. When bowel loops perforate, their walls are inflamed, thin, delicate, and fragile. While performing autopsy, locate site of perforation, number, and size of perforation. Perforating bowel wall can adhere to adjacent viscera. Hence, dissection should be carried out in such a way that anatomy is maintained. This is important especially in postoperative cases. Examine and sample perforated bowel loops. Generally, in presence of perforation, bowel wall is opened on opposite side of perforation. If perforation is on mesenteric border, then bowel opening is done from antimesenteric border so as to visualize perforated site completely. Note down adjacent mucosa or bowel wall if it is showing any pathology such as stricture, ulceration, or malignancy. Majority of times perforation is complicated by peritonitis.

Gastrointestinal Bleeding

Esophageal varices, peptic ulcer disease, Mallory–Weiss tears, Dieulafoy's lesion, NSAIDs, and vascular ectasias are common causes for upper GI bleeding. Ulcerative colitis, septicemia, Crohn's disease, colonic ulcers, NSAIDs, and angiodysplasia are common causes for lower GI bleeding. GI bleeding can be in the form of hemorrhagic mucosal spots, hemorrhagic ulcers, to fresh or altered blood. Note the color, quantity, and probable site for bleeding. Most of the times at autopsy, it is not possible to identify the source of bleeding. Bowel loops filled with blood should be opened under running tap water. Examine underlying mucosa for any pathology.

Bowel Gangrene

Small and large bowel gangrene is not uncommon. Gangrenous loops look dusky bluish red. Bowel loops should be dissected along with mesenteric blood vessels. It is difficult to locate thrombus by naked eye examination. Blood vessels should be palpated while searching for thrombus. Dissection should be extended till you include viable bowel segment at both ends.

Histopathological Examination of Gastrointestinal Tract

Histopathological features of GIT at autopsy are very discouraging. Autolytic changes develop very fast in gastrointestinal mucosa. However, there is no much concern about autolytic changes of GI mucosa as major pathology is rarely a cause of death. Mucosal lining, surface epithelial changes, villous morphology, villi, and crypts cannot be well assessed at autopsy. Hence meticulous gross examination is the key for evaluating gastrointestinal pathology at autopsy.

FURTHER READING

1. Bayer-Garner IB, Fink LM, Lamps LW. Pathologists in a teaching institution assess the value of the autopsy. Arch Pathol Lab Med. 2002;126:442-7.
2. Connolly AJ, Finkbeiner WE, Ursell PC, Davis RL. Autopsy Pathology: A Manual and Atlas, 3rd edition. Philadelphia: Elsevier; 2016.
3. Waters BL. Handbook of autopsy practice, 4th edition. United States: Humana Press; 2009.

5E: Approach in Autopsy of Patients with Liver-related Problems

Ashim Das

INTRODUCTION

Nowadays, a large number of deaths occur as a result of various liver diseases. The increase in liver-related deaths in the hospital are possibly due to liver diseases resulting from increased alcohol intake in our society and due to increase in the number of viral hepatitis of various causes. One can encounter even many pregnancy-related deaths with liver diseases like viral hepatitis. It is very important that a meticulous autopsy is needed to reach a final diagnosis because the etiology of chronic liver diseases is also numerous. A different cohort of liver diseases exists in our pediatric populations; hence a detailed understanding of the disease occurring in different age groups is also needed. An external examination during the time of autopsy with a detailed gross and microscopic examination is a must in all cases of liver related deaths. The liver is usually preserved with the biliary tract, portal venous system, and the spleen (**Figs. 5.38A and B**). The sera should be preserved in all cases of liver diseases for viral serology for future use. The liver tissue should also be preserved for any further molecular biology study to find etiology in these cases (hepatitis A, B, C, D, or E).

EXTERNAL EXAMINATION

An external examination should include the findings of engorged abdominal veins for assessing the portal hypertension, the color of skin for jaundice, and the bilateral

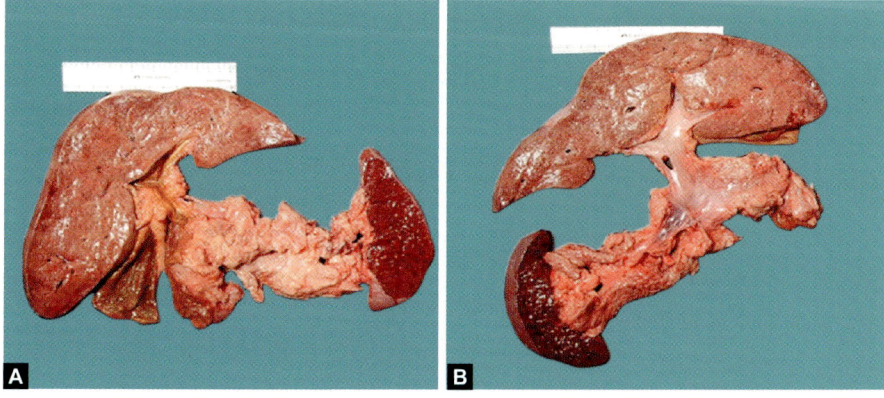

FIGS. 5.38A AND B: (A) A slice of normal liver with normal biliary tract and gallbladder, pancreas, and spleen; (B) Cut surface of liver with normal portal and splenic veins.

enlargement of parotid gland or the testicular atrophy in chronic liver diseases; as these are important clues for chronic liver diseases.

INTERNAL EXAMINATION

- The serosal cavities should be examined thoroughly regarding the amount and color of ascitic and pleural fluids. A turbid ascitic fluid may indicate spontaneous bacterial peritonitis in cirrhosis of liver.
- *Examination of liver:*
  - *Examination of the capsular surface:* The capsular wrinkling may indicate the loss of hepatic parenchyma in massive hepatic necrosis following viral hepatitis. The bile stained and congested liver may be seen in viral hepatitis. The shrinkage of the liver volume may also indicate the loss of hepatic parenchyma. The markedly congested liver may be following due to acute Budd–Chiari syndrome or chronic passive venous congestion.
  - *Color of the liver:* The brown color of the liver may indicate an iron overload state whereas the pale, yellow liver indicates fatty liver (**Fig. 5.39**).
  - *Presence of nodules:* The next assessment should be whether the liver is cirrhotic or noncirrhotic by examining the capsular and cut surface of the liver. The presence of nodules should be diffuse with fibrosis. A diffuse vague nodularity in the liver without any fibrosis may indicate diffuse nodular regenerative hyperplasia.
    – *Assessment of cirrhotic liver:*
      ▪ The size of the nodules is important to determine whether the liver micronodular or macronodular depending on the 3-mm cutoff. It is important to get a clue to the etiology of the cirrhosis. An enlarged micronodular liver without any significant splenomegaly points

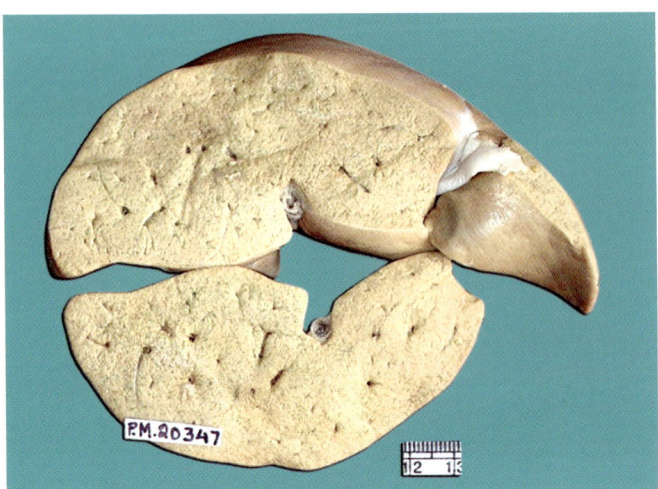

FIG. 5.39: Diffuse yellow discoloration in fatty liver.

toward alcoholic cirrhosis (**Fig. 5.40A**), while the liver of macronodular cirrhosis following viral hepatitis or autoimmune hepatitis may be shrunken with significant splenomegaly (**Fig. 5.40B**).

- *Abnormally sized nodules:* Any abnormality in the size of the nodules warrants for a thorough microscopic examination. The nodules of >1 cm indicate a macro-regenerative nodule (**Fig. 5.40C**), and an abnormally sized nodule may indicate a hepatocellular carcinoma (HCC, **Fig. 5.40D**).
- *Texture of nodule*: It is important to assess any change in color or texture in any of these nodules of cirrhotic liver to identify HCC. Abnormally large regenerative nodules should be identified and sampled for microscopic examination. In this way, one can identify dysplastic nodules and small and well-differentiated HCC. Any cirrhotic nodules with hemorrhagic and necrotic cut surface indicate HCC.
- *An abnormally sized nodule in a background of cirrhosis indicates HCC:* The HCC may be unicentric or multicentric. The unicentric HCC may have one large unicentric nodule with small satellite nodules. On the other hand, multiple small nodules indicate a multicentric HCC. The HCC can occur in a noncirrhotic background. The examination of portal veins and bile ducts is needed as HCC often invades the portal

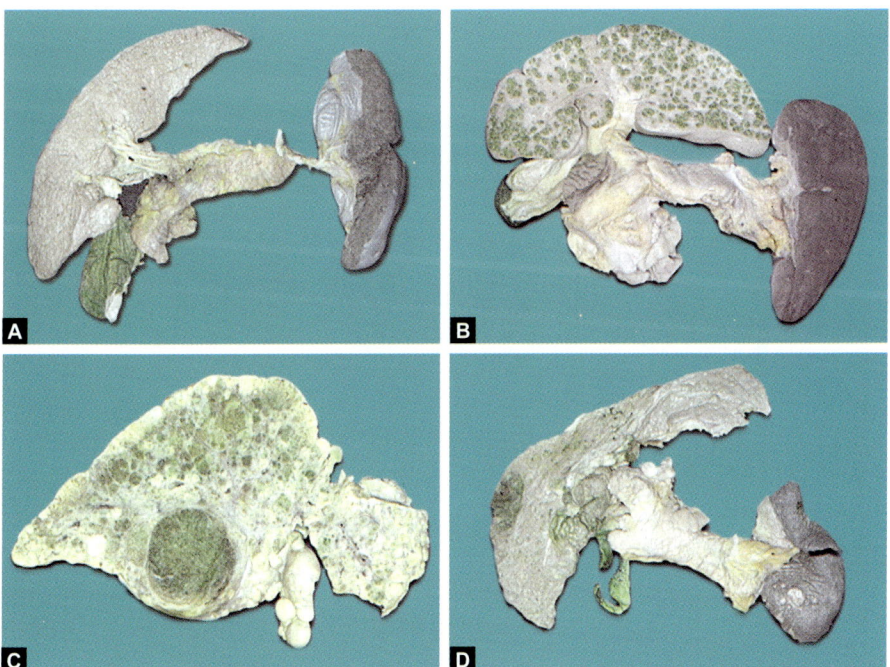

FIGS. 5.40A TO D: (A) Alcoholic micronodular cirrhosis; (B) Macronodular cirrhosis–autoimmune hepatitis related; (C) Macrogenerative nodule in hereditary tyrosinemia; and (D) Macronodular cirrhosis with development of hepatocellular carcinoma.

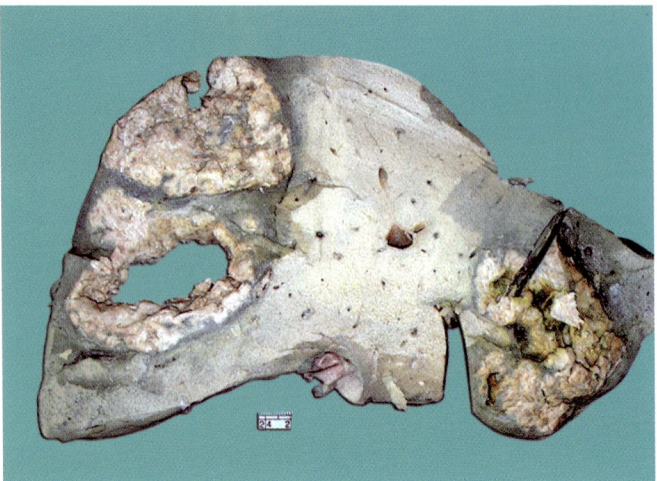

FIG. 5.41: Hepatic amebiasis with multiple abscesses.

vein and bile ducts. The examination of the lymph nodes around the porta and the portal vein is essential to exclude any tertiary metastasis.
– *Assessment of noncirrhotic liver:*
- A large solitary necrotic lesion of the liver in the absence of underlying cirrhosis should be suspected for amebic liver abscess; on the other hand, multiple abscesses should be suspected for pyogenic liver abscesses. There may be exception for this generalization. In case of amebic liver abscess, multiple small satellite abscesses may be seen in addition to a large abscess (**Fig. 5.41**). The examination of the surfaces of the liver and the diaphragm is needed to assess any rupture of the abscess. The amebic liver abscess may rupture into the pleura, lung, or peritoneum; hence, the examination of the lung and pleurae is important. The involvement of small portal veins may lead into hemorrhagic infarcts in amebic liver abscess.
- Multiple nodules in liver are usually characteristic of metastatic liver diseases (**Fig. 5.42A**); however, multicentric HCC or intrahepatic cholangiocarcinoma may be multinodular (**Fig. 5.42B**). The metastatic nodules can show surface umbilication.
- A hemorrhagic infarct in the liver has to be labeled as Zahn infarct, which can be seen in portal vein thrombosis or preeclampsia—preeclampsia syndrome.
- A nutmeg liver is recognized by the presence of hemorrhagic and nonhemorrhagic liver and indicates the presence of chronic passive venous congestion. The presence of nutmeg liver should prompt a thorough examination of the heart to identify any valvular lesions.
- An enlarged hemorrhagic liver should prompt a thorough examination of the hepatic veins.

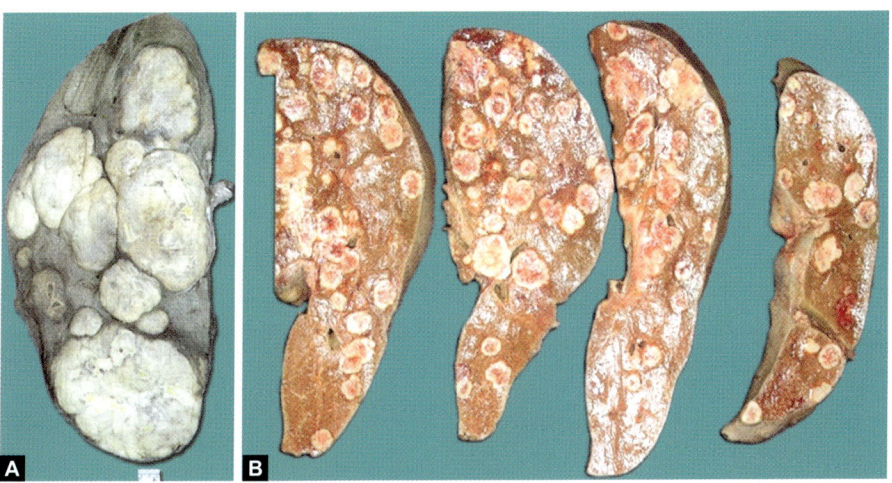

FIGS. 5.42A AND B: (A) Metastatic liver from a small gastrointestinal gastrinoma; (B) Intrahepatic cholangiocarcinoma mimicking metastatic liver disease.

- A thorough examination of portal veins, hepatic veins, and biliary tracts is needed (this part is generally ignored).
  - *Examination of portal veins:* The portal vein should be dissected from its origin to its bifurcation approaching from the posterior aspect. The splenic vein and superior mesenteric veins should be examined. The portal vein should be dissected to identify any thrombus or any extension of HCC into the portal vein. An unusually enlarged spleen may suggest a thrombus in the portal vein or its branches. An atrophic lobe of liver may also suggest thrombosis of one branch of the portal veins. The angiomatous transformation of the portal vein at the hilum with massive splenomegaly suggests a diagnosis of extrahepatic portal vein obstruction (EHPVO, **Figs. 5.43A** and **B**). A patent portal vein with massive splenomegaly will favor a diagnosis of noncirrhotic portal fibrosis (NCPF, **Figs. 5.43C** and **D**) than EHPVO.
  - The examination of hepatic veins is essential when there is a clinical suspicion of hepatic outflow tract obstruction (HPVO) or otherwise. The posterior most slices are to be examined for the hepatic veins. Even the examination of inferior vena cava is essential in HPVO. In the absence of any obstruction in the hepatic veins in an otherwise hepatic venous obstruction may suggest either veno-occlusive disease or congestive heart failure.

    The biliary tract should be examined from the hepatic ducts to the duodenal papilla approaching from the anterior aspects meticulously to exclude extrahepatic biliary atresia in children and any causes of large bile duct obstruction by stone or tumors in adults. The examination of duodenal papilla and the head of pancreas are essential to exclude any other causes of large bile duct obstruction. Many times HCC may infiltrate the biliary tree. In intrahepatic and extrahepatic cholangiocarcinoma, the bile ducts should be traced up to the lesion. The cholangiocarcinoma may

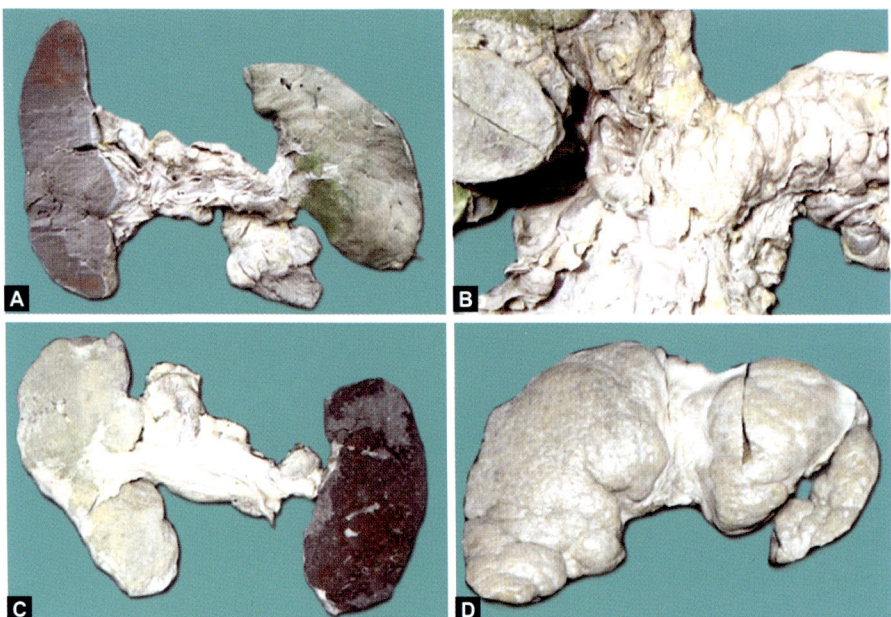

FIGS. 5.43A TO D: (A) Extrahepatic portal vein obstruction (EHPVO) with massive splenomegaly; (B) Tortuous splenic vein with obliterated portal vein and varices; (C) Noncirrhotic portal fibrosis (NCPF) with massive splenomegaly; and (D) Irregularity on external surface of liver in NCPF.

be intraductal producing stenotic lesions or may be periductal without producing obstructive lesions and may be mass forming. The bile ducts and hepatic ducts should be examined for the identification of stricture in primary sclerosing cholangitis (PSC). Multiple strictures in the extrahepatic ducts favor a diagnosis of PSC.

- The status of gall bladder should be noted. Absent gall bladder suggests extrahepatic biliary atresia in neonatal cholestasis syndrome than neonatal hepatitis or any metabolic liver disorders. A small contracted gallbladder is more commonly seen in cystic fibrosis. The gallbladder lumen and the associated biliary tract should be examined for the presence of stones (**Fig. 5.44**). The appearance of the mucosa and thickness of the wall also should be noted. At times, occult gallbladder cancer is associated with distant dissemination.

- *Examination of spleen:* The spleen should be weighed; an unusually enlarged spleen should warrant for an additional diagnosis for any hematological causes. A massively enlarged spleen in alcoholic cirrhosis should raise the suspicion of portal vein thrombosis, as the spleen in alcoholic cirrhosis is not significantly enlarged.

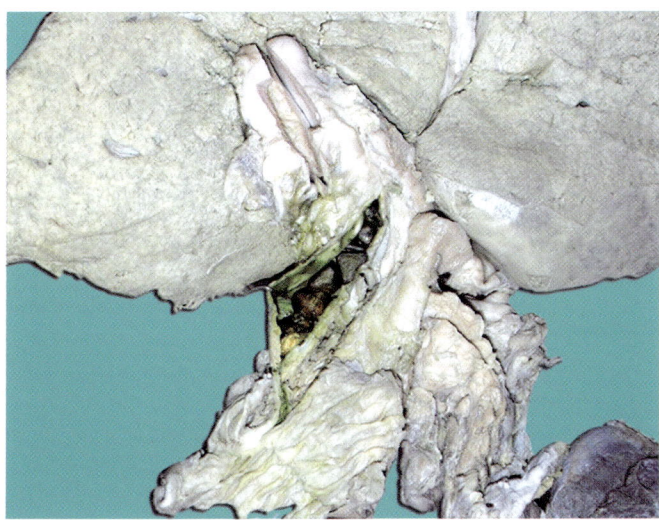

FIG. 5.44: Thick gallbladder with choledocholithiasis.

Examination of the pancreas: It is essential to exclude any evidence of pancreatic disease, which may be associated with alcoholic liver disease or any neoplastic lesions in case of large bile duct obstruction or metastatic liver disorders. The appearance and size of the pancreas is noted. Depending on the pathology, the pancreas may be longitudinally bisected or transversely sliced. Presence of peripancreatic cysts like pseudocyst as a complication of acute pancreatitis is also to be noted.

- *Others:* The esophagus and the stomach should be examined for the presence of varices or congestive gastropathy. Examination of colon is needed for the identifications of amebic ulcers in amebic liver disease and to recognize ulcerative colitis in a case of primary sclerosing colitis. Careful examination of heart is also needed to exclude any cirrhotic cardiomyopathy by demonstrating four-chamber dilatations or by identifying any right ventricular dilatation and hypertrophy due to pulmonary hypertension following cirrhosis.

Microscopic Examination

At last, the sections should be taken from various organs for microscopic examination, which can reveal many unexpected findings. The autopsy is not complete without a microscopic examination.

FURTHER READING

1. Connolly AJ, Finkbeiner WE, Ursell PC, Davis RL. Autopsy pathology: A manual and atlas, 3rd edition. Philadelphia: Elsevier; 2016.
2. Waters BL. Handbook of autopsy practice, 4th edition. United States: Humana press; 2009.

5F: Urogenital Tract at Autopsy

Vinaya Shah

EXTERNAL EXAMINATION OF THE KIDNEYS

The kidneys are preferably taken out with the ureters and urinary bladder as a block. It may also be important to keep the abdominal aortic segment so that the renal arterial ostia are examined for patency (**Fig. 5.45**), the caliber and adequacy of the vessels are established. Aberrant arteries are sought and also their relationship, if any, to kinks of the ureter. One may also keep a segment of the inferior vena cava and the renal veins are also opened. The simplest maneuver is to grasp the kidney in situ through its fat after making a sweeping knife cut outside the lateral border, through the peritoneum and fat. The fingers readily tear through the perirenal tissue, freeing the organ except at the hilar region. One must then identify the ureter and free it all the way down to its entry to the bladder. Next, probe in the preperitoneal tissue in the lower end of the abdominal incision. This liberates the front of the bladder. In the male, in the posterior and lower aspect of bladder is prostate, which is also freed simultaneously. In the female, uterus, tubes, and ovaries are removed with the bladder. It is advisable to free the tubes and ovaries as the first step in the dissection, cutting them loose from the pelvis. Otherwise atrophic ovaries can be lost unaccountably.

The normal weight of kidney in adult males is 100–140 g, while in women the range is 90–130 g. At the center of the medial border is a concavity, which contains a vertical fissure transmitting the vessels and pelvis—the hilum. The anatomical relationship of the structures at the hilum allows one to allocate a separated kidney to its correct

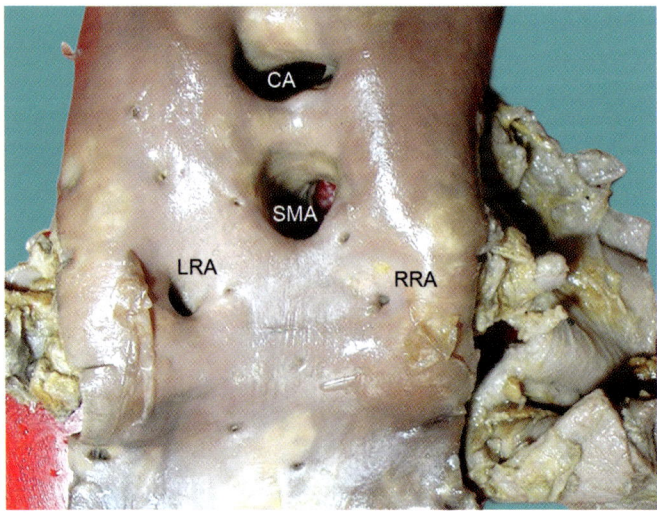

(CA: celiac artery; SMA: superior mesenteric artery; LRA: left renal artery; RRA: right renal artery)

FIG. 5.45: Opened out abdominal aorta showing marked narrowing of the right renal arterial (RRA) ostium.

side, where the renal vein is anterior to the renal artery, while the pelvis and ureter are posterior to both vessels. In children, the surface of the kidney is smoothly lobated by the presence of deep narrow grooves, representing the embryonic lobations (**Fig. 5.46A**). They gradually disappear, but in some adults they persist and should not to be confused with postinflammatory scars.

The usual size of the kidney is 12 × 6 × 3 cm. Decreased size is observed in hypoplasia, atrophy, and end-stage renal diseases. If the size of kidney is small and weighs 50–60 g, the diagnostic difficulty arises whether it is secondarily contracted kidney or a hypoplastic kidney in which inflammatory changes have caused scarring. One must carefully seek out the causes of unilateral renal disease (inflammatory or renal vascular disturbance on that side). If disease is present bilaterally in a pair of small kidneys, the hypoplastic kidney is unlikely. The hypoplastic kidneys are miniatures with fewer calyces than normal. The pelvis may lead directly into minor calyces or else a small pelvis may have only one or two calyces. The presence of single or multiple cysts is also in favor of congenital abnormality. Finally, if the renal artery has a caliber like that serving a normal sized kidney, then the small kidney has probably undergone secondary atrophy. Increased size occurs as a result of compensatory hypertrophy, and many non-neoplastic and neoplastic causes.

The kidneys have a firm consistency. The consistency is tested before the organ is cut. The consistency of a normal kidney is such that when the mid portion of the kidney is held between the thumb and forefinger the two poles fall away in a gentle arc. The consistency of kidneys becomes soft in cases of injury (like acute tubular necroses) or inflammations.

Normal perirenal fat is easily stripped away from the transparent capsule, but some part remains tenaciously attached to the hilar region. Fat attached elsewhere indicates that it is anchored by the remnant of some inflammatory process. After the perirenal fat is removed, the thin, smooth, transparent, and tough capsule is seen. It is stripped away with toothed forceps after the kidney and pelvis is cut open from the convex border of kidney (see later). Generally the capsule is easily removed from the smooth surfaced kidney; it is possible for the capsule to be stripped more easily than usual if there is underlying interstitial edema. Difficulty arises when the cortical surface is scarred by inflammatory or noninflammatory processes. Frequently adhesion is so strong that the capsule cannot be removed or else brings fragments of cortex with it.

The normal external surface is smooth, mottled by slippery blue markings of the stellate veins. Examine the surface for pallor, petechiae or obvious hemorrhagic, diffuse or localized discolorations, fine or coarse granularity, nodularity, and foci of scars and cysts. These changes can be symmetrical or asymmetrical. Large pale white kidneys (**Fig. 5.46B**) are seen usually seen with reversible kidney injury (cloudy change), early phase of fatty change, acute tubular necroses, primary/secondary causes of nephrotic syndrome, and diffuse leukemic infiltrates. Flea-bitten kidney due to multiple petechial hemorrhages (**Fig. 5.46C**) is present in primary/secondary causes of nephritic syndrome, malignant hypertension, acute pyelonephritis/pyemic abscess (when they are small in size), hemorrhagic diathesis caused by infective, and noninfective or neoplastic conditions. Jaundice, malaria, and hemosiderosis impart yellowish/green, gray, and brown discoloration mainly to the cortex of the kidneys,

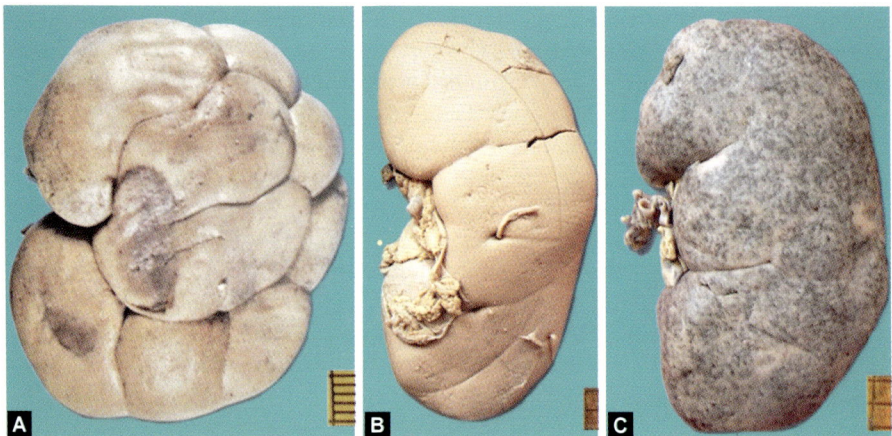

FIGS. 5.46A TO C: External surface of the kidneys showing. (A) Fetal lobulations; (B) Enlargement with diffuse pallor; and (C) Petechial hemorrhages.

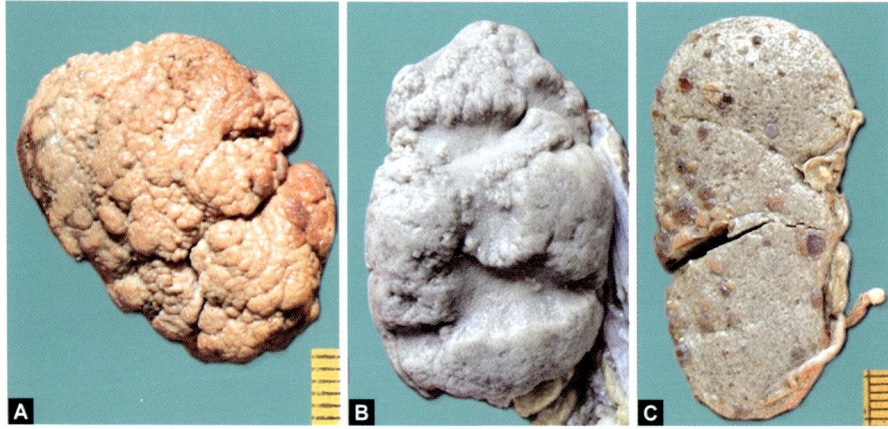

FIGS. 5.47A TO C: (A and B) External surface of the kidneys in chronic pyelonephritis; (C) benign nephrosclerosis with presence of small cysts.

respectively. The kidneys in chronic pyelonephritis are frequently asymmetrically involved. This is the most common disease of the kidney found at autopsy. Two varieties exist. In the diffuse form (**Fig. 5.47A**), there is an irregular coarse granularity of the entire kidney with an adherent capsule and irregular scars as well. Focal chronic pyelonephritis (**Fig. 5.47B**) creates a number of broad, flat or even V-shaped/U-shaped depressions with red-brown granular base

In benign nephrosclerosis (**Fig. 5.47C**), there is fine granularity of kidneys, where the granules are no >1 mm across, are red and very slightly raised. The total reduction in renal size is not great and when the kidney is greatly shrunken, it is still unlikely to be as small as that of chronic glomerulonephritis. Even when severe, the capsule will strip quite easily or there will be mild to moderate adhesions. The consistency is firm and tough. Larger arterioles on the cut surface may be gaping. The kidneys in chronic glomerulonephritis (the end stage of nephritis) are affected equally. This condition and chronic pyelonephritis are the two causes of the smallest kidneys, other than hypoplasia. The capsule is frequently extremely adherent. The granularity is fine but larger than that of benign nephrosclerosis. Each granule is 1–3 mm across, with considerable variation within the range. The kidney is pale yellow-gray rather than red. Two more causes of granular kidney are late stages of diabetic nephropathy and amyloidosis. Four conditions have to be considered whenever there are large or deep scars—chronic pyelonephritis, renal arteriosclerosis, healed infarcts, and polyarteritis nodosa.

EXAMINATION OF CUT SURFACE OF THE KIDNEYS

The kidney is bisected by pressing a layer of wet cotton over the external surface and cutting through the convex border so as to split the kidney in half and open the pelvis. To achieve the latter every time is difficult, as a slight deviation of the knife easily causes one to miss the pelvis entirely. When the kidney is bisected, it will be seen that the hilus immediately expands into the renal sinus. It contains fat in which are the pelvis and its calyces and the renal vessels.

Four features of the cut surface demand separate consideration—cortex, medulla, pelvicalyceal system and blood vessels. In the adult, the cortex is 0.5–0.7 cm thick and is pale gray-brown. On the other hand, the medulla is seen as dark areas, which are wedge shaped or triangular on an ideally bisected kidney. Hence the corticomedullary junction is sharply demarcated with a ratio of 1.6–2:1 in children and 2.5–3:1 in adults. The renal pyramid (which is the part of the medulla) has a base directed toward the cortical surface and an apex that projects into the pelvicalyceal system. There are about 18 dark purple-red pyramids although only five or six will be present on one cut surface. The tip of each pyramid, called the papilla, projects into a calyx. The surface of the papilla has a sieve-like appearance because of openings of the collecting ducts. In between are the extensions of the pale cortex termed as the columns of Bertin. Fine vertical streaks—medullary rays run from the bases of the pyramids, converging upon their apices. They are alternately light and dark and correspond to tubules and vessels, respectively. At the apices the tubules predominate, thereby imparting the pallor. From the pelvis come three or four major calyces into which drain 7–13 minor calyces (not necessarily visible in a single cut). Most are cupped around a single renal pyramid, although occasionally a minor calyx may serve up to three pyramids. The pelvic mucosa is always surrounded by the fat, which in turn is continuous with the fatty tissue filling the spaces of hilum. Having learnt from experience how much fat is normal, one can then appreciate when it is increased as a result of obesity or of atrophy of the kidney. Pelvic mucosa should be smooth, glistening, gray-white, and without visible blood vessels. The renal vessels can be seen as they travel up Bertin's columns as interlobar arteries. Smaller branches passing in the same direction into the cortex are the interlobular arteries, which arise from vessels running parallel to the bases of the pyramids, the arcuate arteries. The important observation to make it that if these vessels are normal they will be collapsed. Gaping vessels are always diseased.

Renal diseases in general produce alterations in the corticomedullary ratio. The cortical width is increased with increasing pallor and blurring of the junction in reversible renal injury, acute tubular necroses, nephrotic syndrome, or leukemic infiltrates. Widening and prominent demarcation are seen with acute inflammations. There is conspicuous decrease with blurring of corticomedullary differentiation in all cases where the kidneys are shrunken.

Coagulative necroses are seen with renal infarctions and cortical necrosis (**Figs. 5.48A** and **B**). In infarcts, the size of the occluded artery determines the shape, position, and size. For example, occlusion of arteria radiate results in triangular cortical infarction. Rectangular-cortical infarction is produced by occlusion of arcuate artery, while a triangular corticomedullary infarction is seen with occluded interlobular artery. Subtotal and total kidney infarction is produced by occlusion of extrarenal branch of the renal artery and of renal artery, respectively. However, infarction is also known to occur as a result of shock. Nearly always a thin rim of about 0.1 cm of subcapsular cortex is preserved by its small extrarenal vessels. The gross appearance of a kidney infarction changes with time, but are usually always pale. Hemorrhagic infarctions are of venous origin and are seen in thrombosis of the main renal vein in infants, especially those with severe gastroenteritis, dehydration, or pneumonia. Bilateral cortical necrosis in its classical form shows swollen kidneys with a dull, opaque, yellow-white, necrotic cortex, a change which usually extends into Bertin's columns and may not even spare the subcapsular zone. The pyramids are not affected by this destruction and may stand out all the more because of intense hyperemia. No changes are to be seen in the renal vessels. This condition is often seen as a complication during pregnancy, infections, poisons, shock, and dehydration.

Both cortex and medulla are affected in acute pyelonephritis/pyemic abscesses (**Figs. 5.49A** and **B**); others include tuberculous inflammation and xanthogranulomatous pyelonephritis. The cut-surface should also be inspected for the presence of cysts. The diagnosis would depend upon the number, size, and location of the cysts and presence of inter-cyst communications, along with alteration in the size and

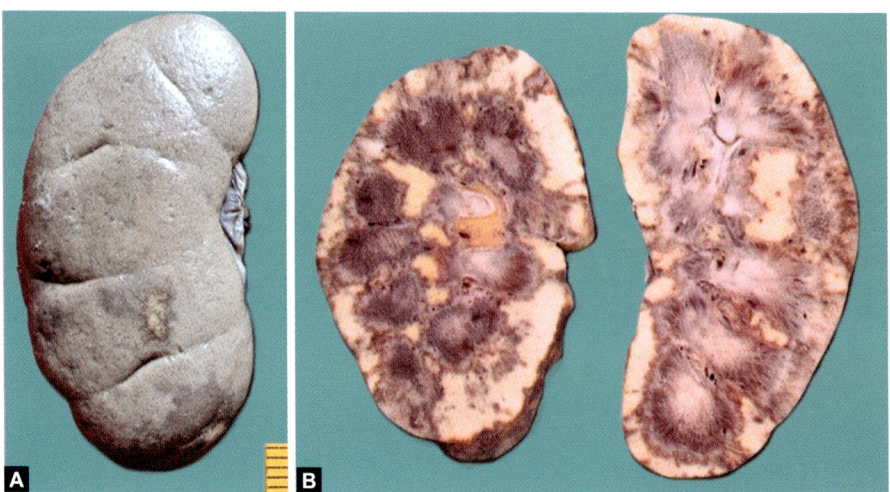

FIGS. 5.48A AND B: (A) External surface of the kidney showing multiple small infarcts; (B) bilateral diffuse cortical necrosis.

Systemic Examination

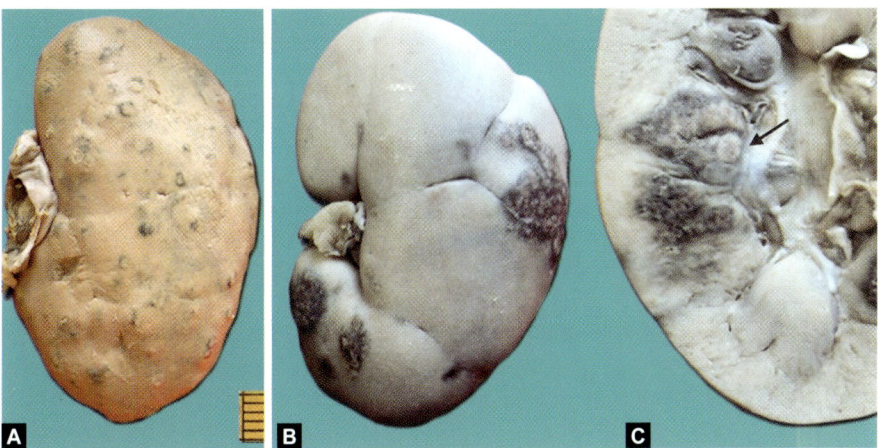

FIGS. 5.49A TO C: (A) Case of acute pyelonephritis characterized by randomly distributed abscesses all of which have hyperemic rims; (B) Conglomerate of abscesses with surrounding hyperemia in a case of pyemia; and (C) This case was also associated with papillary necrosis (arrow).

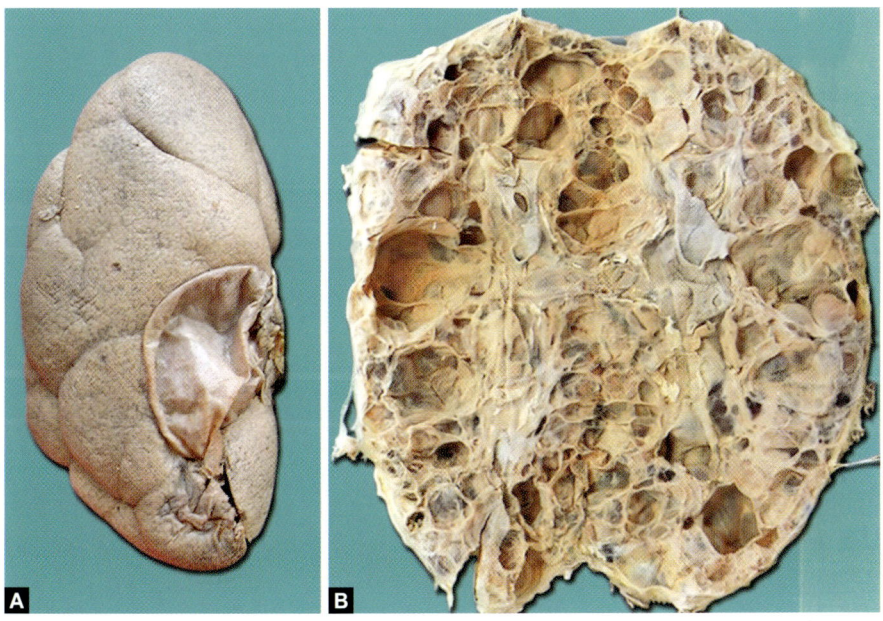

FIGS. 5.50A AND B: (A) Retention cyst; (B) Cysts involving both cortex and medulla in autosomal dominant polycystic kidney disease. Note marked enlargement of the kidney.

shape of the kidneys. Cortical cysts are seen as simple and retention cysts (**Fig. 5.50A**); they are numerous in polycystic kidney disease (**Fig. 5.50B**) with involvement of the medulla as well. Cysts are seen in the medulla and corticomedullary junction in medullary sponge kidney and uremic medullary cystic disease (nephronophthisis).

Multicystic dysplastic kidney is the most common cystic malformation of the kidney in infancy. Parasitic cysts are seen, but rarely.

Changes in the medulla are less numerous than cortical ones. Pyramids may be obliterated by hydronephrosis or partially destroyed by necrotizing papillitis (**Fig. 5.49C**), commonly produced by analgesics or as complication of acute pyelonephritis in diabetic patients or in sickle cell anemia. In some cases, there may be dilatation of the pelvicalyceal system of varying degrees. The long-standing hydronephrosis leads to kidney enlargement with thin rim of compressed and atrophied renal tissue. The dilated pelvis and the calyces contain clear, pale yellow fluid and are lined by thickened, white, smooth mucosa. The causes of hydronephrosis, either bilateral or unilateral may be congenital or acquired. Most often, the disease is complicated by the presence of stones or nephrolithiasis. Superadded infection can lead to pyonephrosis as well.

One can also encounter renal tumors at autopsy as incidental lesions or at times with dissemination (**Figs. 5.51A** and **B**). Capsular tumors are all great rarities, generally described as being incidental autopsy findings and therefore very small. The exception to this is the rare sarcoma which can be very large, invading the renal pelvis and perirenal tissues. Benign parenchymal tumors are quite common at autopsy seen as 0.1–0.2 cm, white or yellow nodules in the cortex (subcapsular or deep) or in the medulla. They are indistinguishable from the miliary tubercles. As age increases, more small tumors are found, particularly in benign nephrosclerosis.

Renal cell carcinoma, the most common renal malignancy of adults, can also be present as incidental tumors with or without dissemination. Necrotic or hemorrhagic areas may be succeeded by cyst formation; few tumors may mimic multicystic disease. Wilm's tumor is the most common abdominal malignancy of children and is seen at autopsy in cases of usually neglected treatment. Metastatic tumors are fairly common in the kidney. Lung is the most common primary site followed by breast, stomach and

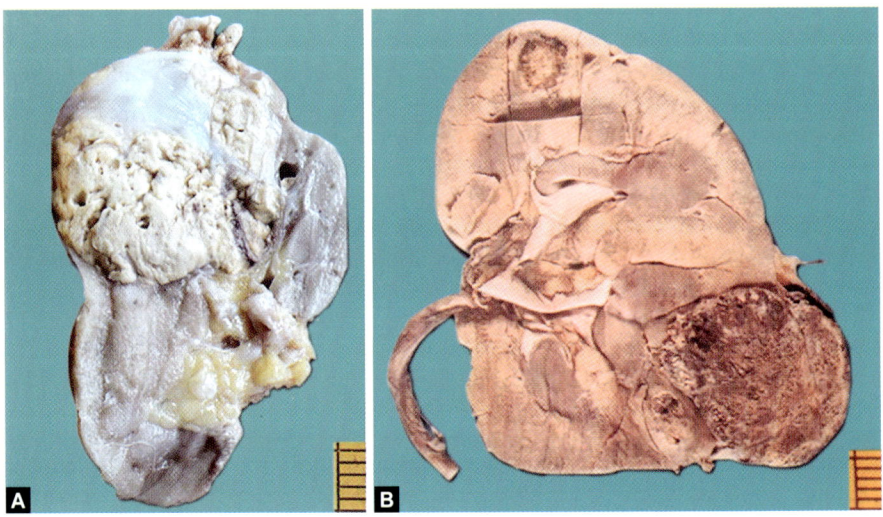

FIGS. 5.51A AND B: (A) Renal cell carcinoma as an incidental autopsy finding; (B) Multiple metastatic choriocarcinoma seen as hemorrhagic nodules.

cervix, colon, and pancreas. The various forms of lymphoma produce one or more well-circumscribed white nodules. Occasionally, more diffusely infiltrating forms appear. Only rarely does leukemic infiltration produce a distinct mass of tumor tissue. Other tumors are urothelial or squamous in nature.

EXAMINATION OF THE URETERS

The adult ureter has a length of about 30 cm and a diameter of about 0.5 cm with a thick wall and small lumen. Three points of embryological narrowing are always present, at the ureteropelvic junction, at the passage over the iliac vessels and at the entry to the bladder wall. The ureter has an entirely retroperitoneal course. In the male, the ureter is in front of the upper end of the seminal vesicles, and the vas deferens is interposed between the ureter and the bladder. In women, the final section of the ureter runs below the lower part of the broad ligament, lateral to the cervix and lateral vaginal fornices and is briefly in front of the vagina just prior to entering the bladder.

Apart from congenital anomalies, there are also acquired ureteral diseases. Inflammation of the ureter (including tuberculous inflammation) is nearly always accompanied by renal infection. When the ureters are transplanted into the colon, there is also a risk of a purulent ureteritis developing with subsequent spread to the kidneys and eventual pyelonephritis. It is also possible for peritonitis, intestinal obstruction, or formation of a urinary or fecal fistula to set in. Chronic infection of the ureter is responsible for ureteritis cystica, in which discrete, gray or translucent, 1-2 mm, cysts appear beneath the mucosa. Stones found in the ureter hardly ever have originate there, except in the cases of diverticulae or ureteroceles. They come from the kidney and usually lodge in the lower third of the ureter or at one of the three points of anatomical narrowing. They are therefore fairly small, 5 mm being an average width. Most stones eventually pass on, but if they become impacted, there is acute inflammation and ulceration. This may be followed by fibrosis and subsequent hydronephrosis. There can be an accidental ligation or tumor-induced obstruction and traumatic, iatrogenic, or disease-induced perforation/tear/rupture of the ureters. Benign tumors of the ureter are extremely rare. A few soft, smooth, or lobulated, fibrous polyps have been reported growing into the lumen on a narrow pedicle. Whatever the type of malignancy, it soon becomes large enough to induce a fusiform enlargement of the ureter. Transitional cell carcinoma can occur in one spot, or may be multiple or even bilateral. Quite often there is also carcinoma in the renal pelvis or the bladder. The only important tumor metastatic to the ureter is carcinoma of the cervix, following invasion of the tissues of the lateral pelvic wall.

EXAMINATION OF THE URINARY BLADDER

The base (fundus) of the urinary bladder faces downward and back toward the rectum. In the males, it is separated by the rectovesical fascia containing the seminal vesicles and the terminal portions of the vasa deferentia and the ureters. In the female, the base is separated above by the uterovesical pouch of peritoneum from the uterus and below by connective tissue from the cervix and upper part of the vagina. The inferior surface of the bladder lies on fat, which separates it from the pubis, and the triangular superior surface is covered by peritoneum. The neck of the bladder is that portion around the internal urethral orifice and in the male is above the prostate. The anterior surface is in relation to the anterior abdominal wall without any intervening peritoneum. In relation to the posterior surface is the rectovesical pouch in the males and uterovesical pouch in the females. On the superior surface of the bladder are three umbilical folds, a median one in continuity with obliterated urachus and two lateral ones which represent the obliterated umbilical arteries.

If bacteriological or chemical examination of contents of the bladder is required, they should be withdrawn by a 50 mL syringe with a wide bore needle while the organ is still in situ. Otherwise bladder is routinely opened in the midline of the superior aspect, using a toothed forceps and scissors. This gives adequate exposure without damaging the trigonal area. In cases of suspected urethral obstruction, the bladder should be opened before removal to allow probing of the urethra. The thickness of the wall and size of the lumen vary with the degree of filling and the effects of any obstruction. The normal capacity is 200 or 300 mL and it can readily be distended to 2–4 L. Frequently, the urine seen at autopsy is cloudy, but this does not necessarily mean infection. It may be precipitated phosphates or urates, or to the desquamation of large numbers of urothelial cells after death. The bladder mucosa is gray white and generally be seen to be ridged and folded. However, a smooth triangular area, the trigone (resembling an equilateral triangle) is always present immediately above and behind internal urethral orifice. The openings of the ureters are slit-like, while that of the urethra is crescentic.

In most autopsies, the mucosa is markedly hemorrhagic (**Fig. 5.52A**), a finding that can usually be related to catheterization. Always observe the mucosa, appearance of residual urine, probe the three orifices, note the thickness of the muscle, look for trabeculations, diverticulosis, obstructions at the bladder neck, stones (**Fig. 5.52B**)/foreign bodies, and tumors (**Fig. 5.52C**); examine for enlargement of the middle lobe of prostate. Blunt trauma to the abdomen may perforate the bladder, especially if it is full, or may merely cause a hemorrhagic contusion of the muscle. Other causes of trauma include that occasionally following catheterization, cystoscopy or endoscopic interventions, following instrumentation in childbirth and that due to perforation by bone spicules in pelvic fractures. The causes of spontaneous rupture are tuberculosis, carcinoma, cystitis, or scars, secondary to urethral obstruction, neurological disorders, and unrelieved reflex retention. When the fluid leaks extraperitoneally from

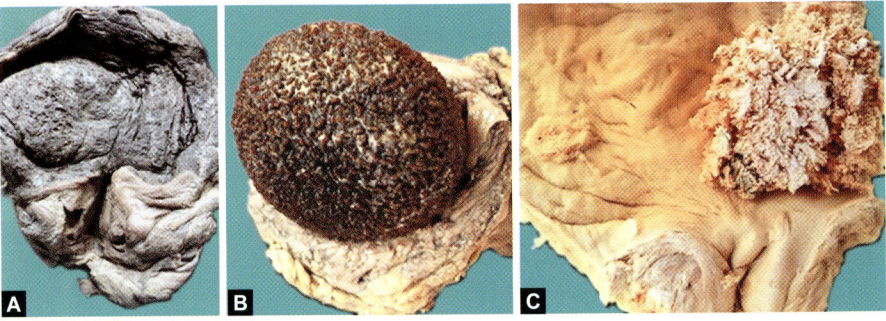

FIGS. 5.52A TO C: (A) Hemorrhagic cystitis with a diffuse reddish discoloration of the bladder mucosa; (B) A very large, speculated bladder stone; and (C) Urothelial carcinoma showing a distinct papillary fronds.

the anterior part of the bladder, it collects in the suprapubic tissues and extends into the thigh, inguinal region, scrotum, and lower abdominal wall. Internally, it passes into the connective tissue of the wall of the pelvis. A perforation closer to the base and neck allows infiltration of urine into the soft tissues around the rectum and vagina. It can also pass upward in the retroperitoneal tissue. Wherever, it is, the urine induces great edema and hyperemia, followed by infection and the formation of abscesses and fistulae to the skin, rectum, or vagina. Presence of fistulous connections (vesicocutaneous, vesicovaginal, or vesicointestinal fistulas) should be looked for and their causes (iatrogenic, traumatic, inflammatory, or neoplastic) should be ascertained.

EXAMINATION OF THE TESTES

The adult testis is ovoid, weighs 10–15 g, and is 4–5 cm wide, 3 cm in anteroposterior diameter. Attached to the posterolateral aspect is the epididymis. The rest of the surface of the testis is free and smooth, being covered by opaque, gray-white tunica albuginea over which are present the visceral and parietal layers of the tunica vaginalis. Between the layers of the tunica vaginalis is a potential space, where fluid (hydrocele) can collect. The epididymis is composed of a coiled mass of tubes connecting the testis to the vas deferens. We can recognize the upper pole of the testis by the head of the epididymis and can assign its laterality with the knowledge that the sinus epididymis, a deep cleft between the epididymis and the testis, is on the lateral side. The head (globus major) of the epididymis is its expanded upper end. The tail (globus minor) is the smaller end from which the vas emerges. The head and tail are fixed to the testis while the intervening body is free, being surrounded by tunica vaginalis. The main artery of the testis and epididymis is the testicular artery, which arises directly from the aorta just above the origin of the inferior mesenteric artery. The veins unite to form the pampiniform plexus, finally draining into the inferior vena cava/renal vein. Lymph vessels from the testis and epididymis ascend in the cord to reach the lateral and preaortic lumbar nodes.

As far as the naked eye is concerned, the testis internally consists only of the stringy yellow to brown seminiferous tubules, which are divided into lobules by fibrous septa. When the cut surface of the mature testis is teased with a needle point or a fine forceps the tubules come away in fine threads (**Fig. 5.53A**). This effect is lost in testicular atrophy, where the testes are smaller, firmer, and paler than normal. The cut surface of the testes is examined for presence of torsion, fluid collections, inflammation, and tumors (**Figs. 5.53B to D**).

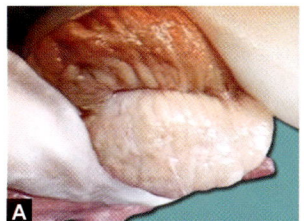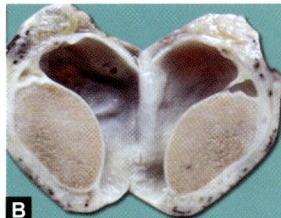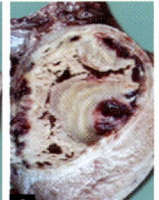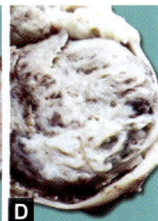

FIGS. 5.53A TO D: (A) The string test for normal testis; (B) hydrocele; (C) hematocele; and (D) Malignant mixed germ cell tumor.

EXAMINATION OF THE PROSTATE

The prostate is well described as being shaped like a chestnut with the base uppermost. Weighing about 20 g in the young adult, its base is continuous with the inferior surface of the bladder neck. In the transverse and vertical diameters, it is about 4 cm and anteroposteriorly it is about 3 cm. Its rounded apex is in contact with the upper surface of the sphincter urethrae; nearly always this part is left behind when the prostate is removed. The only important lateral relationship of the gland is the prostatic venous plexus. Posteriorly, the prostate is bound to the anterior wall of the rectum by a little connective tissue. The prostate has a rubbery to firm consistency with light brown slightly fasciculated cut surface. Apart from several inflammatory and noninflammatory conditions, the prostate is particularly examined for the presence of nodular hyperplasia and carcinomas. The latter becomes particularly important, in cases of clinically disseminated malignancy with occult primary tumors.

EXAMINATION OF THE SEMINAL VESICLES

The paired seminal vesicles lie above the prostate between the base of the bladder and the anterior wall of the rectum, separated from the latter only by rectovesical fascia.

Each vesicle consists of a single tube which is coiled upon itself and forms diverticuli; its size is about 5 by 2 cm. The upper end is blind, while the lower end is a narrow straight duct which unites with the vas deferens to enter the prostate as the ejaculatory duct. The last is 2 cm long. Important pathology in these organs at autopsy is presence of inflammation, which occurs in concurrence with infections of the prostate or posterior urethra.

EXAMINATION OF THE FEMALE GENITAL TRACT

The mode of examination of the female genital tract is no different from the surgically excised specimens. Most of the lesions are usually incidental findings and may not contribute to death, except in cases of maternal mortality (see Chapter 6B). A uterus is a symmetrical, smooth organ, related anteriorly to the bladder, the two being separated by the uterovesical pouch of peritoneum. The level of reflection of the peritoneum is at the isthmus. Posteriorly, the peritoneum covers the whole uterus and passes down to cover the upper portion of the vagina before crossing over to the rectum. This difference of serosal covering allows one to identify front and back of the uterus after it has been removed. The space between uterus and rectum is the rectouterine pouch of Douglas. Loops of intestine are usually present in it.

The size of the uterus depends on whether it is infantile, nulliparous, or gravid. The nulliparous uterus weighs 30–40 g, measuring about 7.5 × 5 × 2.5 cm and is customarily described as having the shape of an inverted flattened pear. A little below the midpoint is a slight constriction, the isthmus, which is the outward mark of the internal os. All below this level is cervix, and all above it is corpus uteri, which widens as far as the level of the insertion of the tubes. The portion of the corpus above this level is the fundus. The cervical canal is narrow and fusiform with a tree-like mucosal pattern on its anterior and posterior walls. The endometrial cavity is flat and triangular, best opened by inserting a probe and cutting along it with a knife. The myometrium is 1-2 cm, thick, pale red brown and is streaked by its muscle bundles. This tissue enjoys the property of being one of the last to succumb to postmortem autolysis. A multiparous uterus is about 10 × 5 × 4 cm and weighs up to 60 g or 70 g. Because it does not quite return to the virginal size; its cavity is larger. The edges of the external os are usually fissured, and the lips are more prominent. The postmenopausal uterus is smaller as compared to the nulliparous state. The uterus enjoys considerable mobility, but the determination of its actual position is more important during life. Anatomically, the uterus is described as being sharply bent forward upon the vagina (anteversion). It may be in fact be found to be anteflexed, retroverted, or retroflexed. Only part of the vagina of removed at autopsy.

From each side of the uterus the broad ligament passes to be inserted into the lateral wall of the pelvis. The broad ligament has anterior and position surface and a free upper border. Fallopian tube travels in the free border and the ovary is attached to the posterior surface. Just anteroinferiorly to the tubes are the round ligaments. These have a length of 10-12 cm. and run below the tubes, between the layers of the broad ligament to the pelvic wall where each enters the deep inguinal ring, passing through it, each ligament reaches labium majus, and then peters out. The most lateral portion of the broad ligament (i.e., lateral to the tube and ovary) is called the infundibulopelvic ligament or suspensory ligament of the ovary, important because it transmits the ovarian vessels, lymphatics, and nerves. Each Fallopian tube is up to 10 cm long. It communicates with the uterine cavity at the cornu by traversing the myometrium. At this point, the lumen is about 0.1 cm. On emerging from the uterus, it forms a short cord-like portion called the isthmus. This gradually broadens to an external diameter of 0.5 cm in the somewhat tortuous ampulla. At its termination, the fimbriated end or infundibulum, it has a diameter of up to 1 cm with a 0.1-0.3 cm opening to the peritoneal cavity. There are fimbriae around this ostium, one of which is larger than the others and is attached to the ovary. The ovary is attached to the posterior aspect of the broad ligament by a short mesovarium, and lies below the tubes. Its medial aspect is connected to the uterine cornu by a cord, the ligament of the ovary (not to be confused with the suspensory ligament of the ovary). This together with the round ligament is homologous with the gubernaculum testis. The mature ovary measures about 3.5 × 1.5 × 1 cm and has a shiny, smooth, and gray surface through which bulge the various follicles and corpora of the ovarian cycle.

The surface of the ovary is germinal epithelium.

FURTHER READING

1. Cooke RA, Stewart B. Renal System and Male Genital System. In: Cooke RA, Stewart B (Eds). Color Atlas of Anatomical Pathology, 2nd Edition. London, UK: Churchill Livingstone;1995.
2. Hill RB, Anderson RE. The uses and value of autopsy in medical education as seen by pathology educators. Acad Med. 1991;66:97-100.
3. JürgenL. Esophagus and abdominal viscera. In: Jürgen Ludwig, Moore TH (Eds.). Text Book of Handbook of Autopsy Practice, 3rd Edition. New Jersey: Humana Press Inc. Totowa; 2002. pp. 53-63.
4. Sandritter W, Thomas C. Kidneys and Urinary System. In: Kirsten WH, Editor. Text Book of Color Atlas and Textbook of Macropathology, 3rd Edition. Chicago: Year Book Medical Publishers, Inc; 1971. pp. 243-84.

5G: Examination of the Lymphoreticular System

Daksha Prabhat, Shubhangi Agale, Subhash Yadav

INTRODUCTION

The lymphoreticular system (LRS), which includes spleen, lymph nodes, mucosa-associated lymphoid tissue, thymus, and bone marrow, plays a major role in immunity and hematopoiesis. Lymphoreticular organs are affected in variety of hematologic disorders, infective diseases, storage disorders, and benign/malignant neoplastic conditions, resulting in enlargement of these organs. Hence, abnormalities of the LRS can be misdiagnosed or underdiagnosed, if careful examination is not done during autopsy.

The lymphoid organs in the body are basically divided into (1) primary lymphoid organs (generative organs), which includes the thymus and bone marrow, and (2) secondary lymphoid organs (peripheral lymphoid organs), which includes the spleen, lymph nodes, and mucosa-associated lymphoid tissue. Thymus and bone marrow allow the lymphoid stem cells to proliferate, differentiate, and mature. They contain either T- or B-cells and have no contact with antigens. The spleen and lymph nodes, on the other hand, allow the lymphoid cells to become functional and contain both T- and B-cells. These organs do come in contact with antigens and thus are able to produce antibodies. As the humans are prone to acquire infections, autoimmune and neoplastic disorders, it is not surprising that abnormalities of LRS are commonly found at autopsy. To achieve accurate diagnosis, the microscopic examination of LRS has to be combined with clinical history and necessary laboratory investigations including microbiology, cytology, histopathology, virology, and genetic analysis to reach a final diagnosis.

SPLEEN

The spleen is the largest lymphoid organ that lies far back on the left side of the upper abdominal cavity behind stomach and hence may not be visible on in situ examination unless it is markedly enlarged in size (**Fig. 5.54**). The spleen may be wedge shaped, tetrahedral, or triangular and it has capsule, which covers purplish, solid to sponge-like, friable parenchyma. The adult spleen measures on an average 13 × 8 × 3 cm and weighs 100–150 g. It has two surfaces: A smooth convex diaphragmatic surface and a visceral surface, which is further divided into anterior gastric surface, and posterior renal surface. The tail of the pancreas abuts the splenic hilum. Due to support by a single vessel and two tiny ligaments (gastrosplenic and the lienorenal ligament), spleen is highly mobile. The splenic artery is the largest branch of the celiac axis of the aorta. It runs tortuously along and above the splenic vein, passing behind stomach and lesser sac, along the upper border of the pancreas. The splenic vein crosses the abdominal aorta and ends behind the neck of pancreas where it joins the superior mesenteric vein forming the portal vein.

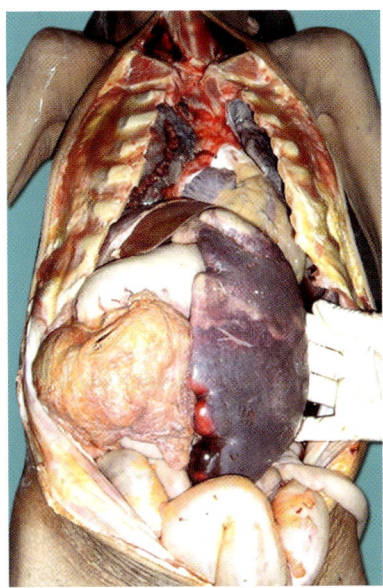

FIG. 5.54: In situ examination shows markedly enlarged spleen with a stretched capsule and presence of pale white (old) and red (recent) areas of infarcts.

The spleen is to the circulatory system as the lymph nodes are to the lymphatic system. It is ingeniously designed by virtue of the red and white pulps to filter the blood and is a site of immune responses to blood-borne antigens. Spleen is also a major repository of mononuclear phagocytic cells in the red pulp and of the lymphoid cells in the white pulp. The major functions of spleen are antibody production, hematopoiesis, sequestration of formed blood elements, and phagocytosis of particulate matter and blood cells.

Removal and Examination of Spleen

Trace the splenic artery to the hilum of the spleen, noting the splenic vein and body, and tail of pancreas as well. Free the spleen by lifting it anterolaterally and dividing its hilar connections. Avoid injury to the hilar structures and tail of pancreas. Examine the hilum and cut the spleen along its long axis in multiple thin slices (at least 1 cm thick) for a good fixation.

The normal weight of spleen is around 100–150 g. Variation in splenic sizes and weights is seen in various conditions. Splenomegaly is classified as mild (200–500 g), moderate (500–1,000 g), and severe (>1,000 g). Mild and moderate splenomegaly have many overlapping etiological factors; however, massive splenomegaly (**Figs. 5.55** and **5.56**) is specifically seen in conditions such as malaria (tropical splenomegaly), kala-azar, chronic myeloid leukemia, hairy cell leukemia, myelofibrosis, amyloidosis, and storage disorders like Gaucher disease. Atrophic shrunken spleen can be seen due to age related changes, repeated splenic infarcts, and autosplenectomy due to sickle cell anemia. It weighs 50–70 g and capsule is wrinkled.

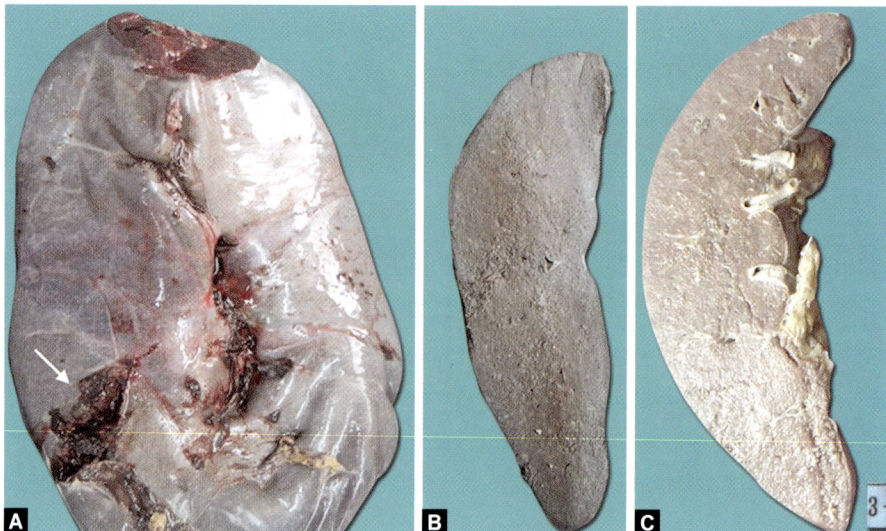

FIGS. 5.55A TO C: (A) Moderate splenomegaly with spontaneous rupture (arrow); (B) cut surface of the malarial spleen shows a prominent slate gray appearance due to accumulation of hemozoin pigment; and (C) enlarged, firm spleen with a gray-white pale and waxy cut surface due to amyloid deposition—lardaceous type.

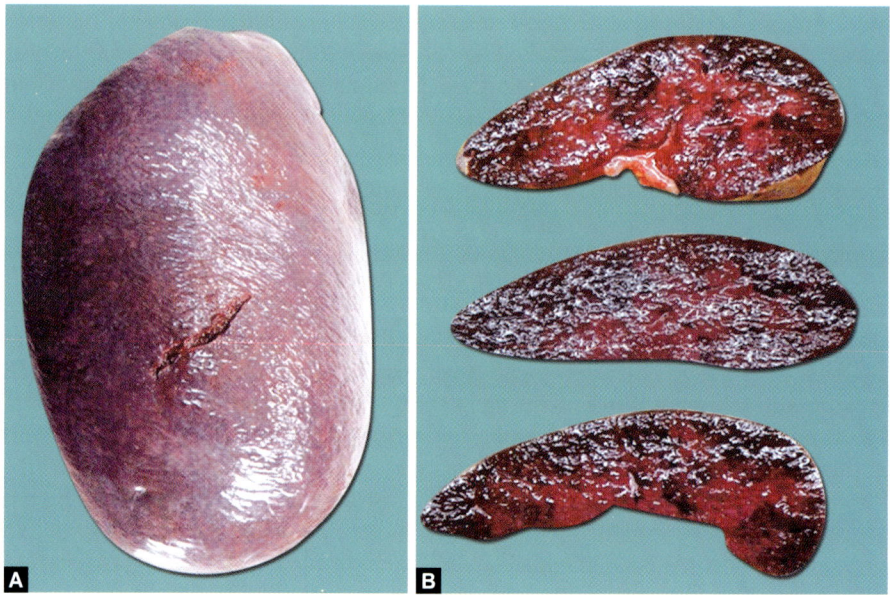

FIGS. 5.56A AND B: (A) Massive splenomegaly (weight 1.4 kg) in a case of chronic myeloid leukemia. The spleen showed tense capsule and (B) congested cut surface.

The hilum of spleen is examined for abnormalities like splenic artery aneurysms and venous thrombosis secondary to portal thrombosis, bacterial endocarditis, etc. Since tail of pancreas is close to splenic hilum, mass lesions of pancreatic tail can cause obstruction of splenic vasculature leading to splenic infarction. Hilum should also be examined for presence of accessory spleen, a congenital disorder, which is found in 10% of population. The typical size is approximately 1 cm but may range from few mm to 3 cm. Hilar lymph nodes should be examined to look for any gross pathology.

The spleen is enclosed in a thin glistening slate gray connective tissue capsule through which the dusky red splenic parenchyma can be seen. Because spleen is a soft, contractile, and highly vascular organ, its shape and size are inconstant and depend upon the structures around it. In case of doubts about the size of the spleen, examine the capsule for wrinkling. Tense shiny appearance with rib imprints on capsule indicates increase in splenic size whereas capsular wrinkling indicates shrinkage of splenic parenchyma. Perisplenitis is seen as creamy yellow to white exudates or firm glistening "icing-like" plaques on the capsular surface, indicating active acute or regressed infection, respectively. It is usually secondary to generalized peritonitis or extension from local infection. Infarcts (**Fig. 5.57A**) produce whitish discoloration, which may be bulging, flush with the normal surface or depressed, depending on their duration. At times, capsular nodularity may be present due to both inflammatory and noninflammatory conditions. Lacerations of splenic capsule are secondary to trauma, while spontaneous rupture occurs (**Fig. 5.55A**) mostly in acute infections especially infectious mononucleosis or typhoid and even in some cases of malaria, leukemias, and lymphomas. The complications of rupture are hemorrhage, hematoma formation, and splenosis. The latter refers to autoimplantation of splenic tissue on the peritoneal surface that can be confused at autopsy with metastatic carcinoma of peritoneum, melanoma, or multiple hemangiomas.

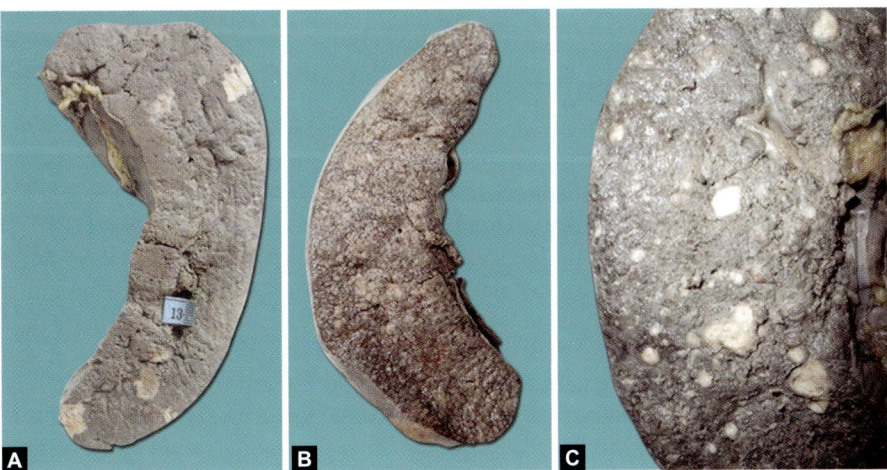

FIGS. 5.57A TO C: (A) An enlarged spleen showing multiple wedge-shaped foci of fresh infarcts; (B) Nodules were seen on the cut surface of the spleen in a case of lymphoma; (C) Small and large well-spaced out and circumscribed gray-white nodules seen in an HIV positive patient due to tuberculosis. Some appear frankly caseous.

The dusky red color of the spleen on the cut surface is due to the red pulp of the spleen, which is traversed by numerous thin-walled vascular sinusoids, separated by the splenic cords or "cords of Billroth". Gray-white specks produced by the splenic or Malpighian follicles stand out against the red background and these are often prominent in children. The cut surface of the spleen is dotted with gray specks. Different diseases produce various changes in spleen size, color, weight, consistency, and appearance on cut surface. Cut surface of the spleen at autopsy gives many clues about the disease pathology. Extremely congested and soft spleen with semifluid consistency of its pulp that sticks over the cutting knife and easily flows away under tap water is known as mushy, diffluent, or septic spleen. This can also be artifactual, if the autopsy has been delayed. Malarial spleen is diffusely enlarged and slate gray in color (**Fig. 5.55B**) due to deposition of hemozoin pigment in the reticuloendothelial cells of spleen. When the malaria is chronic, the spleen is greatly enlarged, firm with slate gray cut surface and the capsule is studded with pearly white thickenings—"ague cake spleen." Conditions like chronic hemolytic anemias, and hemochromatosis causes diffuse brownish appearance. Siderotic nodules (Gamna–Gandy bodies) are seen as focal yellow rusty nodules on the cut surface. In case of amyloidosis, cut surface of spleen may take one of the two forms: Sago spleen which is characterized by whitish deposits, largely limited to the splenic follicles, producing tapioca-like granules on gross inspection, and lardaceous spleen (**Fig. 5.55C**), in which amyloid involves the walls of the splenic sinuses and connective tissue framework in the red pulp giving it a rubbery uniform translucent gray white waxy look on cut surface. A diffuse gray white discoloration with very firm consistency is also seen with chronic myeloproliferative disorders and hairy cell leukemia. Splenic surface may show focal or diffuse nodules in conditions such as abscesses, miliary tuberculosis, hemangiomas, lymphangiomas, lymphomas (**Fig. 5.57B**), inherent, specific but rare splenic primary tumors and metastatic deposits. It is important to remember that in human immunodeficiency virus (HIV) positive patients, tuberculosis (**Fig. 5.57C**) or cryptococcosis also results in large nodular lesions, which are opaque white and white glistening, respectively. Sickle cell disease causes splenic enlargement in initial stages followed by multiple splenic infarcts due to veno-occlusive phenomenon and then finally atrophy of spleen and autosplenectomy. As with other solid organs, infarcts in the spleen are also wedge-shaped and pale. The zone of hyperemia is better seen after fixation. The infarction results from occlusion of the splenic artery or its branches. However, it can be seen in obstruction of the microcirculation which often occurs with massive splenomegaly. If emboli contain bacteria then infarct undergoes rapid softening and suppuration (septic infarct). In uremia, a special type of necrosis is observed as a terminal event. The necrotic areas are of variable size, irregular, white, or yellowish, central as well as peripheral and the cut surface has spotted appearance ("spotted spleen"). On rare occasions, cystic lesions of the spleen can also be seen as incidental findings (**Fig. 5.58**).

Other abnormalities associated with spleen include:
- *Asplenia or absent spleen:* It is important to identify this condition, not only for functional relevance but also to for other commonly associated conditions, particularly complex congenital heart disease.

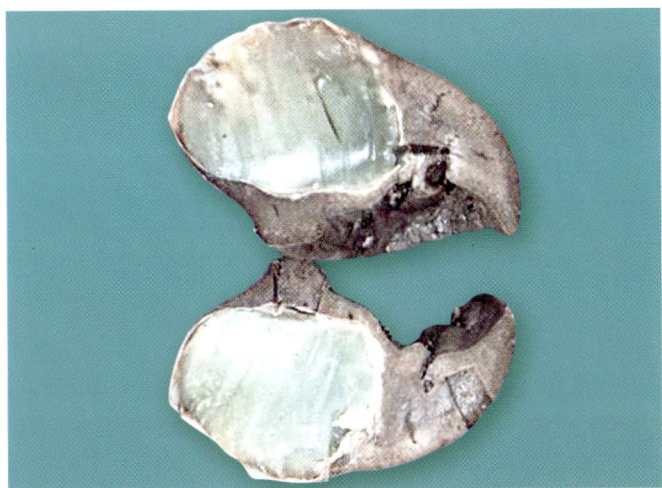

FIG. 5.58: Cut surface of the spleen revealing a solitary cyst with mucoid inspissated secretions.

- In polysplenia, there are several, more or less equal splenic masses instead of a single spleen. These conditions are associated with various other congenital malformations.
- *Wandering spleen and torsion:* Due to its excessive mobility and narrow attachment, they are prone for twisting and splenic infarction.
- Splenogonadal fusion is a rare congenital malformation that results from an abnormal connection between the primitive spleen and gonad during gestation. It is of two types continuous and discontinuous. At autopsy left testis should be examined for splenogonadal fusion as it is common in males.

Splenic touch imprint is an important postmortem investigation to diagnose infiltrative disorders of spleen. The cut surface of the spleen is mopped with a dry filter paper and then glass sides are being touched to its surface gently. Both air dried and fixed slides are prepared and are stained accordingly (hematoxylin and eosin, Giemsa, and other special stains such as Ziehl–Neelsen (Z–N), periodic acid-Schiff, and mucicarmine (**Figs. 5.59A** and **B**). In infective cases swabs for culture have to be collected, and this has to be carried out before cutting the spleen. The capsule of the spleen should be sterilized with hot knife and swabs are inserted through the sterile area and sample collected for culture. If the lesions are focal, then the sections are taken from those areas for histopathological examination but in diffuse splenic involvement three to four representative sections will be sufficient.

Examination of Lymph Nodes

Lymph nodes are an important part of the immune system and are distributed throughout the body. These are located in groups, and each group drains a specific area of body. The major functions of lymph node are lymphopoiesis, filtration of lymph, and processing of antigens. The B- and T-immune cells that are present in these nodes stand ready to attack any bacteria, viruses, or other foreign substances

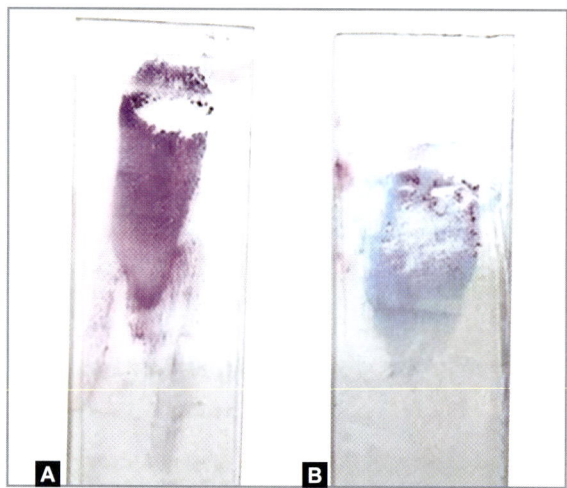

FIGS. 5.59A AND B: Smears made from splenic lesion stained by (A) hematoxylin and eosin and (B) Ziehl–Neelsen stains.

that enter the body. They also represent a site where differentiation of plasma cells, and they are thus major organs of antibody synthesis and secretion. Areas which are thymus dependent, take active role in cell-mediated immune responses and others in which thymus-independent cells abound that participate in antibody mediated cellular immunities and humoral immune responses.

Lymph nodes are small, light brown, oval, or bean-shaped glands with a firm consistency. They range in size from few mm to 1 cm. They have smooth capsule and soft texture. The cut surface of normal node is light gray to tan and has firm consistency. The superficial nodes are palpable in the neck, axilla, groin, and sometimes in the arm (elbow), and back of the knee. These sites should be examined at autopsy during external examination. Also the overlying skin should be examined for redness, puckering, sinus formation, and scarring. The main deeply situated nodes are mediastinal lymph nodes, tracheobronchial lymph nodes, mesenteric lymph nodes, para-aortic lymph nodes, retroperitoneal lymph nodes, and pelvic lymph nodes. These must be examined along with splenic examination.

Significant lymphadenopathy seen during postmortem examination and should be carefully dissected out. The lymphadenopathy in adults is often defined as a short axis of one or more lymph nodes is >10 mm. Lymphadenopathy of >1.5–2 cm increases the risk of malignancy or granulomatous disease as the cause rather than only inflammation or infection. There is no particular special method for removing lymph nodes. The site of the enlarged lymph nodes should be noted. The nodes should be examined for the sizes and number and whether they are single or in discrete groups or as a conglomerate. Occasionally, there is infiltration into perinodal tissue; in these cases the mass of tissue should be removed as completely as possible to assess the extent of the disease process and to sample tissue for subsequent histological characterization of the pathology. It is usually not necessary to weigh the lymph nodes. The pulmonary hilar group of lymph nodes usually shows black anthracotic pigment on its cut surface.

In case of lymphadenopathy, each lymph node should be sliced through to examine the cut surface. The normal lymph node is uniformly light gray/tan. In cases of infections, the nodes are soft with a congested appearance. In tuberculosis, due to marked periadenitis, the lymph nodes are matted with each other, yellowish white foci of caseation necroses (**Fig. 5.60A**). Sometimes this caseation can appear solid and mimic metastases. In cases of lymphomas, the nodes are usually markedly enlarged with a firm fleshy and bulging cut surface. Metastatic nodes are firm to hard with discolored area depending upon the primary tumor (**Fig. 5.60B**). In many diseases, lymphadenopathy is accompanied by splenomegaly and implies a systemic illness such as lymphoma, acute or chronic leukemia, systemic lupus erythematosus, sarcoidosis, toxoplasmosis, or other less common hematologic disorders. The skin lesions in the form of papules and nodules are seen in non-Hodgkin's and Hodgkin lymphomas. Also in cutaneous lymphomas, regional lymph nodes may be involved. HIV/AIDS patients may present with persistent lymphadenopathy and various skin lesions. As each lymph node group drains a specific area of the body; the site of body drained by that enlarged group must be examined to identify the underlying cause. For example, enlarged axillary lymph nodes in elderly females indicate metastasis from breast malignancy. Also lymphadenopathy of the right supraclavicular node is associated with cancer in the mediastinum, lungs, or esophagus. The left supraclavicular (Virchow's) node may signal pathology in the testes, ovaries, kidneys, pancreas, prostate, stomach, or gallbladder.

Imprints of lymph nodes are of diagnostic importance. Imprints are made by cutting the node into two halves and dabbing the cut surface on to clean glass slides, taking care not to press too hard; otherwise the cytological details may be obscured. Air-dried and fixed imprints can be made and stained accordingly (**Fig. 5.61**). In case of necrotic nodes, the necrotic material can be subjected to Z-N stain to rule out tuberculosis. With infections, it may be necessary to identify the infective organism. In such situation, part of the lymph node can be collected in a sterile container and sent for microbiological studies. While dealing with lymphoma it may be necessary to save appropriate tissue (fresh-frozen) for molecular studies.

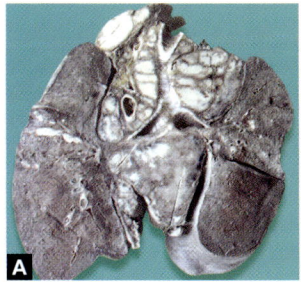
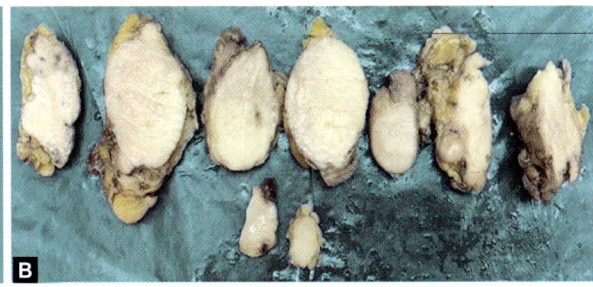

FIGS. 5.60A AND B: (A) Matted group of mediastinal lymph nodes of varying sizes in a case of disseminated tuberculosis. (B) Multiple enlarged axillary lymph nodes in a case of breast carcinoma. Cut surface is grayish white, firm with total replacement of lymph node parenchyma by metastasis.

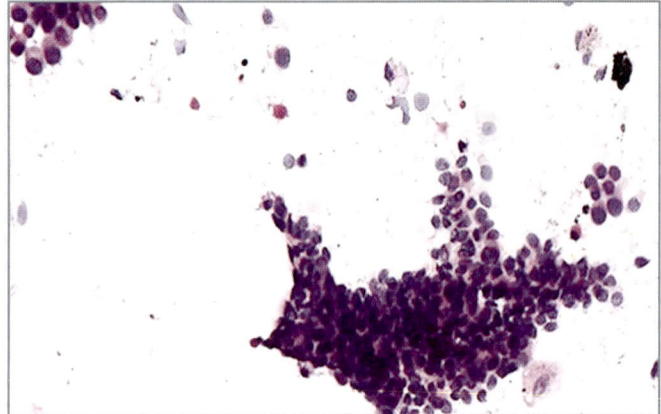

FIG. 5.61: Smears prepared during autopsy from enlarged lymph nodes showed features of metastatic adenocarcinoma (H and E × 250).

THYMUS

Once an organ buried in obscurity, the thymus now has a major role in cell-mediated immunity. The thymus is a specialized primary lymphoid organ of the immune system where the T-cells develop from hematopoietic progenitor cells. The T-cells' cytotoxicity comes from the cytokines it produces. The main function of the thymus gland is to release thymosin hormone that will stimulate the maturation of T-cells.

Embryologically, it is derived from the third and, inconstantly, the fourth pair of pharyngeal pouches. At birth, it is around 10–35 g and grows until puberty, when it achieves a maximum weight of 20–50 g. Thereafter, it undergoes progressive involution to little >5–15 g in older adults. The thymus can also show involution in children and young adults in response to severe illness and HIV infection.

A fully-developed thymus is composed of two well-encapsulated lobes with a fibrous capsular extension dividing each lobe into numerous lobules. The thymus is composed of an outer cortical layer and inner medulla. It can be easily seen during in situ examination (**Fig. 5.62**) as it is located in the superior mediastinum, behind the sternum and over the pericardium appearing as a lobulated, whitish, soft tissue particularly in neonates and children; in them the organ is the largest and most active and hence inspection is important (**Table 5.1**).

At autopsy thymus should be removed completely, weighed, and examined carefully for the lesions. The main disorders which cause thymic enlargement are thymic hyperplasia, thymic cysts, thymoma, and thymic carcinoma. The uncommon thymic neoplasms are thymolipoma, thymic carcinoid, and lymphangioma. In neonates and infants, congenital thymic cysts and true thymic hyperplasia (TTH) are common. Any pathological lesion should be sampled for the histopathological examination.

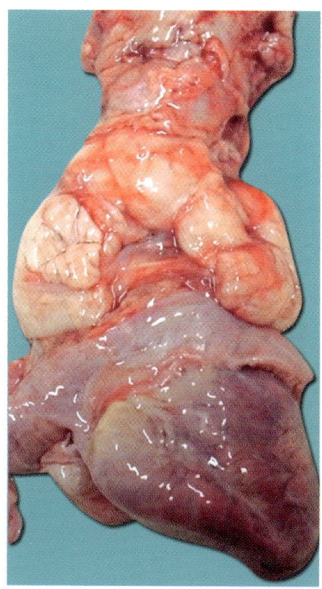

FIG. 5.62: Normal thymus in a neonate.

TABLE 5.1 Thymic lesions with their gross appearance and related conditions.

Thymic abnormality	Gross appearance	Related conditions
Thymic dysgenesis, aplasia, and dysplasia	Ectopic location in neck, diaphragm, and pleura	Congenital immunodeficiency syndrome
Hyperplasia	Weight of the thymus is well above the normal range for the age	Endocrinopathies-thyrotoxicosis and Addison's disease
Acute involution	Weight is less than the normal. Cystic change noted	Pregnancy, lactation, and due to drugs
Tumors	Exaggerated lobulated appearance and large in size	Thymoma and thymic carcinoma

Bone Marrow Examination

Gross abnormalities of the bone marrow are not easily appreciated. Sites of bone marrow examination include sternum, iliac crest, and vertebral bodies. The marrow is examined for its expansion for the age to suspect any infiltrative disorders. Bone marrow imprints give good cytological detail, and provide a rapid diagnosis in suspected cases. A simple technique was described by Kao in which 0.5–1 cm sample of marrow is squeezed out of a rib/sternum with a pressure applied through a bone-cutter; the squeezed out marrow is then transferred onto the glass slide and a thin smear is made. Smears are then stained using Giemsa stain. This is particularly useful for infective and infiltrative diseases.

Examine the appearance of the intervertebral joints and vertebral marrow or the sternal marrow, and test the degree of ossification of these bones by compressing them under your thumb. Using a hammer and bone knife, obtain a thin (1 cm or less) section of bone for decalcification and marrow examination. A vibrating saw should not be used as it would produce lot of bone dust and may affect processing and even cytological details. Even decalcification may affect the histomorphology. If the patient is suffering from hematological disease, rib/sternum should be the site of marrow section as these may not require decalcification.

FURTHER READING

1. Burton J, Saunders S, Hamilton S. Atlas of adult autopsy pathology. 1st ed. London, CRC Press, 2015.
2. Finkbeiner, W. Autopsy Pathology: A Manual and Atlas. 2nd ed. Elsevier, 2009, p.60.
3. Ludwig, J. Handbook of Autopsy practices. 3rd ed. Humana press; 2002, p.59.
4. Sheaff MT, Hopster DJ. Post mortem technique handbook. 2nd ed. London: Springer; 2005:249-56.

CHAPTER 6

Autopsies in Special Situations

Bhuvaneshwari Kandalkar, Pragati Sathe, Ratnaprabha Ghodke, Kusum Jashnani

6A: Pediatric Autopsies

Bhuvaneshwari Kandalkar, Pragati Sathe, Ratnaprabha Ghodke

INTRODUCTION

A pediatric autopsy is of great value to the clinicians and to the kith and kin of the child who has died. Maximum information should be garnered from each and every autopsy so as to reduce mortality and morbidity in other children. Pediatric autopsies include autopsies of the fetus, neonate (age from birth up to 1 month), infant (age up to 1 year), and child, which in many centers is up to the age 12 years, although this limit can be extended to 18 years. In general, like autopsies in adults, autopsies performed in the pediatric age group also help to judge the accuracy of diagnosis, to rule out the differential diagnosis, to document surprise findings and confirm the cause of death. In addition, it provides feedback regarding therapeutic outcomes, diagnostic technologies, and tests. In some cases, it may help study new diseases and their courses, and may also alleviate guilt feelings in parents following the death of their children.

Maternal medical disorders like eclampsia, diabetes mellitus, coagulopathies, and infections contribute significantly to fetal growth and outcome. Likewise, common placental abnormalities like twinning, umbilical cord related lesions, vasculopathies, and abruption can also affect fetal outcome. Fetal autopsy reveals confirms gestational age, maternal/placental problems, and genetic abnormalities which are useful for future counseling for hereditary disorders. Perinatal and neonatal deaths are often due to infections, congenital anomalies, and respiratory complications, whereas in infants and children, infections, inborn errors of metabolism, and tumors contribute to death. There, however can be overlapping or common problems in all of them.

Before commencing a pediatric autopsy, the case history should be thoroughly evaluated and documented for the maternal history and birth history, immunization schedule, and milestones. Particular attention should be paid to all investigations, particularly radiological images. After a careful record of the history, a systematic autopsy has to be performed commencing with a good external examination followed by in situ and internal organ system examination.

EXTERNAL EXAMINATION

Apart from the usual observations performed in an adult autopsy, in a pediatric autopsy, weights, measurements, and photographs are of great importance. The gestational age-wise weights can be compared with the standard charts to decide appropriate or small for gestational age babies, especially in the perinatal period. The important measurements include crown-heel length, crown-rump length, head circumference, abdominal circumference, chest circumference, foot length, distance between nipples, and mid-arm circumference. All measurements can be accurately performed with a measuring tape at various levels. The value should be reported to the nearest 0.01 cm and plotted on a standardized growth chart. Out of these measurements, foot length correlates well with gestational age. It is helpful in disrupted fetuses as well. These measurements also have an internal control, e.g., crown-rump length is equal to two-thirds of crown-heel length and head circumference is approximately equal to crown-rump length. Head circumference is measured in children up to age three, as this is the time of greatest brain growth. Abnormal measurements tell us about abnormality in the growth of the brain inside the skull cavity. These measurements also give us information about the nutritional status, overall skeletal development, and the chronicity of the illness. As per World Health Organization (WHO) guidelines, a mid-upper arm circumference <115 mm is considered to be a significant indicator of malnutrition in children 6–60 months of age. At the extremes of malnourishment, thickness of subcutaneous fat on the chest midway between the nipples and on the abdomen midway between the xiphoid process and the umbilicus serve as rough indicators of nutritional status (<3 mm fat at abdominal level and <2 mm fat at the chest level indicates severe wasting whereas >25 mm at the abdominal level and >12 mm at the chest level are indicative of obesity).

Photographs are important for documentation of external abnormalities and can also serve as material for future reference. The important planes include full image of the front and the back of the body and a close-up view of the face from front and profile. Signs of maceration vary with the time spent intrauterine after death and thus help in deciding the time since death (**Table 6.1**). Signs of prematurity are important to investigate the gestational age of the fetus (**Box 6.1**). Abnormal facial appearance and maldevelopment of ears, hands (**Fig. 6.1A**), feet, rib cage, vertebral column, and genitalia (**Fig. 6.1B**) may suggest a syndromic association and hence should be carefully documented. The skin color should be examined. Meconium staining may be seen in cases of asphyxia.

Bruising, fractures, and hemorrhages may suggest birth injuries that could have directly or indirectly contributed to death. Position of umbilicus and the cord structures should be noted as vascular anomalies like single umbilical artery may indicate internal anomalies.

Autopsies in Special Situations

TABLE 6.1 Grades of maceration in relation to time since death.

Time since death	Grades of maceration
Intrapartum death	None
Less than 12 hours between death and delivery	*Slight:* Skin slippage (on rubbing of skin the epidermis is detached from the underlying tissues), rare bullae (blisters), little (e.g., scrotum only or single spots of skin loss elsewhere) or no denudation (due to rupture of bullae)
About 12–24 hours between death and delivery	*Mild:* Focal denudation of multiple regions without other changes
One to a few days between death and delivery	*Moderate:* Generalized skin maceration/denudation but without significant compressive changes
More than a few days between death and delivery	*Advanced:* Compression and/or mummification and/or internal liquefaction

BOX 6.1 Common signs of prematurity.

- Lanugo hair
- Maldeveloped ear cartilage
- Absent breast bud
- Undescended testes
- Length of finger nails (the nails are identifiable after 17 weeks and reach the finger tips by 32 weeks)
- Rugose scrotum
- Poorly developed palmar/plantar creases

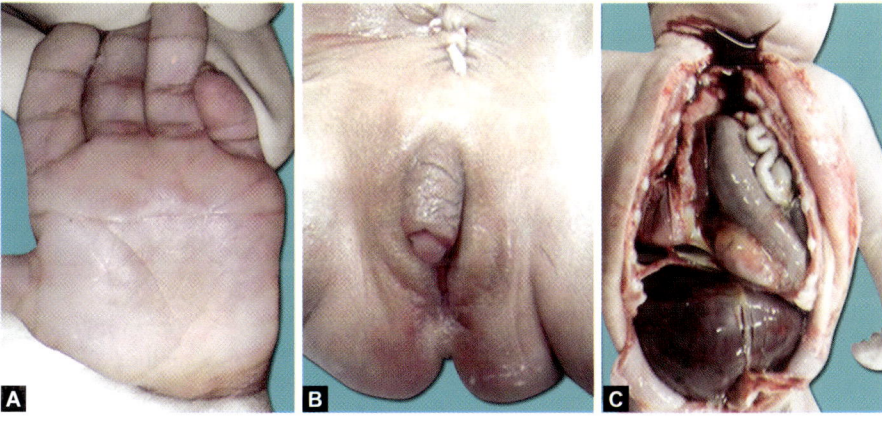

FIGS. 6.1A TO C: (A) Simian crease in a baby of Down's syndrome; (B) Ambiguous genitalia. Micropenis is seen along with labia majora; (C) Congenital diaphragmatic hernia. Note the intestinal loops in left thoracic cavity.

INCISIONS AND IN SITU EXAMINATION

In contrast to opening of the cranium in adults and older children, Beneke suture-splitting technique is used to open the cranium of fetuses and infants. This is possible as the sutures are not closed and cranial bones are still soft. One has to look for cephalohematomas and hemorrhages in subgaleal, subdural subarachnoid or intracerebral locations as they may be related to birth trauma. Record of hemorrhages especially extradural in location is also important in cases of battered baby syndrome.

The thoracic cavity is best examined before the peritoneal cavity is opened so as to avoid possible contamination by intestinal organisms when lung tissue has to be sampled for culture. The chest should be opened after aspirating the pleural cavities for air to identify a possible pneumothorax that may have occurred during attempted resuscitation. One has to look for effusions, positions, and shapes of organs namely the heart, lungs, great vessels, thymus, and for any abnormal presence of abdominal organs within the thoracic cavity like in cases of diaphragmatic hernia (**Fig. 6.1C**). After removing the thymus and pericardial sac, the external configuration and vascular connections of the heart are checked while the heart is still in situ. Procedure of dissection is similar to adults except that the venous and arterial connections of the heart must be determined before removal of heart-lung en bloc. When the abdominal cavity is opened, one should check for situs, organomegaly (**Fig. 6.2A**), masses, and the nature of ascitic fluid, if present. Marked dilatation of a loop of intestine may suggest atresia in the segment distal to it.

SYSTEMIC EXAMINATION

All major organs need to be weighed and compared to published data. However, there are variations in individual as well as racial and pathological conditions. Hence, weight ratios are more reliable.

For example, lung: heart = 3:1, brain: liver = 3:1, liver: heart = 6:1, and thymus: spleen: adrenals = 1:1:1.

The gyral and sulcal patterns of development of the cerebral hemispheres should be compared with published diagrams that indicate increasing complexity with advancing gestational age, as this is a relatively reliable tool for determining gestational age in preterm neonatal deaths. The pituitary could be in a defective position in cases of anencephaly. Various anomalies like absent corpus callosum, holoprosencephaly, etc., may be incompatible with life and have to be documented. The brain would be edematous in cases of perinatal hypoxia. As a consequence of ischemia or hypoxia, hemorrhages most often occur in the germinal matrix of the ventricles (**Fig. 6.2B**), cerebellum, and around small blood vessels (ring hemorrhages).

Periventricular leukomalacia is a form of coagulative necrosis with tissue lysis, edema, cyst formation, and gliosis, indicating an intrauterine ischemic event most commonly seen in prematurity. When present, kernicterus is usually recognizable on the cut surfaces of the peduncles as deep yellow staining. A single midcoronal cut through the hemisphere will also show yellowish discoloration of the basal ganglia (**Fig. 6.2B**).

The heart and lungs should be eviscerated together with the tongue, pharynx, submandibular salivary glands, esophagus, larynx, and trachea. Usually the thoracic and abdominal block can be dissected after separation. However, the blocks need to be dissected in continuity in congenital heart diseases when there is pulmonary arterial or particularly venous malformations (where one might severe the connections due to lack of awareness) and in the heterotaxy syndromes. The esophageal hiatus should be examined in situ. The esophagus should be opened from posterior aspect

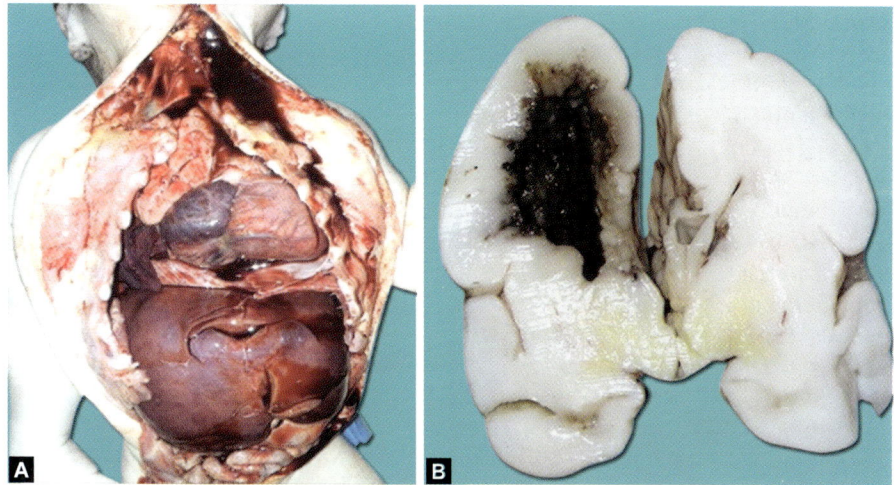

FIGS. 6.2A AND B: (A) Enlarged liver is seen to occupy almost the entire abdominal cavity; (B) Yellowish discoloration of thalami in a case of kernicterus. There is a large periventricular hemorrhage as well.

so that esophageal atresia or tracheoesophageal fistula may be detected. Gross examination and sampling of the larynx and vocal cords in young infants should be done particularly when dealing with sudden unexpected death in infancy. The intact larynx, trachea, and main bronchi should be opened along their posterior surface. Also check for plugging by mucus, meconium, or aspirated material. The heart has to be checked for position, size, external appearance, and relation to great vessels. The opening of heart is along the flow of blood as done in adults. Complex congenital cardiac anomalies are likely to manifest early and should be looked for in all neonatal hearts. The lungs have to be checked for their size and shape, number of lobes and position, abnormalities in the form of hypoplasia, atelectasis/collapse, congestion and hemorrhage pneumonia/abscesses, and bullae/cystic lesions.

The mesentery has to be kept intact till intestinal atresia or stenosis examined. There can be incomplete mesenteric fixation, which renders the cecum excessively mobile, with displacement of the vermiform appendix to the right upper quadrant.

One has to look for intussusceptions, atresia, bands, and volvulus, besides the usual inflammations, infections (**Fig. 6.3A**), and infestations. Frequently mucosal polyps like Peutz-Jeghers polyp are found at the tip of the intussusception. The liver is frequently slightly enlarged in preterm babies as it is a site for extramedullary hematopoiesis. Hepatomegaly in neonates, infants, and young children commonly occurs due to cholestatic and metabolic diseases; it may be greenish in cholestatic disorders, cirrhotic in diseases like Wilson disease, slate gray as in malaria, nodular (**Fig. 6.3B**) or even focally cystic at times (**Fig. 6.3C**). The patency of the extrahepatic biliary tree has to be checked by confirming the flow of bile at the ampulla of Vater. The gallbladder in these cases is shrunken, atretic, and does not contain bile. The bile

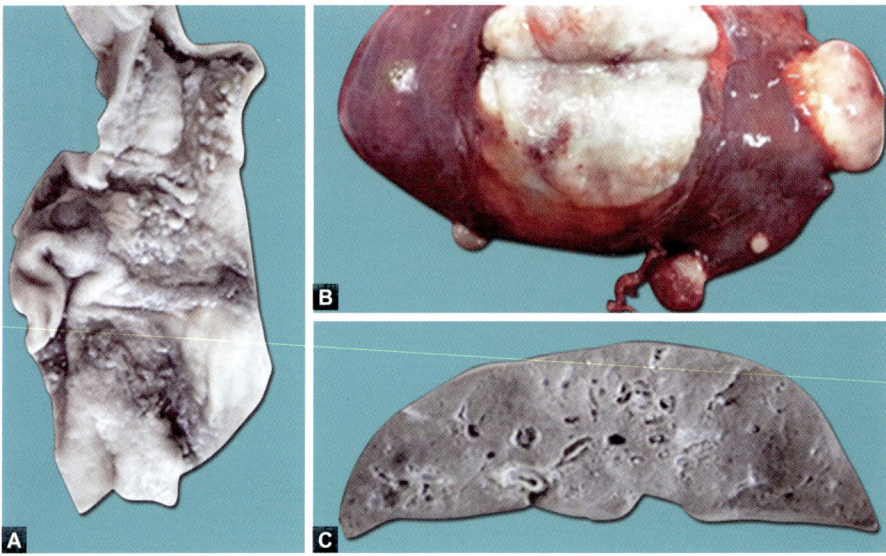

FIGS. 6.3A TO C: (A) Transverse ulcers of ileal tuberculosis; (B) Multiple gray white lesions of metastasis of Wilms tumor in the liver; (C) Multiple tiny cysts distributed throughout the liver parenchyma. The patient also had autosomal recessive polycystic kidney disease.

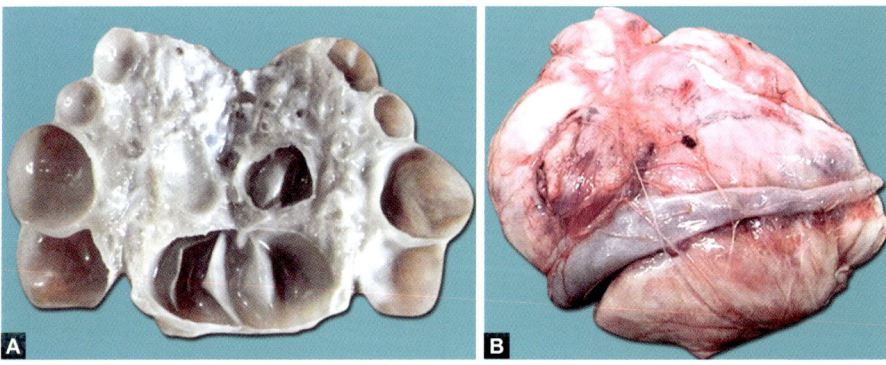

FIGS. 6.4A AND B: (A) Multicystic renal dysplasia in a newborn; (B) A large Wilms tumor with intestinal loop stretched over it.

duct may be reduced to just a fibrous tract. It is advisable to perform a hepatobiliary dissection for better demonstration of the biliary tract. The other causes of obstructive biliary disease like choledochal cysts are common in older children.

Anomalies of urinary tract such as renal agenesis/hypoplasia, horse-shoe shape, cystic anomalies (**Fig. 6.4A**), ureteral, bladder and urethral abnormalities, and tumors (**Fig. 6.4B**) should be looked for. Presence of undescended testis and observation of internal genital organ development are important in cases of ambiguous genitalia. It is important to remember that adrenal glands are large in children and are usually one-third the weight of the kidneys. They can be decreased in size in anencephaly and growth retardation and can be enlarged in Rh isoimmunization, hemorrhage, hypoxia, necrosis, abscess, and congenital infections. In stillborn babies with complex congenital anomalies, asplenia is common. Spleen may be enlarged in infants and young children due to infections, metabolic disorders, and hemolytic anemias. Mildly enlarged reactive mesenteric lymph nodes are frequently seen in pediatric population and may not be of diagnostic significance.

POSTMORTEM INVESTIGATIONS

Routine microbiology cultures should be taken from turbid peritoneal fluid, abscesses, cerebrospinal fluid, and rectal stools in cases with diarrheal disease. Cerebrospinal fluid should be collected by cisternal puncture. Blood culture is performed from blood collected from the heart after searing the right ventricular surface in cases of sepsis. Swabs should be collected from bronchial secretions after opening the trachea with flamed scissors to avoid contamination.

Hematological and histochemical investigations should be ideally performed within 12 hours after death for reliable results. Immunological tests [e.g., toxoplasma, syphilis, rubella, cytomegalovirus, and herpes simplex (TORCH) titers, human immunodeficiency virus (HIV) antibody] should be completed by 24 hours after death. A blood spot on a Guthrie card can be useful for potential future deoxyribonucleic acid (DNA) analysis. When there is suspicion of an inborn error of metabolism, and in forensic cases, samples of blood, urine, bile, gastric content, and vitreous humor should be taken for biochemical or toxicologic analysis. Portions of liver and kidney may also be kept in a freezer until histology is complete. Presence of zonal necrosis in the liver may suggest poisoning and in such cases toxicologic analysis can be performed further. Material for viral culture (suspected organ of involvement like lung, kidney, and liver) has to be collected in virus transport medium. For chromosome assays, if leukocytes of blood are used for culture then it has to be performed within 12 hours of death. If skin or amnion fibroblasts are used for culture, then the test has to be performed within 3 days of death. For electron microscopy, especially in cases of inborn errors of metabolism, remove representative portions of the organ (cortex and medulla for kidney, parenchyma, and peribronchial/perivascular tissue for lung) and place in glutaraldehyde. The optimum tissue size is 1 mm^3.

SAMPLING FOR HISTOPATHOLOGY

Microscopic examination of tissues helps to assess maturation, may help to observe changes occurring during the period immediately preceding death, and of course determining the pathologic process that led to death. Thus, routine sampling of the following tissues should be regularly undertaken. Following tissues should be sampled in addition to routine sections:
- Thymus to evaluate for small hemorrhages (as stress reaction), and involutionary changes.
- Rib costochondral junction to assess the duration of terminal stress and possible underlying rickets and/or scurvy.

- Adrenal glands to evaluate the cortical lipid content, pseudoacinus formations, necrosis, hemorrhages, and retention of fetal cortex. Midportion of adrenal should be sampled.
- Kidney should be sectioned at right angles to capsule to count glomerular generation. Do not strip the capsule.
- Lungs should be sampled midway between the hilum and the most distant periphery of each lobe to discern whether or not patchy pathologic findings are sufficient to explain death. Hilar and pleural surface also has to be sampled.
- The paraventricular area of the brain below the corpus callosum should be sampled for demonstration of germinal matrix hemorrhages.
- Sections from both papillary muscles of the heart should be taken for demonstration of vacuolated myocardial fibers in perinatal asphyxia.
- Any abnormal finding should be sampled for histopathology for confirmation.

When all the tissues have been examined and the results of laboratory investigations are available, a final autopsy diagnosis is given. An opinion should be given whether the microbiological test findings are of clinical significance keeping in mind the interval between time of death and autopsy. The final diagnosis should list all the abnormal gross and microscopic findings, and ancillary abnormalities that contributed to the death of the patient in order of their importance. In addition, the pathologist should provide a clinicopathologic correlation of the sequence of events leading to death. If any special requests or queries were made by the concerned party wanting the autopsy it should be especially mentioned. There are occasions when the pathologist should recommend that particular corrective action be taken to avoid recurrences of harmful events, such as inborn errors of metabolism. The final report should indicate the number of paraffin blocks that have been processed and their organ of origin. The report should be dated and signed by the concerned pathologist.

FURTHER READING

1. Newton D, Coffin CM, Clark EB, Lowichik A. How the pediatric autopsy yields valuable information in a vertically integrated health care system. Arch Pathol Lab Med. 2004;128:1239-46.
2. Siebert JR. Perinatal, fetal and embryonic autopsy. In: Gilbert-Barness E (Ed). Potter's Pathology of the Fetus, Infant and Child, 2nd edition. Philadelphia: Elsevier; 2007. pp. 695-739.
3. Stocker JT, Macpherson TA. The pediatric autopsy. In: Stocker JT, Dehner LP (Ed). Pediatric Pathology, 2nd edition. Philadelphia: Lippincott Williams & Wilkins; 2001.pp. 5-17.
4. Wainright HC. My approach to performing a perinatal or neonatal autopsy. J Clin Pathol. 2006;59:673-80.

6B: Autopsy in Maternal Deaths
Kusum Jashnani

INTRODUCTION

Maternal mortality is an important event to assess the quality of healthcare system, as it is not only a health issue but also a matter of social injustice. Maternal deaths are defined as "deaths occurring during pregnancy or within 42 days of childbirth or of an abortion from any cause related to or aggravated by pregnancy or its management". Maternal deaths are subdivided into direct, indirect, and coincidental. Direct causes are related to obstetric complications occurring during pregnancy, labor, delivery, and the postpartum periods. Indirect causes are related to preexisting or newly developed medical conditions that may be aggravated by the physiologic demands of pregnancy. Coincidental causes include deaths due to homicide, accidents, illicit drug toxicity, and suicides. A list of the causes of maternal death is available in comprehensive review of this subject (**Tables 6.2** and **6.3**). The medicolegal aspects of autopsies in maternal death will not be dealt here.

TABLE 6.2 List of common causes of maternal death.

Direct causes	Indirect causes	Coincidental causes
Hypertensive diseases of pregnancy	Venous thromboembolism	Homicide/suicide (particularly burns)
Obstetric hemorrhage	Hepatitis/hepatic necrosis	Road/railway accident
Peripartum dilated cardiomyopathy and some cases of acute aortic dissections	Preexisting congenital or acquired heart diseases	Illicit drug toxicity
Amniotic fluid embolism	Tuberculosis, malaria, and HIV/AIDS	
Puerperal sepsis	Anemia	
Ruptured ectopic pregnancy	Stroke	
Acute fatty liver of pregnancy	Cancer	

(AIDS: acquired immunodeficiency syndrome; HIV: human immunodeficiency virus)

TABLE 6.3 Causes of obstetric hemorrhage.

Early pregnancy bleeding	Antepartum hemorrhage	Postpartum hemorrhage
Abortion	Placenta previa	Tone: Atony
Ectopic pregnancy	Abruptio placentae	Tissue: Retained, accreta
Gestational trophoblastic tumor	Uterine rupture	• Trauma: Rupture, laceration • Thrombosis: DIC, sepsis, HELLP

(DIC: disseminated intravascular coagulation; HELLP: hemolysis, elevated liver enzymes, and low platelet count)

Delay in deciding to seek care may be one of the reasons for maternal death. It is common in developing countries, to see women die at home from maternal complications, not knowing where and when to ask for health care. Also women who do ask for care may not receive effective treatment. Studies have shown that half of the deceased women were taken to at least two facilities, causing fatal delays in receiving appropriate care. Maternal Death Review is a tool used to analyze the reasons for maternal deaths for appropriate local intervention. The Government of India introduced Maternal Death Review guidelines in 2010 and hence it is important for all administrative staff (medical and nonmedical) to implement and follow the guidelines. For example, since then, each and every maternal death in the city of Mumbai is reviewed by a committee of members appointed by the Municipal Corporation of Greater Mumbai (MCGM). Maternal mortality ratio (MMR) is the number of women who die from obstetric complications in a given year per 100,000 live births in that year. Maternal mortality rate is defined as the number of maternal deaths to women in the ages 15–49 per lakh of women in the same age group.

ROLE OF AUTOPSY IN MATERNAL DEATHS

Autopsy still plays an important role in healthcare and educational programs, in spite of declining autopsy rates. Despite advances in imaging and laboratory diagnostic services, an autopsy remains the most accurate way to identify the cause of death. Maternal autopsy is not different from any other adult autopsy, provided that one remembers that certain lethal complications of pregnancy are either unique [amniotic fluid embolism (AFE) and eclampsia] or unusual in nonmaternal autopsies (air embolism and pituitary necrosis) for which one must positively identify their presence or absence. Also, maternal death autopsies assume greater significance than most other deaths as recommendations for improving the obstetric practice can be based on these reports.

IMPORTANCE OF CLINICAL RECORDS

The first step in performing an autopsy is the thorough review of the medical records. The pathologist must obtain a clear understanding of the mother's present and past medical history, place and type of delivery process or abortion, transfer/s from one healthcare center to the other, therapeutic interventions if any, and the terminal events leading to death.

Fetal/neonatal information is also relevant, e.g., infected peripartum, small-for-dates, etc. It would be preferable if the pathologist can get in touch with the obstetrician/physician to discuss the case before beginning the prosection. The clinical team should be invited to visit the autopsy room during or after the autopsy (if no negligence is suspected).

EXTERNAL EXAMINATION

Look for signs of pallor, icterus, edema feet, anasarca, and any injuries. External signs of disease should be sought, e.g., vaginal discharge (genital tract infection and possible systemic sepsis), generalized bleeding from multiple sites [disseminated intravascular coagulation (DIC)], and examination of external genitalia for signs of injury which may be related to medical intervention, e.g., use of forceps and episiotomy. After external assessment and before evisceration proceeds, samples required for microbiological analysis should be collected with swabs from localized septic sites.

IN SITU EXAMINATION

Blood samples after right atrial puncture should be taken for hematological, biochemical, and serological investigations (particularly in acute febrile illnesses, if not already performed antemortem). AFE, air embolism, pneumothorax, and pulmonary thromboembolism (PTE) need to be tested on in situ examination. The buffy coat of blood sample from the pulmonary artery may reveal evidence of telltale fetal squames in patients suspected of death from AFE, although this procedure is not commonly performed. Close inspection of the uterus, cervix, vagina, and adjacent soft tissue for tears or rupture is mandatory to identify macroscopic evidence of AFE. The final diagnosis of AFE requires histopathological examination of lung vasculature for presence of squames, fat, mucin, and lanugo hairs (**Fig. 6.5**). It may be necessary to perform special stains like Alcian blue to demonstrate amniotic acid mucin and high molecular weight keratin immunohistochemistry to demonstrate the squames. Sudden cardiorespiratory arrest resulting in acute hypoxia, occurring during or just after labor or cesarean section is the classic presentation of AFE. This condition is often used as a defense against claims of clinical negligence where there has been fatal peri- or postpartum hemorrhage (PPH). It therefore achieves a medicolegal angle and should therefore be looked properly, to prove or exclude it.

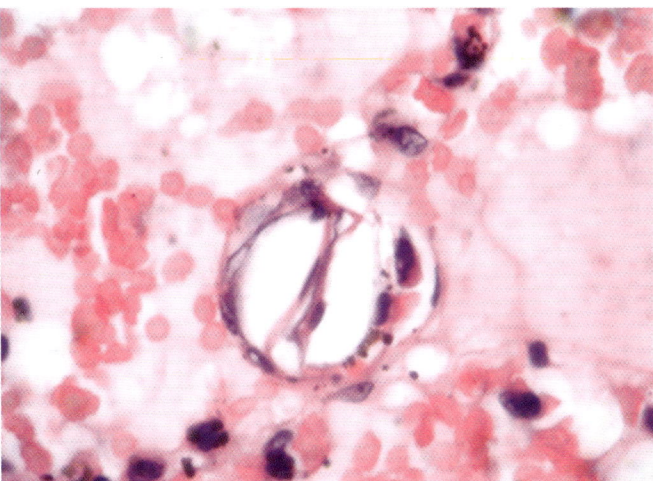

FIG. 6.5: Tiny blood vessel in the lung shows presence of few fetal squamous cells [hematoxylin and eosin (H&E) × 400].

The skin over the neck and anterior chest should be palpated for evidence of crepitus and soft tissue emphysema. The techniques for checking for pneumothorax, pulmonary embolism, and air embolism are discussed in Chapter 5C.

INTERNAL SYSTEMIC EXAMINATION

Examination of all the systems does not differ from any other autopsy. Particular attention must be paid in view of maternal death in all the following systems.

Central Nervous System

Look for intracranial hemorrhage consequent to the toxemias of pregnancy. Histologic examination is mandatory, since these hemorrhagic lesions can be a manifestation of metastatic choriocarcinoma. Infarction, sagittal sinus/cerebral venous thrombosis, and meningitis are other lesions to be looked for.

Pituitary gland necrosis/Sheehan's syndrome is a common cause of hypo-pituitarism in the postpartum period. Sections should be taken from the pituitary gland routinely.

Cardiovascular System

The heart should be weighed and inspected for cardiomegaly, which may occur with toxemias of pregnancy, preexisting heart diseases or in some instances peripartum cardiomyopathy. In the latter condition, there are no characteristic histological features, but focal fibrosis, variability in myocyte caliber, and scattered chronic inflammatory cells; it may be viral in etiology. Dilated cardiomyopathy (**Figs. 6.6A and B**) is also recognized increasingly in association with HIV infection as this pandemic increasingly affects women. The valves should be examined for possible infective endocarditis and appropriate swabs taken for microbiological studies. Chronic rheumatic heart disease with mitral stenosis is often a surprise finding.

Respiratory System

The upper air passages and laryngeal inlet should be examined for trauma consequent upon intubation. Stomach contents may be present in the upper air passages; this finding needs to be interpreted with caution since regurgitation can occur during resuscitation measures and even after death by movement of the body. A more reliable guide to assess aspiration is a thorough histological examination of the lungs. Vegetable matter may be seen within the bronchioles or alveolar spaces along with bacterial colonies in the absence of pneumonia. Look for varying morphologic lesions of tuberculosis and angry red boggy lungs of acute respiratory distress syndrome. Pregnancy, being a hypercoagulable state, often shows massive PTE as a cause of sudden collapse and death. Hence, it is critical to examine the entire length of pulmonary artery tree thoroughly to show or exclude massive thromboembolism.

Gastrointestinal System

In situ, the stomach and intestines should be examined for gaseous distention which may indicate misplacement of the endotracheal tube. Hemorrhagic gastritis may be a finding in a case of DIC (**Fig. 6.6C**).

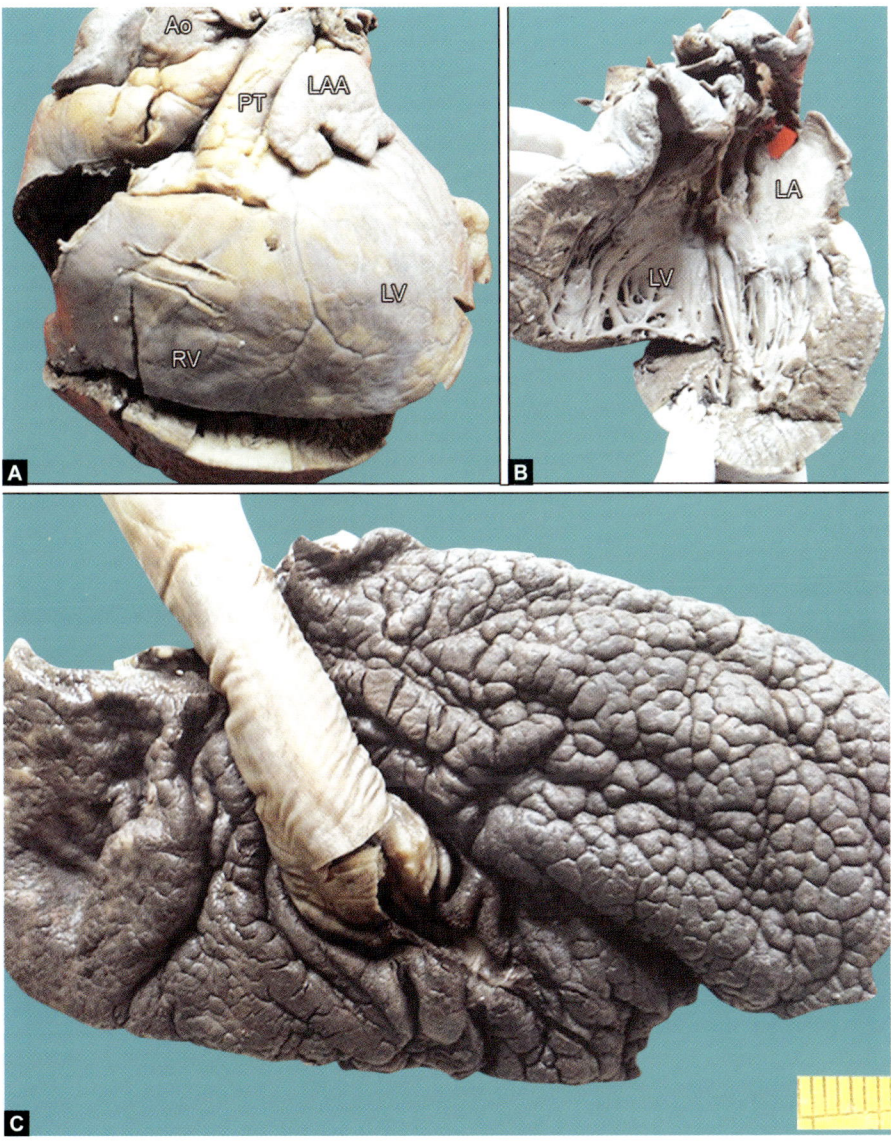

(Ao: aorta; LA: left atrium; LAA: left atrial appendage; LV: left ventricular; PT: pulmonary trunk; RV: right ventricular)

FIGS. 6.6A TO C: (A and B) Markedly enlarged and flabby heart with dilated left ventricle in a case of peripartum dilated cardiomyopathy; (C) Gross specimen of stomach showing extensive mucosal hemorrhages in a case of disseminated intravascular coagulation.

Hepatobiliary System and Pancreas

The liver can be involved in a number of disease processes during pregnancy, including intrahepatic cholestasis, toxemias particularly eclampsia, acute fatty liver of pregnancy (AFLP), and submassive to massive hepatic necrosis, especially in hepatitis E infection. Frozen section of the liver with Oil Red O staining for fat may be essential in AFLP, which is commonly seen in third trimester of pregnancy and can be fatal. It shows yellow greasy liver on gross with microvesicular fatty change in centrilobular hepatocytes and normal periportal hepatocytes on histopathologic (HP) examination (**Fig. 6.7**). Necrosis is not a feature. Hepatitis E infection is usually a self-limiting infection but may develop into fulminant hepatitis in pregnant women (**Figs. 6.8A to C**). The cause may be reduced immunity or altered hormonal status in pregnancy promoting increased viral replication and hepatic dysfunction. This also explains occurrence and dissemination of other infections, including tuberculosis.

Urogenital System

The kidney can be affected by several disease processes in pregnancy. The kidney may show features of acute pyelonephritis, hypertensive disorders, and renal cortical necrosis due to a number of causes. Appropriate histological examination is essential in all cases including diabetic mothers. Fibrin thrombi in the glomerular capillaries are an important histopathological finding in DIC. Special stain Martius scarlet blue (MSB) for fibrin can be used to highlight these thrombi. The lesion of glomerular endotheliosis is characteristic and unique to hypertensive disease of pregnancy. The endothelial cells are swollen, making the glomerular capillaries appear bloodless.

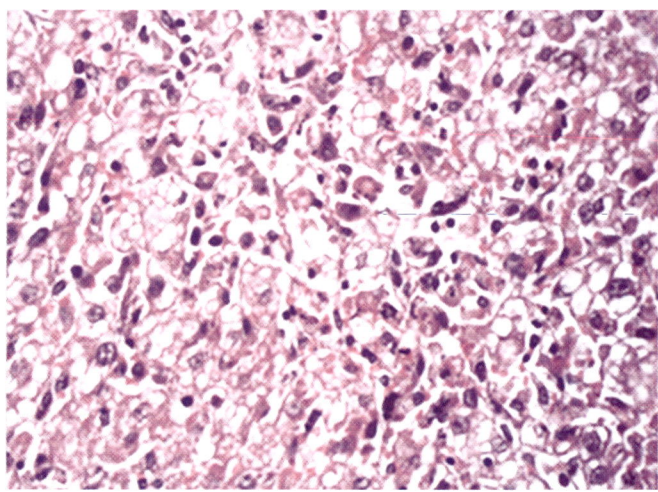

FIG. 6.7: Microvesicular fatty change in acute fatty liver of pregnancy [hematoxylin and eosin (H&E) × 400].

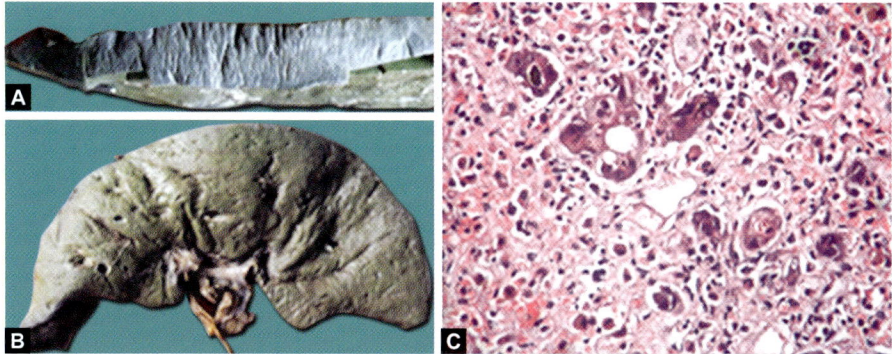

FIGS. 6.8A TO C: Slice of liver in a fatal case of hepatitis E showing (A) wrinkled capsule and (B) soft foldable parenchyma suggestive of massive necrosis, which is confirmed on (C) histopathologic examination.

In any event, the cervix, vagina, uterus, and placental site should be examined. Evidence should be sought for retained products of conception, abnormal placental adherence (accreta), placenta previa, rupture of uterine scar, retroplacental blood clot, etc. It should be remembered that endometrial congestion and/or hemorrhage; cervical congestion and/or hemorrhage; as well as similar findings in the vagina are not to be taken as pathologic/abnormal findings. These findings are normal physiologic findings seen in almost all cases of vaginal delivery. These changes result from the passage of the entire fetus through the birth canal. HP examination of cervix and vagina in vaginal deliveries also shows dilated and congested blood vessels in their wall along with multiple tiny foci of hemorrhages.

Uterine atony is the most common cause of PPH, but shows no definable pathology. Other important causes are the placental disorders.

Abruptio placentae are partial or complete separation of a normally implanted placenta from the uterine wall, before delivery, after the 20th week of pregnancy (**Fig. 6.9A**). Maternal hypertensive diseases, cocaine, and vasoconstrictive drugs, cigarette smoking, multiple pregnancies, premature rupture of membranes (PROM) and chorioamnionitis are some of the risk factors for abruptio placentae. Retroplacental hematoma is a pathologic lesion of the clinical condition of placental abruption. Activated neutrophils in cases of inflammation, secrete cytokines, and tumor necrosis factor. There is upregulation in the production and activity of matrix metalloproteinases in the trophoblasts. This leads to the destruction of extracellular matrices and cellular connections of the placenta, causing premature detachment.

Placenta creta, a life-threatening obstetric condition, is divided into accreta, increta, and percreta distinguishable by the depth of penetration. All these conditions are characterized by deficiency or absence of decidua basalis and incomplete development of the Nitabuch's layer. The placenta attaches strongly to the myometrium, but does not penetrate it in a case of placenta accreta. Placenta increta occurs when the placenta penetrates the myometrium. Placenta percreta is the worst form of the condition in which the placenta penetrates the entire myometrium to reach the uterine serosal aspect leading to uterine perforation. If placenta previa is suspected,

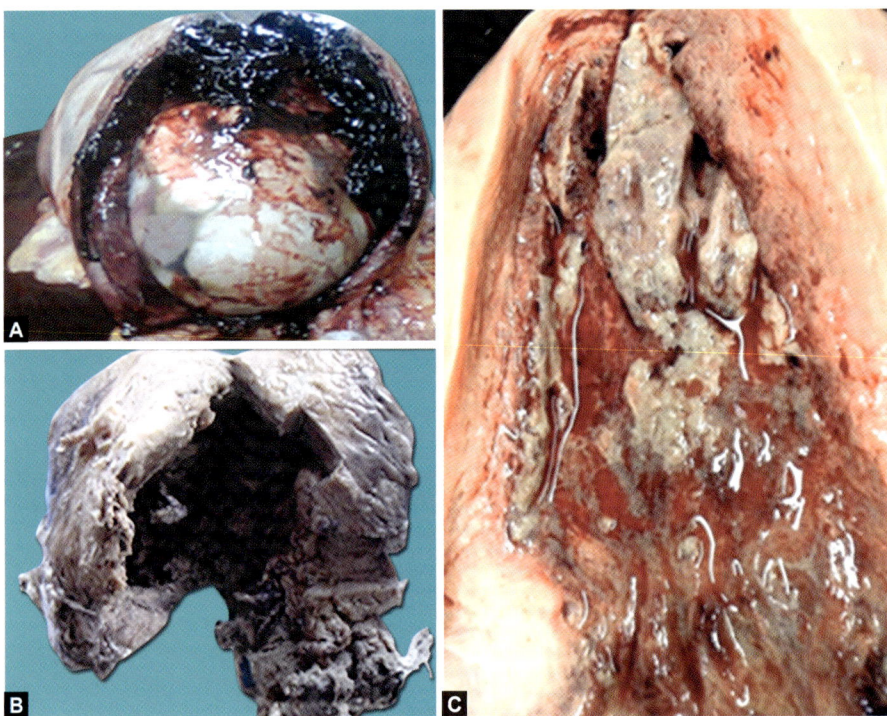

FIGS. 6.9A TO C: (A) Extensive intrauterine hemorrhage in a case of complete abruptio placentae. This woman had been admitted with cold clammy extremities and other symptoms of shock. There was no evidence of per vaginal bleeding—a case of concealed abruptio placentae; (B) Rupture of uterus is seen along the anterolateral border. Histopathologic examination showed adherent placenta invading through the full thickness of myometrium (placenta percreta). The dead fetus was lying partly outside the uterus; (C) Yellowish exudate seen over the endometrial surface. This was a case of home delivery followed by complaints of fever and abdominal pain few days postpartum.

antemortem ultrasound data should be sought in the notes before autopsy, and the uterus opened away from the site of placental attachment.

In cases of uterine rupture (**Fig. 6.9B**), the extent, size, and weight/volume of blood clot/hemorrhage should be documented. The majority of uterine ruptures happen at the site of a scar, and ruptures tend to occur during labor because a scar is most likely to give way under the stress of contractions. The size and site of rupture; whether lower segment cesarean section (LSCS) scar, previous myomectomy scar, etc., should be noted. Rupture of unscarred uterus may occur in women with overtly distended uterus (from too much amniotic fluid or carrying twins or more), or due to contractions that are too frequent and forceful. Grand multiparity, neglected labor, malpresentation, and uterine instrumentation are some other causes of unscarred uterine rupture. There may be other albeit rarer causes for hemorrhage such as vascular malformations.

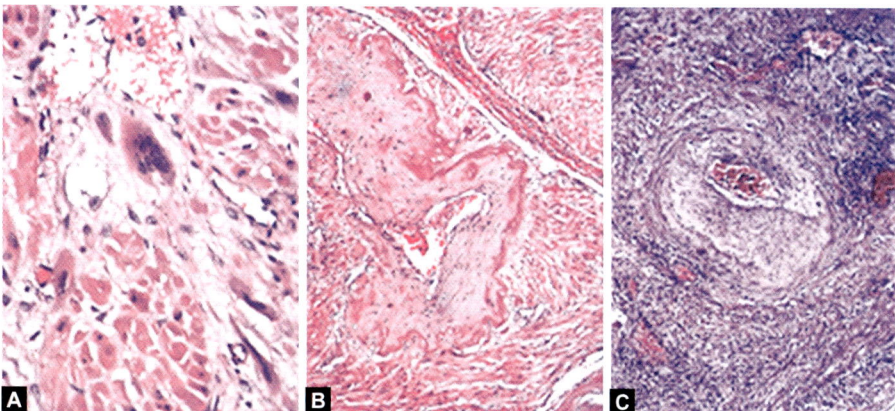

FIGS. 6.10A TO C: (A) Mono- and multinucleated intermediate trophoblasts with hyperchromatic nuclei invading the myometrium; (B) Loss of muscle in the vessel wall due to fibrinoid deposition in the wall; (C) An artery is seen with retained muscular wall and presence of lipophages in the wall (atherosis).

On cut surface of uterus, the endometrial surface should be examined for any greenish yellow purulent exudate suggestive of puerperal sepsis (**Fig. 6.9C**). The myometrium and the serosal aspect should be examined for any yellow white areas of abscesses. The causes of death in such cases may vary from septic shock to DIC. Obstetrical hemorrhage, puerperal sepsis, and preeclampsia form the lethal triad of causes of maternal death. Postpartum birth canal remains susceptible to invasion for several days after delivery. The fallopian tubes and ovary need to be examined properly in cases of ectopic pregnancy. Ruptured ectopic pregnancy is one of common causes of maternal mortality.

Sections from the placental bed (site where the placenta was implanted) of the uterus show physiologic changes of trophoblastic invasion of the decidua and myometrium as well as of the vessel wall, thinning of these vessel walls with deposition of fibrinoid material. These changes are referred to as "placental site reaction" (**Fig. 6.10A**). These normal vascular physiologic changes are not seen in cases of pregnancy-induced hypertension (PIH). The vessels show muscular wall retained and presence of lipid macrophages in the wall [atherosis (**Figs. 6.10B and C**)]. Thus in every case of PIH, it is essential to take sections from the uterine placental bed. Placental dysfunction, triggered by poorly understood mechanisms-including genetic, immunologic, and environmental—also plays an early and primary role in the development of preeclampsia. The damaged placenta in turn secretes the antiangiogenic factors into the maternal circulation. These factors lead to impaired vascular endothelial growth factor (VEGF) and transforming growth factor-β (TGF-β) signaling, resulting in systemic endothelial cell dysfunction. Endothelial dysfunction, in turn, results in the systemic manifestations of preeclampsia. Similarly in puerperal sepsis, endometritis usually begins from the placental bed.

Examination of Products of Conception

These include the placenta, membranes, fetal material and occasionally, molar tissue and other products of gestational trophoblastic disease.

Placenta, if available should be subjected to standard examination, with measurements and weight, and histopathology for inflammation, infection, and placental bed arterial lesions.

Fetus present in the mother need not be autopsied as it will not help in understanding the mother's cause of death. However, examination findings like gender of fetus, fetal weight, crown-heel length, crown-rump length, presence of any external congenital anomalies, etc., are noted and documented in the autopsy records.

Sometimes, maternal death occurs after some surgery (obstetric hysterectomy, resection anastomosis in case of gangrenous bowels, etc.). Review of the histopathology report in such cases will help immensely in giving the final cause of death. A provisional cause of death is given on completion of the autopsy after gross examination of various organs and clinicopathological correlation. Sections are taken from each and every organ for HP examination followed by final cause of death. The final autopsy report should be completed in 30 calendar days or less. Clinicians should receive their autopsy report while the clinical issues of the case are still fresh in their minds.

Anesthetic Deaths

These include those related to biochemical, toxicological or oxygenation problems which may not give rise to specific gross or microscopic findings even after thorough examination. Anaphylaxis and hyperthermia are other anesthetic complications leading to death.

Criminal (Unsafe) Abortion

India has in place all legalities of safe abortion. Still it sees increased numbers of deaths due to unsafe abortions. One of the reasons may be nonaccessibility to safe abortion services. WHO has listed unsafe abortion as one of the easiest preventable causes of maternal death. Death due to unsafe abortion accounts for approximately 13% to one-third of maternal deaths; however, much of it goes undocumented; figures are therefore estimates.

Hemorrhage, infection, sepsis, genital trauma with uterine perforation, and necrotic bowel are the different causes of death in such cases.

Negative Autopsy

Occasionally, after a thorough gross and HP examination has been performed, no satisfactory cause of death can be found. In fact if no specific gross findings are found, the provisional cause of death is given as "after HP examination". We may find a cause after a thorough HP examination. Sometimes no cause of death is found even after HP examination. This does not imply that the pathologist has failed in the autopsy investigation: negative findings are just as valid as positive ones. Such a case should be discussed in detail during the multidisciplinary meeting with the treating obstetrician, physician, intensivist, anesthetist, etc., who then may give a consensus opinion on cause of death based on clinical circumstances.

FURTHER READING

1. Christiansen LR, Collins KA. Pregnancy-associated deaths: A 15-year retrospective study and overall review of maternal pathophysiology. Am J Forensic Med Pathol. 2006;27:11-9.
2. Jashnani KD, Rupani AB, Wani RJ. Maternal mortality: an autopsy audit. J Postgrad Med. 2009;55:12-6.
3. Confidential Enquiry into Maternal and Child Health. (2007). Saving Mothers' Lives: Reviewing maternal deaths to make motherhood safer-2003-2005. [online] Available from https://www.publichealth.hscni.net/sites/default/files/Saving%20Mothers%27%20Lives%202003-05%20.pdf. [Last accessed March, 2020].
4. Lucas S. Maternal death, autopsy studies, and lessons from pathology. PLos Med. 2008;5:e48.
5. Lucas S. The maternal death autopsy. In: Pignatelli M, Gallagher P (Eds). Recent advances in Histopathology. London: JP Medical Publishers; 2014. pp. 17-30.
6. The Royal College of Pathologists. Guidelines on Autopsy Practice; Scenario 5: Maternal Death. [online] Available from https://www.rcpath.org/uploads/assets/827a1a8c-5ed4-4203-9eb336e0de0f7d2d/G100Autopsypracticesection5maternaldeathFINALOct2010.pdf. [Last accessed March, 2020].
7. Jashnani KD, Chandekar SA, Pawar A, Dalal AR, Wani RJ. Hepatitis E infection and pregnancy: A fatal combination. Int J Basic Appl Med Sci. 2015;5(2):264-9.

CHAPTER 7

Autopsy and Law

Shailesh Mohite

INTRODUCTION

Medicolegal or forensic autopsy is a type of examination of a dead body carried out in accordance with laws of the state. It is for the protection of its citizens and for identification of individuals and assisting in the process of dispensing justice in cases of unnatural deaths. It is a special type of examination of a dead body to find out the cause and nature of death, by examining all the body parts, all the organs, and all the body cavities and to corroborate with the evidences of eye witnesses as per laws of the land toward administration of justice and prosecution of guilty. The differences between a clinical or pathological autopsy and medicolegal autopsy are given in **Table 7.1**.

The objectives of a medicolegal autopsy are:
- To determine the cause of death
- To determine the manner of death
- To find out the circumstances of death
- To estimate time since death

TABLE 7.1 Differences between forensic and clinical autopsy.

Features	Forensic autopsy	Clinical autopsy
Synonyms	Postmortem examination or medicolegal autopsy	Pathological or academic autopsy
Consent of relatives	Not required	Consent of relatives is a must
Conducted	Under legal authority	Not so
Requisition	From legal authority is necessary	Not required
Procedure	Always complete	May be complete or incomplete (partial) depending upon the consent

- To establish identity of unidentified dead body
- To document injuries and to deduce how the injuries occurred
- To collect the evidences to identify the object causing death and to identify criminals
- To obtain relevant viscera/organs, samples of tissues/body fluids for examination/analysis wherever necessary
- In case of newborn infants, to determine the issue of live birth and viability
- To obtain photographs and video films wherever necessary

The pre-requisites for clinical autopsy are:
- Requisition from the concerned clinician mentioning specific dilemmas or doubts, so that better clinicopathological correlation can be achieved. If any new emerging finding observed during treatment/in case of new emerging diseases following emergence of new strains of organisms then for correlating it.
- Written informed consent from the next of kin or near relative in presence of hospital administrator. The consent should be signed by the relative with date and time. Consent should mention the extent of autopsy as required by the treating doctor and agreed by the relative. One of the clauses of the consent may be that if after restricted postmortem, a definite cause of death is not found, the autopsy can be converted to a complete one.
- Detailed clinical record (medical case sheet) of past illness with detailed treatment, investigations and follow-ups.
- Detailed clinical record (medical case sheet) of present illness—including all investigation reports, treatment sheet, etc.
- Collection of material (fluids, swabs, etc.) and specimens for any investigation.
- It has to be performed by an authorized qualified pathologist holding at least a postgraduate diploma.
- A medical graduate is usually not considered qualified to carry out a clinical autopsy.
- In medical colleges, a postgraduate in pathology as part of the training can conduct autopsies under supervision of senior qualified faculty.
- In hospitals where a pathologist is available, he can perform autopsy in the mortuary if facilities for postmortem are available.
- For conducting medical autopsies, no authorization and approval from any health authority is required. However, disposal of biomedical waste should be done as per biomedical rules 2018.

On the other hand, the prerequisites for medicolegal autopsy are:
- It can be undertaken only when there is an official and written order/request from the appropriate legal authority, i.e., usually a police officer not below the rank of a police sub-inspector or an Executive Magistrate and head constable in periphery.
- It can be performed only at the authorized center and preferably be done by a person of experience and knowledge in that particular field.
- Occasionally, it may have to be conducted at the site, particularly when the body is in the advanced stage of putrefaction and materials of evidentiary value may be lost during its transportation or where the District Magistrate desires it to be conducted at the site due to some law and order problem.

Autopsy Practices

- All registered Medical Practitioners in Government Service are authorized to conduct the medicolegal autopsy.
- The private medical institutions can undertake the medicolegal examination of living as well as of the dead, provided they possess resources and approval of the concerned State Government. In India, certain states such as Karnataka and Maharashtra have permitted medicolegal autopsies to be conducted at certain private medical colleges.
- With the requisition, a copy of the inquest or preliminary investigation report prepared by the investigating officer (IO) at the scene of death, a dead body *challan*, hospital record and any other relevant paper are necessary as to enable the doctor to concentrate on the organ or the part of the body most suspected and likely to serve as a guide to retain and send the appropriate tissue/blood/fluids to the Forensic Science Laboratory (FSL).
- When the death has occurred during or shortly after the operation or procedure, the surgeon or clinician who operated, treated or anesthetized the deceased prior to death, should provide complete and detailed clinical notes before the autopsy is performed.
- The autopsy surgeon should always carefully go through the inquest report, case sheet or accident register, if available to obtain all the important details of the case, so that the attention can be directed to the salient points, while performing the autopsy.
- The autopsy should always be held at the earliest, after receipt of the requisition paper without any undue delay.
- The examination should preferably be conducted under natural sunlight. However, under circumstances of urgency, it may have to be carried out at night with the help of the adequate and good quality artificial light.
- Identification of the dead body should always be done before the doctor by the police constable who brought it to mortuary before the autopsy is started. If necessary, the body can also be identified by relatives before the autopsy surgeon. In case of unknown, unidentified bodies, the police will always take the photograph as well as the finger prints and foot prints (in case of newborn babies). In case of decomposed bodies, the Medical Officer on request from police, will either preserve the skin over the palms and fingers, if that comes out like a glove then dissect the entire thickness of skin from terminal phalanx of each finger and of the palm and preserve them in 10% formalin in separate vials.
- No unauthorized person should be permitted to enter the mortuary.
- No police official should be present while the autopsy is being conducted.
- The exact date and time of receipt of the dead body at the mortuary should always be noted by the autopsy surgeon, in postmortem report, along with place (station), date and hour of holding of the autopsy. The dead body is brought in the mortuary by police.
- All the details should be noted there and then in the postmortem register. If there is an assistant, it may be better to dictate the notes to him as the autopsy proceeds step by step and then to read, verify and attest the report. Where dictaphone or tape recorder is available, he can make use of it. All correction should be initialed and dated. Nothing should be erased or mutilated or left to memory. Few states

(Punjab and Maharashtra) and union territories (Chandigarh) have made it mandatory to use software to enter postmortem notes to overcome problem of illegible handwriting.
- Viscera, blood or any other medicolegal exhibits are preserved after performing the autopsy, these should be properly noted and labeled, packed, signed and sealed before the autopsy surgeon and then handed over to the police for sending to FSL for further examination. Every article removed from the body and preserved, should be noted in postmortem report. All these items comprise "chain of evidence".
- Video recording has to be done in cases of custodial deaths as per guidelines of National Human Right Commission (NHRC). The video cassettes/CDs/DVDs should be sent to the Chairman, NHRC, New Delhi, by doctor himself and one copy of which should be retained by autopsy surgeon. In cases of exhumation, requisition by relatives or officer conducting inquest may request for video recording.
- It is desirable to visit the crime scene before starting of autopsy or after completion of autopsy, depending upon the need and the circumstances. If law and order problem exists or persists; it may be visited subsequently or another team of doctors may be deputed for collection of evidences and photographs at the time of autopsy being conducted. The team visiting the crime scene must prepare a detailed report on following points: Facts and observations, conclusions drawn, samples collected, names and number of people present—police officers, relatives, photographers, etc., names of the people interviewed and facts/statements noted from them. The team should also note in their report whether the crime scene was secured, nontampered, cordoned off, under lock and seal when they visited.
- A doctor should not perform a medicolegal autopsy: (1) In cases where the doctor does not feel competent to perform the autopsy; or (2) Where more than one doctor is required for conducting autopsy, e.g., in dowry deaths; or (3) When a panel of doctors are recommended by government rules, e.g., in negligence cases. The doctor on duty should suggest to the IO the nearest, equipped and authorized higher center for referring the case. Preliminary external examination (especially injuries) and findings that would suggest time since death should be noted before the referral. At times, while transportation of body to another center with qualified competent and experienced doctors for conducting autopsy, there may be undue delay leading to decomposition and addition of artifacts thereby defeating the whole purpose.
- Every medicolegal autopsy should always be performed with utmost care and immediately; it should always be complete, thorough and most carefully performed.

The scenario in the country is changing with many states making it mandatory to conduct autopsies round the clock. In metropolitan and other major cities there is movement of people for education, trade and other activities. If a body has to be transported to another city, state or country and if it needs to be autopsied, facilities for conducting postmortems round the clock should be made available. If body is to be handed over the next day due to delay in conducting postmortem examination on the same day, it would lead to the loss of many working human hours especially in developing countries. The delay in handing over bodies adds to the psychological stress on the grieving relatives. Also, some states such as Karnataka are offering incentives for conducting autopsies after sunset. In the earlier days, as far as possible, postmortem examinations were to be performed in natural daylight. In most of the autopsy centers even during day time autopsies are conducted under artificial light. The objections raised were verification of color matching which is more accurate in natural light than in artificial light in different injuries. However, recently various State Governments have issued orders to introduce night postmortems, e.g., Government of Maharashtra. However, there are different set rules in some of the states regarding medicolegal autopsies performed at night, for examples,

- The Government of Gujarat does not permit night autopsies in cases of poisonings (actual or suspected), mutilated bodies and deaths of women below 30 years of age, particularly if the incident has occurred in her husband's or in-laws place of residence.
- Medicolegal autopsies in the state of Kerala are performed from 8 am to 5 pm only and such instructions have been given to the relevant authorities.
- Similarly, in Tamil Nadu, such autopsies are performed from 6 am to 6 pm, unless there has been a clear-cut accidental death.

It should be noted that medicolegal autopsies are performed for legal issues and cannot be viewed as an "emergency" procedure.

INDIAN LAW RELATED TO MEDICOLEGAL POSTMORTEM

A brief description of Indian law related to medicolegal postmortem are as follows:
- Criminal Penal Code 1973 (CrPC) deals with the procedure of investigations and trial of offences.
- Inquest is an enquiry or investigation in the cause of some unnatural death done under CrPC in India.
- There are four types of inquest, which are as follows:
  1. Coroner's inquest which was held in certain parts of Mumbai and Kolkata, but later on it has been abolished since July 1999.
  2. Police inquest is the most common inquest done in India done under 174 CrPC.
  3. Magistrate inquest is done by District or Subdivisional Magistrate in some specific cases under 176 CrPC.
  4. Medical examiner's inquest, which is done by the doctor himself but is not practiced in India.

174 CrPC: Police to inquire and report on suicide, etc.
- When the officer-in-charge of a police station or some other police officer, especially empowered by the State Government in that behalf, receives information that a person has committed suicide, or has been killed by another or by an animal or by machinery or by an accident, or has died under circumstances raising a reasonable suspicion that some other person has committed an offence, the officer shall immediately give intimation thereof to the nearest Executive Magistrate empowered to hold inquests. Unless otherwise directed by any rule

prescribed by the State Government, or by any general or special order of the District or Subdivisional Magistrate, the officer shall proceed to the place where the body of such deceased person is. There, in the presence of two or more respectable inhabitants of the neighborhood shall make an investigation, and draw up a report of the apparent cause of death, describing such wounds, fractures, bruises, and other marks of injury as may be found on the body, and stating in what manner, or by what weapon or instrument (if any); such marks appear to have been inflicted.
- Such report shall be signed by the police officer and other persons, who have prepared the same, and shall be forthwith forwarded to the District Magistrate or the Subdivisional Magistrate.
- When (i) the case involves suicide by a woman within 7 years of her marriage; or (ii) the case relates to the death of a woman within 7 years of her marriage in any circumstances raising a reasonable suspicion that some other person committed an offence in relation to such woman; or (iii) the case relates to the death of a woman within 7 years of her marriage and any relative of the woman has made a request in this behalf; or (iv) there is any doubt regarding the cause of death; or (v) the police officer for any other reason considers it expedient so to do, he shall, subject to such rules as the State Government may prescribe in this behalf, forward the body, with a view to its being examined, to the nearest Civil Surgeon, or other qualified medical man appointed in this behalf by the State Government, if the state of the weather and the distance admit of its being so forwarded without risk of such putrefaction on the road as would render such examination useless.
- Magistrates who are empowered to hold inquests, are, any District Magistrate or Subdivisional Magistrate and any other Executive Magistrate, especially empowered in this behalf by the State Government or the District Magistrate.

176 CrPC: Inquiry by the Magistrate into cause of death:
- When any person dies while in the custody of the police or when the case is of the nature referred to in clause (i) or clause (ii) of sub-section (3) of section 174, the nearest Magistrate is empowered to hold inquests, and in any other case mentioned in sub-section (1) of section 174, any Magistrate so empowered may hold an inquiry into the cause of death either instead of, or in addition to, the investigation held by the police officer; and if he does so, he shall have all the powers in conducting it which he would have in holding an inquiry into an offence.
- The Magistrate holding such an inquiry shall record the evidence taken by him in connection therewith in any manner hereinafter prescribed according to the circumstances of the case.
- Whenever such Magistrate considers it expedient to make an examination of the dead body of any person who has been already interred, in order to discover the cause of his death, the Magistrate may cause the body to be disinterred and examined.
- Where an inquiry is to be held under this section, the Magistrate shall, wherever practicable, inform the relatives of the deceased whose names and addresses are known, and shall allow them to remain present at the inquiry. Explanation—in this section, the expression "relative" means parents, children, brothers, sisters and spouse.

Second Autopsy

A medicolegal autopsy is usually conducted for various reasons, as enumerated previously. At times the purpose of autopsy is defeated due to various reasons, e.g., nonqualified or inexperienced doctors, misinterpretation of facts, improper preservation of samples, improper wording of cause of death, etc. In such times, another autopsy is requested and conducted on an already autopsied body at some other center (preferably a tertiary-care facility) where qualified experienced doctors are available. At times an autopsied buried body maybe exhumed, if there is a suspicion raised by the relative regarding the cause and manner of death. Such autopsies are labeled as a repostmortem examination or a second autopsy. Authorization for second autopsy is given by Court order or by Magistrate Inquest. However, there are certain exceptions, e.g., if already autopsied body arrives in our country in such cases, the inquest is conducted by police officer above the rank of sub-inspector of police, if relatives have a suspicion regarding the cause and manner of death or at times even without suspicion by relatives, out of national interests, e.g., international terrorists, gangsters, undercover agents, police inquest maybe conducted and body sent for autopsy.

There are certain conditions that are confused as second autopsy but do not come under the ambit of second autopsy. These include request by an autopsy surgeon for assistance from doctor of same or another specialty related to the matter of contention in that particular case, psychological autopsies and expert opinions based on photographs, radiographs, records of the autopsy, postmortem investigations, clinical notes if any and police records. Even exhumation per se always does not include a second autopsy, at times the cause of death might have been missed at first postmortem due to lack of experience of Medical Officer or due to performance of incomplete autopsy.

In recent years, there has been an upsurge in demand for a second autopsy, though it may not fully satisfy the purpose for which it is carried out. It may not clear the relatives' suspicion but may confuse them further. Also, second autopsy may sometimes be erroneous due to artifacts from the first autopsy, effects of cremation, burial, embalming, etc. Also, some poisons get destroyed with passage of time and are not detectable from the samples collected during the second autopsy. Many times the organ block is completely retained by the autopsy team during the first autopsy, hence collection of samples for chemical analysis or histopathology are not available. This poses problems in concluding the exact cause of death at the end of the second autopsy.

The second autopsy is advantageous in clearing the suspicions arising in the minds of the unsatisfied relatives following the first autopsy, when the cause of death remains unchanged even after second examination. In cases of incomplete first autopsy, a subsequent meticulous autopsy may be of significance in estimating all factors leading to the real cause of death. Wherever the identity of the deceased is in question and the second autopsy is being conducted all vital data such as the hairs, teeth, congenital or acquired deformities, implants, dentures, condition of organs, closure of skull sutures, etc., will be of immense help.

In India, the reasons for second autopsy are:
- Relatives are not satisfied (because of personal bias) with the findings of the first autopsy, though they are genuine, e.g., firm belief of the relatives that it is a case of strangulation when in fact, it is a case of hanging.
- Expert opinion requested by unsatisfied investigating agencies, following unanswered queries.
- Lack of faith or doubt that certain vital facts and clues maybe concealed by the doctor conducting the first postmortem or feeling that the doctor maybe bribed or maybe hand in glove with the offenders.
- Lack of faith or doubt in the investigating agency (police) is suspected in concealing facts, the request for a second autopsy is being asked after the body has been shifted out of the jurisdictional area of the investigating authority where the first autopsy has been conducted.
- Most of the medicolegal autopsies in India are done at primary and secondary health centers by Medical Officers having the basic MBBS qualification. They do not have adequate hands-on training in autopsy techniques during their medical training and also the lack of induction course after joining government service. There is lack of availability of adequate basic facilities for conducting of an autopsy, e.g., autopsy room, instruments, protective gear, autopsy table, trained assistants and no supervisory authority to guide and train. In such circumstances the autopsies tend to be incomplete and inaccurate, leaving the relatives unsatisfied and disgruntled. The inexperienced doctor may not do a thorough autopsy and may at times not open all the cavities or collect all necessary investigations. These things come forth during the second autopsy, which is usually thorough and all things are meticulously recorded, all evidences are preserved and dispatched to the laboratories with a purpose to reach the precise cause of death and give justice to the relatives.

Occasionally the second postmortem examination is conducted at the same autopsy center, particularly in rural areas, where tertiary centers or medical colleges are located far away from the place where first examination was conducted. This leads to persistence of doubt about the reliability of the second autopsy in the minds of the requesting party. Unfortunately, there are no clear-cut national guidelines on the jurisdictional boundaries where a body should be referred for re-examination; however, some states have guided control where the second autopsy can be performed. Procedural delays are widespread, and with the absence of storage facilities, inadequate transport and high temperatures, most bodies begin to decompose and organs autolyze, making it hard to obtain a correct opinion at second autopsy. In India, sending whole organs for examination particularly for histopathology is a common habit. In such cases, no opinion about these missing organs can be obtained. In certain occasions, organs/tissues are retained for academic purposes as teaching material, without the requisite consent/information. Such an organ or tissue is most often, or might be, the one with the case's most important findings. The doctor's assessment conducting the second autopsy is thus focused entirely on the information made available to him for examination, which might not necessarily be the right or absolute opinion. The doctor must always take in to account, before giving an opinion, the findings of the investigations conducted after the first autopsy. The most prevalent method of disposal of dead bodies in India is by cremation. If suspicions develop, when demanding a second autopsy, only the available ashes are often submitted for expert opinion.

There has been another recent trend where the party requesting a second autopsy wishes one of its members to be present during the second autopsy. In India, no outsiders are permitted to witness any medicolegal autopsy; however, there are no written rules for the same. As a result, several times, during the second autopsy, an outsider is allowed to be present in the autopsy room, which is an undesirable and unpleasant practice. The permission for an outsider to be present is given by IO. The doctor conducting the autopsy should know the precise reason why the outsider needs to be present. If no justifiable reason is given, the doctor should refuse permission for the outsider to attend the autopsy. If the outsider is a non-medical person or a doctor not trained in pathology or forensic medicine, then it appears that this could be a mere pressure tactic and doubting the integrity of the autopsy surgeon. If the relatives have any doubt about the manner in which the autopsy is conducted and samples collected, they may approach the police requesting them to photograph and videograph the whole procedure. The relatives may subsequently obtain a copy of the CD/DVD recorded during the autopsy.

There is a need to frame guidelines for second autopsy. The suggestions are:
- The reason for requisition for second autopsy should be genuine and justifiable.
- There must be gross mismatch between the history of the case and postmortem findings where justice appears to be miscarried.
- The IO must forward all the papers, i.e., accidental death report (ADR), *panchanama* of body and spot, statements of witnesses, report of first autopsy and copy of complaint of relatives to the concerned Executive Magistrate.
- Only Executive Magistrates should be empowered to order a second autopsy after perusal of all documents and holding discussions with aggrieved relatives.
- In no case should the police be allowed to take a decision regarding the conduction of a second autopsy. The police if not satisfied with the first autopsy findings should specify, in writing through an officer of the rank of ACP, the reasons for second autopsy. They should approach the designated Executive Magistrate of that area with such a request.
- The Magistrate, after perusal of all case papers including autopsy report and after holding discussions with the police and autopsy surgeon, should come to a conclusion whether second autopsy is necessary or otherwise. This will help in avoiding unnecessary second autopsies. Otherwise, what may start as a "one-off case" may set precedence and not before long, second autopsy would become a routine practice.
- Only the Magistrate could eradicate the component of arbitrariness by determining which cases need a second examination on the merits of each case. This decreases the number of needless second autopsies. Furthermore, the lack of guidelines for the referral center to which an autopsy body is to be re-examined may lead to allegations of unfairness and may lead to an unnecessary request for a third examination. For this rationale, jurisdictional limits should be formulated in such a way that one is clear where to go for a second autopsy. This helps to reduce

administrative delays and also helps to prevent the decomposing of bodies/ organs. Specific criteria for the execution of a second autopsy should be laid down with regard to the authorization document, reliability of the first autopsy report, etc. The second autopsy should not be allowed to happen at the same center where the first autopsy was performed.

The second autopsy should be conducted under the chairmanship of a senior doctor, preferably of the rank of Professor of Forensic Medicine of a Government/ Corporation Medical College. It would be best if a panel of doctors is formed, that includes a pathologist and doctors of the concerned specialties, etc., depending upon the case, especially in cases of alleged negligence. Only those organs or part of the organ showing disease process should be preserved for histopathology, instead of the usual practice of sending the entire organ. Only appropriate organs/material and in prescribed quantity should be sent for chemical analysis or microbiological examination. Whatever investigations advised and organs/material forwarded in relation to it must be documented in the autopsy report. Also, carbon copy of the forwarding letter/form bearing the receivers signature should be preserved along with the PM report.

Custodial Deaths

The NHRC guidelines in respect of custodial deaths/rapes, "encounters", and other related issues require determination of time since death, cause and manner of death. The time since death can be determined by examination of core body temperature, state of rigor, extent of postmortem lividity and signs of decomposition, if any. The same can be determined by the doctor certifying the death immediately after the dead body is noticed.

The guidelines for video-filming and photography of postmortem examination in custodial deaths have been laid down by the NHRC. A detailed format of the postmortem report has also been prescribed by the NHRC. It is the duty of the doctor conducting the autopsy to send the video film and photographs to the commission. The aims of video-filming and photography of postmortem examination are as follows:
- To record the marks of injury and violence, which may suggest custodial torture.
- To corroborate the findings of postmortem examination, by video graphic evidence, so as to rule out any undue influence of seniors or suppression of facts.
- To facilitate an independent review of the postmortem examination report at a later stage by inquiry committee/commission or the court if required.

Following precautions should be taken before conducting postmortem examination:
- Both hands of the deceased need to be wrapped in white paper bags before transportation. The dead body afterwards should be covered in special body bags having zip pouches for proper transportation.
- Clothing on the body of the deceased should not be removed by the police or by any other person. It should be collected, examined as well as preserved and sealed by the doctor conducting the autopsy, and should be sent for further examination at the concerned FSL. A detailed note regarding examination of the clothing should be incorporated in the postmortem examination report by the doctor conducting the autopsy.

- In case of alleged firearms deaths, the dead body should be subjected to radiological examination (X-rays/CT Scan) prior to autopsy.
- In firearm injuries while describing, the distance from heel as well as midline must be taken in respect of each injury which will help later in reconstruction

Video-filming and photography of postmortem examination should be done in the following manner:
- At the time of video-filming of the postmortem examination, the voice of the doctor conducting the postmortem examination should be recorded.
- The chairmen of the committee should introduce the team of doctors and other assistants who will be conducting the autopsy. He should also record the IO handing him over the papers for autopsy. The recording should include the IO and the next of kin/nearest relative identifying the body and also, the first page of the requisition papers.
- The doctor should narrate his prima-facie observations while conducting the postmortem examination.
- A total of 20–25 colored photographs covering the whole body should be taken. Some photographs of the body should be taken without removing the clothes. The photographs should include the following: (1) Profile photo-face (front, right lateral and left lateral views), back of head; (2) Front of body (up to torso-chest and abdomen) and back; (3) Upper extremity—front and back; (4) Lower extremity—front and back; (5) Focusing on each injury/lesion—zoomed in after properly numbering the injuries; (6) Internal examination findings—two photos of soles and palms each, after making incision to show absence/evidence of any old/deep seated injury.
- Photographs with scale should be taken along with label depicting postmortem number, date of examination, ADR number, name of police station, and autopsy surgeons.
- While taking photographs, the camera should be held at right-angle to the object being photographed.
- Video-filming and photography of the postmortem examination should be done by a person trained in forensic photography and videography. The videographer should be from a panel of approved videographers. A good quality digital camera with 10X optical zoom and minimum 10 mega pixels should be used.

FURTHER READING

1. Agarwal SS, Kumar L, Chavali KH. Legal Medicine Manual, 1st edition. New Delhi: Jaypee Brothers Medical Publishers (P) Ltd.; 2008.
2. Bardale R. Principle of Forensic Medicine and Toxicology, 1st edition. New Delhi: Jaypee Brothers Medical Publishers (P) Ltd.; 2016. pp. 120.
3. Department of Home, Government of Kerala, circular no. 18023/H1/86/Home, dated 4 September 1986.
4. GO Ms No. 289. Health and Family Department, Government of Tamil Nadu, dated June 13, 1996.
5. GO Ms No. 629. Health and Family Department, Government of Tamil Nadu, dated 27 September 1995.
6. Government of Kerala, vide circular no. 18023/H2/86/Home dated 4th September 1986.
7. Indiankanoon. Sections, Chapter XII (Information to the police and their powers to investigate); The Code of Criminal Procedure, 1973. [online] Available from https://indiankanoon.org/doc/445276/. [Last accessed August, 2020].

8. Kannan K, Mathiharan K. A textbook of Medical Jurisprudence and Toxicology, 24th edition. Nagpur: LexisNexis Butterworth's; 2012. pp. 293, 295, 297, 360.
9. Khandekar I, Murkey PN, Tirpude BH. Retrieval of organs, body parts and tissue from the medico-legal postmortems for mounting and research purpose: Some legal and ethical aspects. J Indian Acad Forensic Med. 2009;31:171-4.
10. Millo T. Second postmortem: a need for medico-legal guideline in India. J Indian Acad Forensic Med. 2008;30:176-7.
11. Ministry of Home Affairs, Government of India, letter no. 4/4/72-DD/CPA-1, dated 11 June 1987.
12. Parikh CK. Parikh's Textbook Of Medical Jurisprudence, Forensic Medicine and Toxicology, 7th edition, New Delhi: CBS Publishers and Distributors Pvt. Ltd.; 2016. pp. 87.
13. Patnaik AK. Nocturnal forensic autopsy eludes the foot prints of the dead: an explanatory note. Paper presented in the XVI Annual Conference of the Indian Academy of Forensic Medicine at Salem (Madras), 27 February 1995.
14. Reddy KSN, Murty OP. The Essentials of Forensic Medicine and Toxicology, 33rd edition. New Delhi: Jaypee Brothers Medical Publishers (P) Ltd.; 2014. pp. 6-7.
15. The National Human Rights Commission of India. (2014). The guidelines issued by the National Human Rights Commission for video filming and photography of post-mortem examination in cases of custodial deaths and encounter deaths (Circular No.03-Home of 2014 dated 09.04.2014). [online] Available from https://nhrc.nic.in/sites/default/files/Guidelines_for_video_photography_of_PME_death_in_police_action.pdf. [Last accessed August, 2020].
16. Vij K. Textbook of Forensic Medicine and Toxicology, Principle and Practice, 6th edition, Gurugram: Reed Elsevier India Private Limited; 2014. pp. 15-6.

CHAPTER 8

Design of Autopsy Room

Smita Divate, Dhaneshwar Lanjewar

INTRODUCTION

Setting up and designing an autopsy room has specialized, unique, functional, and biosafety demands, which can be particularly challenging. The layout of autopsy workstations should be targeted toward increasing efficiency and, at the same time, toward a reduction of biohazards. The setting of mortuary depends on the availability of space. The autopsy suites in the previous years were often located at the back of hospital, particularly on the ground floor, away from the hospital wards. Such an isolated autopsy block solves problem of offensive smells and the sight of the body transit. However, in some hospitals, they are located in and around the hospital near the wards. In and around the mortuary, the smell is important consideration. In the context of protection against biohazards, the autopsy work area will have to meet Biosafety Level 3 (BSL-3) standards to prevent transmission of virulent organisms including *Mycobacterium tuberculosis*, human immunodeficiency virus (HIV), and hepatitis (particularly blood-borne) from cadavers. Alternately, the main autopsy room could be designed to meet BSL-2 required for protection against less virulent microorganisms (causing only mild disease to humans), while a separate isolation room is designed to meet BSL-3 standards. Walk-in refrigerated morgue rooms and other facilities should be within easy reach. Comprehensive planning of autopsy rooms also needs to consider strategically placing other facilities such as specimen storage and grossing or computed tomography (CT) scanners and other diagnostic imaging equipment for virtual autopsies close to the autopsy rooms.

BASIC FUNCTIONAL AREAS

An autopsy facility comprises various basic functional areas such as the autopsy room, an isolation room for infectious autopsies, storage areas (storage of specimens), separate areas delineated for demonstration tables, cleaning, and disinfection of instruments after use and a distinct "clean" corner for specimen photography, wash-rooms, rooms for administrative purposes, and optionally a separate viewing area in addition to walk-in morgues with facilities for cold storage of cadavers.

Main Doorways

The entire autopsy area should have at least three main doorways for entrances/exits: One for staff, one for acceptance and delivery of the bodies, and one for visiting relatives and friends, which should lead into a visitors' waiting room. The external entrance for collection and delivery of bodies should be screened so that they are not taken in and out of the autopsy area within sight of patients and/or visitors. Communication devices for summoning the attention of mortuary staff and visitors should be provided at all the visitor entrance. Doors to the autopsy room should be provided with a door closure. The doors should also have a locking system to control entry of persons into the room and warning signs prohibiting unauthorized entry should be posted outside the doors. All doors, windows, and ventilation systems should be adequately sealable for decontamination by fumigation.

Size of the Autopsy Room

The number of autopsies expected to be performed annually and, most particularly, the numbers that are expected to be performed simultaneously need to be primarily considered when deciding the size of the autopsy room. Further, it is also necessary to consider the number of medical staff, students, and other interested persons, who are expected to be observing autopsies.

Autopsy Tables

The evisceration and dissection areas need autopsy tables and work surfaces ergonomically designed for efficiency and biosafety. Two autopsy tables should be provided for a 400-bedded hospital. There are many models of autopsy tables available. Tables need to be at a comfortable working height. In this context, adjustable tables may be very convenient. Autopsy tables should be made of stainless steel, be adequately long and wide with a raised edge all around to prevent spillage. The table should have a sufficient tilt to allow free drainage of water from top to bottom provided with built-in liquid waste sinks at the bottom. It should also have a spray nozzle with on/off thumb control and adequately long flexible tubing that will provide a strong stream of water for rinsing instruments and work surfaces. However, pressurized water sprays should not be used in the autopsy room because of the danger of generation of contaminated aerosols. Attached containers for biowaste disposal and vacuum breaker system may be incorporated into the sinks, are additional optional features recommended.

Dissection Area

The dissection area should also have a working surface made of stainless steel or other suitable material for efficient cleaning. Sinks of adequate numbers with hands-free taps and preferably with a vacuum breaker system should be located within the easy reach. The size of the dissection area would depend on the number of autopsies expected to be performed simultaneously. There should be sufficient space for convenient and safe placing of dissection instruments. There should be small wooden boards for cutting and dissecting the removed organs.

Instruments

There is a need of adequate tools such as dissecting knife, brain knife, scissors (8 inches in length), a smaller pair of double sharp pointed scissors about 5 inch in length, manual and/or electric saw, skull key blunt and toothed forceps, probe, chisel, and enterotome. In neonatal and pediatric autopsies, instruments of smaller size are required. Weighing scales for weighing adult and infant bodies, weighing balance for weighing organs, and measuring scale for measuring length of cadaver are also required. There is also a need of suction apparatus for removing fluids from the body fluids present in pleural and peritoneal cavities. There should be a graduated container for measuring the fluid volumes. During dissection, sponges are also required. For an efficient mortuary work, regular care and maintenance of equipment are essential. There should be provision for sharpening of knife and scissors, sharpening and resetting of saw and disinfection of instruments by autoclaving. Storage cabinets, made of metal and preferably with glass doors, should be adequate in number for systematic storage as well as safe and easy retrieval of instruments.

Walls, Floors, and Doors

All walls of the autopsy room should be tiled with durable material that is washable and easily scrubbed, impervious to liquids and resistant to disinfectants. Tiling should be ideally up to the ceiling. To avoid the collection of dirt in cracks, it is important that the flooring is smooth but nonslippery and made of hard material that will be easy to clean, and not crack easily, be resistant to damage from chemicals and corrosives. The floor should also incline toward the drainage point to facilitate easy draining. Joints in flooring those between floors and walls should have waterproof seals. The ceiling should also be washable, impermeable, and nonporous. Doors to the autopsy room should be provided with a door closure. The doors should also have a locking system to control entry of persons into the room and warning signs prohibiting unauthorized entry should be posted outside the doors. All doors, windows, and ventilation systems should be adequately sealable for decontamination by fumigation.

Lighting, Plumbing, and Ventilation

It is essential that the autopsy room should be well-lit with illumination that is independent of daylight. Adequate overhead fluorescent lamps plus at least one lamp with a flexible metal neck that can shine at an angle into the base of the skull and into the thorax and abdomen should be provided. Nevertheless, it should be noted that reports have demonstrated the beneficial effects of natural sunlight in boosting worker efficiency, productivity, and morale, possibly through maintenance of psychological well-being. The autopsy tables and dissection areas should have a good drainage system and all plumbing-related leakages should be promptly repaired.

Due to the extensive use of reagents such as formaldehyde and for the removal of odors and infectious aerosols produced during procedures, it is essential that the autopsy room should be well ventilated with an efficient negative airflow exhaust system. Laminar air flow with a high-efficiency particulate air (HEPA) filter at or near the exhaust fan and a canopy (type A) exhaust hood above the dissecting tables are additional biosafety features that may be incorporated. Sufficient protected electric points should be available throughout the autopsy room for electric saw and X-ray equipment. Many postmortem rooms have fixed audio recording apparatus so that the pathologist can dictate his postmortem report while he is dissecting the organs.

Additional Facilities

A separate office room should be provided to the autopsy surgeons for their paperwork, storage of registers, and supplies. This should open directly into the postmortem room. It should contain an office desk, hand basin with liquid handwash, alcohol-based hand-sanitizers, antiseptics, waterproof bandages, first-aid supplies and adequate storage facilities for keeping stationery, equipment, and other utilities required for performing autopsies. There should be separate area for staff washrooms with toilets, shower and changing rooms, and lockable storage spaces should be available for use of autopsy servants/morgue attendants as well as autopsy surgeons of both genders.

Isolation Room for High-risk Autopsies

High-risk autopsies of cadavers with known or suspected infections such as hepatitis, HIV, influenza, leprosy, meningococcal meningitis, multidrug resistant bacteria, plague, prion disease, rabies, and tuberculosis, need a separate isolated autopsy room designed to meet BSL-3 standards in order to decrease the potential spread of pathogens. This room should have its own autopsy table, sink, dissection area, washing facilities, and a storage place for keeping a separate set of instruments. It is also preferable that the ventilation system of this room is separate from the rest of the morgue facility.

Autopsy Staff

The staffs (assistants and attendants), who have been assigned duties in the autopsy room should be a full-time permanent staff of the hospital. The number of assistants/attendants should be adequate as services in the autopsy room are provided for 24 hours. An assistant (who is generally unwilling) sent for few days from some other department of the hospital should not be assigned duties in the postmortem room.

Recordkeeping

In the mortuary, cadavers are brought for two reasons. The first reason is for preserving before disposal, while other reason is for postmortem examination. The most crucial documents are registers, which record movements of cadavers in and out of the mortuary whether a postmortem is to be done or not. In mortuary, an appropriate identification of the body before disposal is an important issue and problems in this aspect can be avoided by proper documentation. The register should have a strong binding as it gets used a lot and it should be as large as possible so that it does not easily get mislaid or taken away by mistake. Following records need to be entered in the register for each cadaver: Full name and address, hospital registration number, date and time of admission and expiry, date and time of admission to mortuary, date and time of removal from mortuary, countersignature of mortuary technician, address, mobile phone number, and signature of next of kin who takes possession of the body for funeral. If postmortem is to be performed, then it is usual practice to number each postmortem from the start of each year, usually with consecutive number starting from number one and then last four figures of the years. For example, postmortem number one of the year 2015 will be numbered as 1/2015. The same number will be used for labeling all specimens obtained from the particular postmortem. The postmortem register should include the following entries: Full name of the deceased, hospital registration number, date and time of admission and expiry, clinical specialty and the unit-in-charge, names of the autopsy surgeon and his/her assistants, and provisional cause of death.

Other records are often kept in the postmortem room, where specimens of blood and other body fluids and organs are sent for special analysis. These can be recorded in simple exercise book, so that the dates of dispatch can be proved later if there is any problem. Similarly, it is also important to keep a record of all large organs and tissues retained in fixation, awaiting further histopathological examination. It is essential that an "Accident Book" be kept in every mortuary and that every injury, no matter how small, is recorded, with date and type of injury and cause of injury.

Refrigeration

Important component of postmortem section is the cold storage. The refrigerators are the vital part of mortuary and it requires vigilance. Temperature of refrigerators should be checked at the beginning and at the end of the day. For every 100 beds in a hospital, there is a need of four body-storage cabinets. In developing countries like India, where free care and treatment are provided in the public hospital, the bed occupancy is more than available bed and therefore, there should be more provision for body storage. In serious accidents and mass casualties, the simultaneous arrival of cadavers over and above the usual daily quota can also present difficulties. In situations such as railway/bus accidents, jumbo jet air crash, accidents in coal mine, earthquake, explosion of bomb blast, terrorist attacks, riots, death due to adulterated alcohol, accidents in industries, etc., a large number of cadavers are brought in mortuary, an issue of management of cadavers is often neglected. Additional provision of mortuary for such disasters, over and above the normal situation, should be made. The cadavers must be moved under cover, both for the sake of decency and to provide a place for identification.

Restoration of the Body

One of the most important jobs of postmortem technician is to restore the body to as good a condition as possible. All body cavities should be dried out with sponge. The neck and body cavity should be packed with cotton. It is also usual to stuff pelvis with cotton. Any blood on external surface of cadaver must be removed. The skin edges are then sewn together by continuous undersewing. At the end, cadaver must be washed using sponge and water.

Relation with Relatives

To some extent, a hospital is judged by the behavior and attitude of the mortuary staff. Mortuary staff should have a helpful, fairly firm, and sympathetic attitude. The waiting room for relatives should be kept clean, tidy, and free from any smells. There should be no way in which the relatives should be able to wander from the waiting room into the working area.

CONCLUSION

Designing of autopsy rooms has come a long way from the older era, where autopsies were conducted in neglected, badly lit, poorly ventilated, unhygienic rooms away from windows and without protection against transmission of infections from cadavers to the autopsy rooms, where respect of cadaver is maintained, relations with relatives are good, and appropriate care of autopsy staff is taken.

FURTHER READING

1. Parmed. Autopsy Room Design. [online] Available from http://www.parmed.com.au/ index.php?option=com_content&task=view&id=61&Itemid=136 [Last accessed November, 2019].
2. Burton JL, Rutty GN. Autopsy suite design and construction. In: Burton JL, Rutty GN (Eds). The Hospital Autopsy, 2nd edition. London: Arnold Publishers; 2001. pp. 37-41.
3. Thermo Shandon. Morgue/Autopsy Room Planning. [online] Available from http://www.thermo.com.cn/Resources/200802/productPDF_17802.pdf [Last accessed November, 2019].
4. Centre for Disease Control and Prevention, Atlanta, USA. Recognizing the Biosafety Levels.. [online] Available from http://www.cdc.gov/training/quicklearns/biosafety/ [Last accessed November, 2019].

CHAPTER 9

Autopsy Safety Precautions

Smita Divate

INTRODUCTION

Pathogenic microorganisms continue to be infective even after the infected persons die and the autopsy room is, thus, a potential source of infections both blood-borne as well as those induced by aerosols. In some patients, the infections may be asymptomatic and not yet diagnosed or not revealed, hence all dead bodies should be considered to be potential carriers of infectious organisms. It is, therefore, mandatory that standard universal biosafety precautions should be strictly adhered to in the autopsy section at all times by all persons entering the autopsy room for performing or attending autopsies (including medical residents, students or other hospital staff), photographing bodies as well as all mortuary staff handling and/or transporting bodies. The chief biological risks faced by employees in autopsy sections and mortuary are infections caused by hepatitis B virus (HBV), hepatitis C virus (HCV), human immunodeficiency virus (HIV), *Mycobacterium tuberculosis*, rabies, tetanus, plague, meningococcal meningitis, hemorrhagic fever viruses, anthrax, and prions that are responsible for Creutzfeldt–Jakob disease and other transmissible spongiform encephalopathies.

Infections in autopsy room may be acquired by one or more of the following routes:
- Needle-stick injuries or wounds due to blood or body-fluid contaminated sharps or other objects.
- Splashes of blood or other body fluids onto open wounds and dermatitis involved skin.
- Contact of mucous membranes of the eyes, nose or mouth with blood and/or body fluids that include amniotic fluid, cerebrospinal fluid, pericardial fluid, peritoneal fluid, pleural fluid, synovial fluid, and semen and vaginal secretions.
- Inhalation or even ingestion of aerosolized particles.

GENERAL RULES FOR AUTOPSY BIOSAFETY

- All autopsies and fresh autopsy tissues must be considered potentially infective and should be handled using proper protective clothing and stringently employing universal or standard precautions.
- The autopsy room should be designed keeping infection control in mind. The entire autopsy area should be designated as a biohazard area and appropriate warning signs should be prominently posted.
- Entry into the postmortem room should be restricted to workers trained in biosafety precautions pertaining to handling potentially infected autopsy material.
- Although all autopsies should be performed using universal precautions to reduce the risk of infection/contamination, autopsies of bodies known to harbor pathogenic microorganisms (high-risk autopsies) are ideally performed in a separate room specially designed so as to isolate and contain any infective material.
- Eating, drinking, smoking, storage of food, applying cosmetics or handling contact lenses is strictly not permitted in the autopsy room and areas where specimens are either processed or stored. Appropriate instructions should be posted for the same.
- Postmortem examinations should preferably be carried out during normal working hours by well-trained staff because it has been shown that the risk of accidental exposure is greater among the inexperienced and when autopsies are performed under conditions of physical fatigue.
- If multiple autopsies are to be performed sequentially, those with the greatest infective risk should be done first, before the staff becomes fatigued and thus prone to errors including those related to biosafety.
- It is helpful to have a "clean" circulating assistant/circulator who will not have direct contact with potentially infected tissues, fluids, and surfaces and so remains "clean" to record weights and measurements, label specimens or containers, fetch any supplies, adjust overhead lighting, liaison between the prosector, clinicians and administrators (including making or taking phone calls), etc.
- Immunodeficient individuals should not perform autopsies or even enter the autopsy area.
- Cuts, abrasions, open wounds or skin lesions of dermatitis should be covered with an occlusive, waterproof bandage.
- All procedures are carried out taking due precautions to reduce the risk of generation of splashes, spills or aerosols.
- All contaminated equipment, instruments, containers, swabs, clothing, etc., should be confined to designated areas.
- Paperwork leaving the autopsy area must not be contaminated with blood or body fluids. Any paperwork, thus contaminated, should be discarded into appropriate garbage bag-lined disposal bins and replaced by uncontaminated copies of the paperwork before it leaves the autopsy room.
- Telephone calls should not be taken by the autopsy surgeon or assistants during the autopsy.

ISOLATION ROOM FOR SPECIFIC TYPES OF HIGH-RISK AUTOPSIES

- Autopsies of bodies that harbor pathogenic microorganisms like hepatitis, HIV, influenza, leprosy, meningococcal meningitis, multidrug-resistant bacteria, plague, prion disease, rabies or tuberculosis are best performed in a separate, specially designed autopsy room.
- While performing these autopsies, personnel should be limited to only those necessary—generally three staff members, including at least one experienced pathologist and a "clean" assistant who avoids direct contact with the deceased but assists with handling of stationery, specimen containers.
- The isolation room should have all the infrastructural aspects required for a general autopsy room and all biosafety precautions should be strictly enforced.
- A separate set of instruments should be dedicated for high-risk autopsies.

SAFE USE OF SHARP INSTRUMENTS

During autopsies, injuries may occur not only from knives, scissors, scalpels, needles, and saws but also from unknown sharp objects in the body itself like bone fragments and fragments of needles in subcutaneous tissues and even myocardium of intravenous drug users, etc. Care should also be taken during dissection or trimming of tissues for microscopy to minimize the risk of injury from such sharps. The frequency of sharp injuries that could occur while performing autopsies can be reduced by some simple practices (**Appendix 1**). In particular, if a needlestick or scalpel injury occurs while performing an autopsy, the injured person should immediately stop dissecting. The injury should be allowed to bleed freely, immediately washed with soap and water and a disinfectant should be applied to the wound. The injury should then also be immediately reported to concerned authorities and postexposure prophylaxis (PEP) should be followed, if advised.

LIMITING THE GENERATION OF AEROSOLS

While tuberculosis is the most common aerosol-transmitted infection in India, other infections that may also be acquired by autopsy-generated aerosols include meningococcemia, plague, rabies, viral hemorrhagic fevers, anthrax, coccidioidomycosis, legionellosis, and rickettsioses. Many autopsy procedures such as opening of the chest cavity or even from compression of the chest while moving the body can generate respiratory droplet aerosols. Even cutting infected lungs with a knife has been shown to generate small particle aerosols. Hence, performing the procedure carefully is necessary in every case. Immunosuppressed cases with disseminated tuberculosis pose a greater risk for acquiring tuberculosis at autopsy as such cases are likely to have more numerous tubercle bacilli. Aerosols formation may also occur with the use of saws (especially power saws) and through opening of the stomach and intestines. **Appendix 2** summarizes strategies for reducing aerosol generation.

PERSONAL PROTECTIVE ATTIRE/EQUIPMENT FOR AUTOPSIES

Personal protective attire/personal protective equipment (PPE) that need to be used while performing all autopsies include double sets of properly-fitting rubber gloves (double gloving), full-length gowns, disposable plastic aprons, caps, and N-95 particulate masks/respirators. Additionally, eye protection goggles with solid side shields or chin-length face shields are mandatory in all suspected/confirmed high-risk autopsies. Plastic aprons should not to be used as a sole source for protection. All PPE should be disposed of in appropriately designated containers before leaving the autopsy room. Finger rings, watches, bangles, bracelets or other items worn on the fingers/hands/wrists should be removed before wearing gloves because when these are not removed multiple perforations could form in the gloves. Should the same personnel perform multiple autopsies consecutively, frequent change of outer gloves and also preferably other PPE is recommended.

HANDWASHING

Hands should be washed thoroughly with liquid soap and after removing gloves, before leaving the autopsy area, after completing any cleaning procedure with water, and immediately whenever hands are soiled with blood, body fluids or tissues.

CLEANING AND DECONTAMINATION

The disinfectant used is 1:10 dilution of sodium hypochlorite (household bleach) and it should be freshly prepared daily. All clean-up procedures should be performed after wearing personal protective attire.

Instruments and autopsy devices should be immersed in a detergent solution for 10 minutes, rinsed with water and then soaked in a disinfectant such as 1:10 solution of sodium hypochlorite or 2% aqueous glutaraldehyde for another 30 minutes. Glutaraldehyde has an advantage that unlike bleach it does not damage aluminum and steel.

Work surfaces should be rinsed with hot water followed by a 1:10 solution of bleach that should be poured on that surface and kept for at least 30 minutes and then rinsed with water. Splashing should be avoided. Floors and walls in the autopsy work area should also be cleaned with a detergent solution, decontaminated with 1:10 solution of sodium hypochlorite and lastly mopped with water. All work surfaces, floors and walls should be decontaminated, as described above, after completion of any autopsy-related procedures, immediately after any spillage of blood or other potentially infectious materials and again at the end of each shift.

Fumigation or fogging of the autopsy room is to be done with 20% Ecoshield/Virkon fog or other suitable aerosol disinfectant using a fogging machine (fog spraying machine). The autopsy room should be adequately sealed during the fogging procedure for this process to be effective. Ultraviolet light may be used as an additional secondary method for decontaminating room surfaces and air of the autopsy room.

All laundry should be considered as potentially contaminated and thus need to be disinfected. Before transport, all reusable laundry, including towels and wet clothing, should be placed into leak-proof biohazard bags.

Contaminated disposables should be discarded into appropriate biowaste disposal containers as stated in the infection control policy of individual hospitals.

A cleaning logbook should be maintained to document cleaning of the autopsy room, equipment, and laundry.

HANDLING OF CADAVERS

Before the Autopsy

All bandages should be removed and put into appropriate garbage bins. A 2% bleach solution should then be used to wash off visible blood on body surfaces.

After Autopsy

The cadaver should be stitched properly so that no fluid can come out. It should then be washed with a detergent solution followed by an antiseptic such as a 1:10 solution of sodium hypochlorite. The nose and mouth should be plugged with cotton swabs soaked with the sodium hypochlorite solution. The body should then be rinsed with water and placed in a disposable leak-proof plastic body bag. This is especially necessary in known HIV seropositive cases but should preferably be done for all cadavers. It is also recommended to place a warning label on the outside of the body bag, alerting the possibility of leaking fluids.

STORAGE AND TRANSPORT OF TISSUES

Fresh tissues or specimens to be preserved should be placed in 10% formalin fixative in nonbreakable plastic containers with water-tight lids, immediately after retrieval from the cadaver. Specimens for storage in refrigerators/cold rooms must be covered with a leak-proof lid and clearly labeled for that purpose. The outside of all containers should be free of blood and body fluids from the autopsy. Before transporting tissue outside the autopsy suite, the container should be placed in an impermeable plastic bag and securely tied. Uncovered tissue of any kind should not be stored in morgue coolers or left out on counters. No tissue containers should be stored out on the floor.

For adequate fixation, the amount of 10% formalin required is at least 10 times the volume of the tissue; this destroys or inactivates all important infective agents except prions and mycobacteria. Mycobacteria have been shown to be viable in tissues for many days as these organisms are difficult to kill with standard formalin fixatives or embalming fluids. However, it has been reported that mycobacteria are killed when tissues are immersed in a fixative containing a mixture of 10% formalin in 50% ethyl alcohol.

For fixation of HIV seropositive tissues, the entire organ block and the brain are immersed in adequate quantity of 10% formalin for at least 1 week before dissection of the organs/viscera.

DEMONSTRATION OF ORGANS AT MEETINGS

Fresh organs should not be shown at meetings. All organs must be formalin-fixed for at least 24 hours and then washed thoroughly before the meeting in order to minimize formalin exposure. It is advised that the organs are first rinsed in one or preferably two large buckets of water and then rinsed in running tap water for 30 minutes.

BIOWASTE DISPOSAL

Waste for disposal should be kept in specially designated biohazard waste bags, secured, and stored in metal or plastic canisters until removal. The waste should be disposed daily and its record should be maintained in an "autopsy waste disposal" log.

PHOTOGRAPHY

Photography of specimens involves the risk of moving possibly infected tissue around the room. Hence, photography of fixed specimens is preferable especially when an infective agent is known to be present. Photography of fresh specimens requires the same precautions that are recommended to be followed for doing the autopsy. Whether the specimen is fresh or fixed, a separate corner should be delineated for the photography and the organ or tissue should be transported to the photography area in pan. The camera should be handled using a fresh pair of clean gloves or preferably by a "clean" circulating assistant. The photo stand should be cleaned with disinfectant after photographs have been taken. Even the cameras, lenses, and other photographic equipment may be disinfected with a variety of germicidal substances without compromising their functionality. A hands-free camera system would also help to reduce the risk of contamination and thereby the acquisition of infections.

EMPLOYEE HEALTH

Personnel performing autopsies, assistants and all employees working in the autopsy section are strongly recommended to get themselves vaccinated against hepatitis B and tetanus. In areas endemic for tuberculosis all such personnel should have yearly purified protein derivative (PPD) skin tests and chest X-rays. Persons with open wounds or dermatitis lesions should not perform autopsies or assist in autopsy-related procedures unless the injured skin or lesions can be completely covered with a waterproof dressing. Such personnel should also consult the PEP department and undergo PEP, if so advised.

Cuts or needlestick injuries involving exposure to blood or body fluid: The injured person should immediately stop dissecting. The injury should be allowed to bleed freely, immediately washed with soap and water and then a disinfectant should be applied to the wound. Injured personnel should then immediately go to the PEP department and if advised then PEP should be undertaken.

If conjunctival splashes occur: The eyes should be washed immediately at the nearest eyewash station in the autopsy section. The PEP procedure recommended for cuts or needlestick injuries should be immediately followed.

FURTHER READING

1. Autopsy biosafety. In: Finkbeiner WE, Davis RL, Ursell PC (Eds). Autopsy Pathology: A Manual and Atlas, 2nd edition. Philadelphia, PA: Churchill Livingstone; 2009. pp. 25-34.
2. Burton JL. Health and safety at necropsy. J Clin Pathol. 2003;56:254-60.
3. Draft DGAFMS Memorandum on Autopsies on Cadavers Infected with the Human Immunodeficiency Virus. [online] Available from http://www.indianarmy.gov.in/writereaddata/Documents/DraftDGMemo-HIVAutopsy.pdf.
4. Flavin RJ, Gibbons N, O'Briain DS. Mycobacterium tuberculosis at autopsy—exposure and protection: an old adversary revisited. J Clin Pathol. 2007;60:487-91.
5. AIDS Info. Guidelines for Prevention and Treatment of Opportunistic Infections in Adults and Adolescents with HIV. [online] Available from https://aidsinfo.nih.gov/guidelines/brief-html/4/adult-and-adolescent-opportunistic-infection/0. [Last accessed March, 2020].
6. Hall L, Otter JA, Chewins J, Wengenack NL. Use of hydrogen peroxide vapor for deactivation of Mycobacterium tuberculosis in a biological safety cabinet and a room. J Clin Microbiol. 2007;45:810-5.
7. Nichols WS, Geller SA. High risk autopsy cases. In: Collins KA, Hutchins GM (Eds). Autopsy Performance and Reporting, 2nd edition. Northfield, Illinois: College of American Pathologists; 2003. pp. 93-104.
8. Nolte KB, Taylor DG, Richmond JY. Biosafety considerations for autopsy. Am J Forensic Med Pathol. 2002;23:107-22.
9. Nolte KB. Survival of Mycobacterium tuberculosis organisms for 8 days in fresh lung tissue from an exhumed body. Hum Pathol. 2005;36:915-6.
10. Sharma BR. Autopsy Room: A Potential Source of Infection at Work Place in Developing Countries. Am J Infect Dis. 2005;1:25-33.

APPENDIX 1

Strategies that Reduce Injury from Scalpels and Other Sharp Autopsy Instruments

- In general, prosectors should limit their activities to the autopsy table and dissecting area and shut out distractions while using sharp instruments.
- While performing the autopsy or other autopsy-related procedures, the equipment for use should be kept to the minimum. Knives, scissors, scalpels and other sharp instruments should be placed in clear view of the prosector and other personnel at a reachable but safe distance.
- Use of scalpels for tissue dissection should be minimized. Wherever possible, a pair of scissors should be used instead of a scalpel, including during evisceration. Use of blunt-tipped rather than pointed scissors is advisable.
- Scalpel blades should be removed only with a special safety scalpel blade remover.
- Scalpels/knives should never be passed on directly from hand to hand; the instrument should be placed on a flat surface for transfer.
- When making slices of large organs with a long knife, the prosector should use a thick (3-inch) gauze/sponge to stabilize the organ with the noncutting hand.
- When cutting coronary arteries, a thick pad of gauze or cotton should be placed between the heart and the noncutting hand.
- When dissecting with sharp implements, tissue should not be held with the fingers of the noncutting hand, instead a long-handled tissue forceps should be used to hold the tissues.
- Steel-mesh lined gloves or some other scalpel-resistant material can be used for high-risk cases. Obtaining sections for histopathology, which requires the use of a scalpel, should preferably be done a day or two after an autopsy, after the tissue intended for sectioning has been fixed adequately.
- When suturing the body wall at the end of the autopsy, skin flaps should be held with a large-toothed forceps or toothed clamp and suture needles should be held with forceps rather than with a hand.
- Blunt needles and bulb syringes should be used to aspirate fluids in most situations.
- Needles, syringes, scalpel blades and any other sharps should be disposed immediately after use/detection, directly into puncture-resistant "sharps bin" containing a suitable disinfectant. The "sharps bin" should be kept within easy reach of the prosector.
- Many needlestick accidents occur during disposal of needles; hence, needles should never be recapped, removed from syringes, purposely bent, clipped, or otherwise manipulated by hand after use.

Additional Measures to Enhance Safety in the Autopsy Room Even Further

- A plastic bag or tent may be placed around the mechanical saw while it is being used to cut the skull and spine.
- Surgical towels may be placed over the cut edges of the rib cage while the chest is being eviscerated and the thoracic spine and spinal cord cut.
- For autopsies on patients where a transmissible spongiform encephalopathy (TSE)/slow virus infection is suspected, disposable instruments should be used.

APPENDIX 2

Strategies that Reduce Aerosol Generation

- Aerosolization of bone dust while cutting the skull or vertebral bodies can be reduced with a plastic cover on the saw. Bone surfaces should be moistened before sawing to cut down the dispersal of bone dust. Bones should be cut with a handsaw and under plastic covering rather than with electric saw.
- *Specimen handling*: All specimens are to be handled gently to avoid splashing and aerosolization of infectious material while removing, washing or otherwise handling organs. High-pressure water sprays should not be used.
- Some authors have recommended eviscerating the infected body organ-by-organ, rather than with the more traditional technique in which the organs are removed en bloc.
- Clear plastic bags can be placed over the head while eviscerating the brain.
- The stomach and intestines should be opened under water.
- If the presence of pulmonary tuberculosis has already been documented, the lungs may be insufflated with formalin before sectioning.
- Screw cap containers are preferable to snap-top, rubber-stoppered, or cork-stoppered containers for storing samples of blood or body fluids. When opening capped containers, cover the opening with a plastic bag to contain aerosols and splashes.
- Down-draught ventilation tables reduce the particle transmission of micro-organisms (and have the added advantage of reducing odors).
- To avoid spattering, do not sear (burn) tissue to sterilize it before obtaining a culture. Instead, swab the organ surface centrifugally with an iodine solution and incise centrally before a sample is removed.

10 CHAPTER

Autopsy Audit

Jaya Deshpande

INTRODUCTION

The universal decline in autopsy rates is a cause of concern and today even in reputed medical centers worldwide, <15% cases of hospital deaths are autopsied. A major reason for the disinterest in autopsy by both clinicians and pathologist in institutions is the poor outcome of clinicopathological meetings and the inordinate delays in completing autopsy studies. Most autopsies are performed by junior most staff of the department with disinterest at all levels. Many questions are left unanswered particularly due to lack of progress in techniques and investigative tools.

The most important aspect of autopsy quality is the clinicopathological correlation. This measure is not a reflection of how well an autopsy is done or to find faults but to use the potential of autopsy in driving improvements in overall clinical care. Traditionally, the most effective way of training the young medical professionals and even established physicians was at the autopsy table. Today this is carried out in the form of clinicopathological meetings or morbidity/mortality meetings. This also serves as a method of quality assurance of medical services and diagnostics.

The need to invest in autopsy services therefore, means to improve the clinicopathological meetings and to make it more meaningful. For this to be achieved a quality management program should be in place. The quality monitors include surveillance of preanalytical, analytical, and postanalytical phases, using available benchmarks. In most laboratories, autopsy quality management is a part of surgical pathology quality management program. A timeline for reporting results should be prepared and specific responsibilities need to be fixed. To help evaluate the results, external benchmarks may be used though they are hard to come by.

PREANALYTICAL PHASE

This includes:
- Proper identification of the body
- Examination of the autopsy permit signed by the appropriate authority

- Availability of appropriate clinical and demographic details
- Adequacy of clinical information
- Inclusion of any specific requests/questions by the clinician
- Any discussion with clinician should be recorded

Patient identification is the most important aspect of the preanalytical phase. Attempt should be made to achieve 100% compliance.

ANALYTICAL PHASE

This includes:
- *Safe practices in performing autopsies:* Use of adequate protective personnel gear.
- Gross and microscopic examination, use of ancillary testing methods, and histological processing.
- Attendance of the clinical team during autopsy is also a part of the quality check.

Clinicopathological correlation is part of both analytical and postanalytical phase. In the analytical phase, it is of great educational value. Clinicopathological correlation is important in accurately interpreting autopsy findings.

Gross examination and dissection should deal with the following aspects:
- Use of appropriate protective gear.
- Were autopsy limitations adhered to?
- Was examination adequate to demonstrate findings?
- Were organs weighed and measured appropriately?
- Did the provisional cause of death reflect the gross findings?
- Were appropriate tissues processed for sectioning?

Microscopic examination and correlation with gross findings should be a key factor in finalizing the autopsy report.

The key factors in microscopic examination should be:
- The microscopic features should reflect the histological diagnosis.
- The diagnosis should reflect the gross findings.
- Use of consultations.
- Use of special stains and ancillary tools should be used appropriately.
- A key of blocks and slides for major lesions should be available.

POSTANALYTICAL PHASE

The monitors in this phase include:
- Postautopsy care of the body up to its disposal
- Correlation with previous pathology and other tests
- Clinicopathological conferences/meetings or presentations
- Autopsy report adequacy is an important aspect of this phase.

Clinicopathological correlation is a form of audit to assess whether autopsy findings altered the clinical understanding of the case or resolved clinical differential diagnosis. It assesses the appropriateness of treatment and adequacy of care but does not reflect on the pathologist's accuracy of diagnosis. One may also include an expert outside the field of pathology in complex cases.

AUTOPSY CLINICAL AUDIT MONITORS

The best monitor in autopsy audit is the agreement classification. The following points are to be noted.
- Major and minor unexpected findings contributing to patient's death. In the category of minor findings are those related to diagnostic procedure and interventions related to the underlying disease.
- Major and minor unexpected finding not contributing to patient death but eventually would have required treatment.
  - A key indicator of overall function and quality of autopsy service is the turnaround time (TAT). The College of American Pathologists (CAP) recommends a TAT of 2–4 days for gross examination and final reports to be released within 60 working days. All laboratories need to prepare a log of both performance and final TAT for each autopsy. About 90% cases need to meet the preliminary (provisional) anatomic diagnosis in 4 days and final diagnosis in 60 working days. Satisfaction survey is a tool to monitor the expectation and satisfaction with the autopsy service. Such survey should be an ongoing process for each autopsy. The clinician's survey should use the following parameters to evaluate satisfaction levels:
    – Overall autopsy quality
    – Communication
    – *TAT:* Preliminary report, final autopsy report
    – Did autopsy answer specific questions?
    – Did autopsy provide educational inputs?

In western world, autopsy information needs to be conveyed to the immediate family members. This is also included in autopsy audit. The goal of any form of autopsy audit and clinicopathological correlation is to provide inputs which can results in improved patient care.

FURTHER READING

1. Bamber AR, Quince TA. The value of postmortem experience in undergraduate medical education: current perspectives. Adv Med Educ Pract. 2015;6:159-70.
2. Jackett L, McLean C. Hospital autopsy audit: discordant primary clinical diagnoses are found in 20% of cases in a reducing autopsy case load. Selection bias or significant findings? Pathology. 2015;47:499-502.
3. Kusum DJ, Jaya RD, Gayathri PA. Medical autopsy: whose gain is it? An audit. Indian J Pathol Microbiol. 2006;49:188-92.
4. Turnbull A, Osborn M, Nicholas N. Hospital autopsy: Endangered or extinct? J Clin Pathol. 2015;68:601-4.

CHAPTER 11

Embalming

Deepak S Joshi

INTRODUCTION

Embalming is the science involving a process in which special techniques are used to forestall the decomposition of the body. It is a delicate artwork to preserve human or animal remains. The goal is for long-distance transportation, public display at funerals, medical or scientific experiments, or anatomical researches.

HISTORY

More than 5,000 years ago, Egyptians developed embalming ritual which was the utter necessity for preserving dead bodies during civil war. The process was practiced in Egypt for religious and sanitation reasons. Ancient Ethiopian tribes, aboriginal inhabitants of Canary Islands from 900 BC, Peruvians in early 16th century practiced mummification. In Europe, the knowledge and practice of artificial preservation has spread from the earliest known evidence of artificial preservation found in Osborne (Spain), then becoming widespread by about 5,000 BC. In China, artificially preserved remains have been recovered from the Han dynasty (206 BC–AD 220). The anatomist period of embalming, which is known as the period of the middle ages and the Renaissance, is characterized by an increased influence of scientific developments in medicine and the need of the bodies for dissection purpose, fostering the scientific progress.

MODERN EMBALMING

In this modern technique, unlike the other traditional methods, various chemical solutions are injected into the blood vessels of cadaver, mainly arteries, which prevents decomposition. It is then used for various purposes. The first detailed anatomy of the circulatory system was documented by William Harvey using solutions of the different colors which were injected into the cadaver. This technique was first applied for the process of embalming by William Hunter. He not only used this as a part of mortuary practices but also gave a detailed report of the appropriate method. This report was widely cited and helped in preservation of bodies for burial. In another instance dated 1805, at the time of funeral of Lord Nelson, his dead body was found in excellent condition for 2 months which was preserved after his death in the battle of Trafalgar with a solution made using mixture of brandy and spirits with camphor and myrrh. The other alternate methods available included the use of extreme low temperature surrounding the ice packing or cooling board.

After the discovery of preservative properties of formaldehyde, invented by August Wilhelm von Hofmann in 1867, it took place as the principle component of modern embalming techniques and replaced all the prior techniques. Dr Thomas Holmes (1817–1900) is the father of this modern embalming practice. He reportedly embalmed over 4,000 soldiers and officers in civil war. This modern technique helps in storing the corpse in a good condition.

PRINCIPLE OF EMBALMING

Embalming changes the protein colloidal nature and forms a lattice network of inert, more stable, longer lasting firm substances that can no longer act as food for bacteria. The newly formed proteins cannot be broken down by enzymes of body cells or bacteria. There is destruction of all pathogenic and nonpathogenic bacteria. The three essential components of embalming solutions are disinfectants, preservatives, and restoratives. In combination, the three components are biocidal, preserving the natural colors and preventing putrefaction and contamination with insects (especially maggots).

Approximately, 6 L of embalming fluid is required for a body and it is composed of formalin (1–1.5 L), ethyl alcohol (0.5–1 L), phenol/carbolic crystals (800 g), glycerin (500 mL), tap water (2–3 L), oil of wintergreen (10 mL), eosin solution (5 mL), sodium citrate/oxalate, and sodium borate.

- *Formalin* acts by denaturation. It is a disorganization of molecular configuration of proteins. Proteins are converted to a high molecular, cross-linked latticework and the inert solid materials that can no longer serve as food for bacteria or as a substrate for enzyme action. The inert structures lose their ability to retain water and their stability is maintained by the presence of a little uncombined formaldehyde. Hence, cadavers and/or body parts are immersed in 10% formalin-filled tanks.
- *Ethyl alcohol or ethanol:* It is a good solvent. It stabilizes the formaldehyde in formalin solution. It has a unique capacity to penetrate and diffuse readily into tissues.
- *Phenol/carbolic acid* acts as a powerful fungicide and germicide.
- *Glycerin* acts as wetting agent. It makes the organs soft and supple.
- *Sodium citrate/oxalate* acts as anticoagulant.
- *Sodium borate* acts as a buffer.
- *Tap water* acts as a vehicle.
- *Perfumes/dyes*—oil of wintergreen, eosin or vermillion red.

The standard ingredients mentioned above are normally used. There is little variation from institute to institute, but the principle is the same.

PRE-EMBALMING STEPS AND THEIR LEGAL ASPECTS

- The cadaver must be properly identified in the presence of close relatives or a person lawfully in possession of dead body and the consent of the relative must be obtained.
- Death certificate or postmortem certificate (if postmortem done) issued by a registered medical officer is must. The cause of death must be written properly on the death certificate.
- No objection certificate (NOC) from the police is essential in all medicolegal cases. The embalming should not be done prior to autopsy as it can destroy medicolegal evidences.
- Information to concerned authorities is essential if the diseased was suffering from notifiable diseases such as acquired immunodeficiency syndrome (AIDS), hepatitis B, septicemia, rabies, tuberculosis, etc. All "universal precautions" must be taken in handling such bodies.
- The cadaver is to be labeled with five tags on wrists, ankles, and neck.
- The cadaver is then washed with antibacterial solution, e.g., betadine.
- All the surface hair must be shaved from the body.
- All joints must be manipulated to increase flexibility.
- Embalming certificate must be issued, which clearly mentions the type of embalming done, type of fluid used, and the time period for which body can be kept before exemption.
- Permission from police is required to transport the embalmed body from one place to another.
- A clearance from embassy/high commission may also be required if embalming is done in foreign nationals, so as to avoid future complications.

EQUIPMENT REQUIRED FOR EMBALMING

- *Cadaver injector or embalming machine:* It is a simple device where pressure is generated to force fluid from an injection tank into the vascular system. The pump provides steady and high pressure. It delivers 6 L of fluid within 10 minutes. This method provides better perfusion and ensures uniformly good embalming results.
- *Gravity tank method:* It is a traditional, simplest, safest and least expensive of the injection methods. The embalming tank is filled with preservative fluid and is kept at a height of about 4–6 feet from the embalming table and the fluid passes through the vessels under pressure. It takes 30 minutes to 24 hours to complete.

METHODS OF EMBALMING

Arterial Embalming

Major arteries are used for injection of embalming fluid because they do not have valves. Major veins are used as drainage vessels. The following methods can be used for injection and drainage:

- *One-point injection*: Only one site is used for both drainage and injection. One point injection method is easy and less time consuming but perfusion may remain incomplete. They include common carotid artery and internal jugular vein, femoral artery and femoral vein, external iliac artery and external iliac vein, and axillary artery and axillary vein.
- *Split injection*: The injection is given in an artery at one site and the drainage is undertaken at another location. This gives a complete perfusion. They include femoral artery injection and internal jugular vein drainage or common carotid artery injection and femoral vein drainage (drainage technique—it has been estimated that after death, 85% of blood is found in capillaries, 10% in veins and 5% in arteries. The amount of blood in the vascular system depends on the cause and the manner of death. To obtain good embalming results, it is necessary to obtain good drainage. The main purpose of drainage is to make room for the embalming fluid).
- Multiple injections are used in autopsied bodies, especially those with generalized edema or contagious diseases because vessels can be easily procured for injection.
- The artery selected for injection should be sufficiently large to allow proper insertion of a cannula. It should be superficial enough to avoid unnecessary dissection and must be as close as possible to both the aorta and the right atrium. The most commonly used vessels in nonautopsied bodies are the right common carotid, left common carotid, right femoral arteries, and left femoral arteries. In cases of infants and children below 5 years of age, the vessel of choice is abdominal aorta.

   For exposing the common carotid artery, place a wooden block under the shoulder to elevate it and lower the head, so that the whole length of the neck is exposed. The common carotid artery runs vertically from the sternoclavicular joint to the thyroid cartilage. A vertical incision about 1.5–2 inches long is made in skin, the artery is identified and a nick/slit is given to it. A cannula is inserted through this slit, and care is taken not to push the cannula beyond the bifurcation and embalming fluid is injected in it. The advantage of this method is proper distribution of fluid to the face. When carotid artery is raised with aneurysm hooks, two pieces of ligature are placed around the artery with forceps to hold the cannula in place while embalming. The fluid is then injected downward by withdrawal of cannula and reinserted in downward direction so the lower part of body gets perfused.
- The femoral vessels are located in the upper one-third of the thigh. They run from the mid-inguinal point to the adductor tubercle of the femur. A vertical incision

about 2.5 inches long is made near the mid-inguinal point to expose the artery. Fluid can be injected by inserting the cannula in both upward and downward direction.

Cavity Embalming

In this process, the organs in the abdominal and thoracic cavities are treated with the preservative solution. The preservative solution is injected by a trocar or long needle into the abdominal or thoracic cavity.

Hypodermic Embalming

In this method, preservative solution is injected beneath the skin by syringe and needles of 18–20 gauges.

Surface Embalming

In this method, cotton or gauze pieces are soaked in preservative solution and applied to the skin. For example, surface lesions (such as ulcers, bed sores) burnt skin within mouth and eyelids. These methods of embalming are generally used to preserve the local areas of the body that have not received or insufficiently received preservative fluids.

The signs of good embalming are oozing of fluid from orifices, i.e., nose and mouth, firm feeling of skin, and erection of hairs at the end.

PACKING AND TRANSPORTATION

Embalmed body for transportation must be packed in a coffin. The coffin must be labeled with identification of deceased, transport destination, chemical used for embalming and up to what time the body can be preserved.

PLASTINATION

Dr Gunther von Hagens from Germany developed a unique technique of preservation of specimens using polymers such as silicon, epoxy, polyester, etc. These polymers are subsequently hardened after replacing the water and lipid in the biological tissue. It makes the specimen dry and odorless which can be stored for a longer duration.

To maintain the natural look of the body and organs which are thick, silicon is the preferred polymer; for a thin and transparent ones, epoxy is used; whereas, for gray-white matter differentiation in brain, polyester is exclusively used.

The principle of the plastination process includes fixation, dehydration, forced impregnation and hardening. For fixation, formalin in concentration between 5% and 20% is used. Ethanol dehydration is used for embalmed tissues containing standard embalming fluid, because it cleanses of the polyvalent alcohol (glycerin, ethylene glycol) or phenols, thus specimens are defatted. Compound such as acetone readily mixes with variety of resins used in this process. It has properties of causing dehydration, defatting and acting as intermediary solvent, making it the agent of choice for dehydration. At a very low temperature (–25°C), acetone will substitute the water molecules in the cell resulting in dehydration. This is followed by the process of forced impregnation in vacuum which is the most important step in this process. The vacuum causes extraction of acetone from the cell and fills it with the polymer. To complete the plastination, the specimen filled with polymer is subjected for the process of hardening. This is achieved with the help of gaseous hardener such as silicon, ultraviolet A light radiation or heat. This is also known as curing.

This process gives better learning experience and opportunity in neuroanatomy. Silicone gives long-lasting specimens of brain. As mentioned earlier, the polyester plastinated brains provide a great understanding of gray–white matter. The longevity of the specimen and better orientation makes the process of high importance in academic practices. Because of this, it is a well-practiced and followed process throughout the world at various teaching centers. Correlation with imaging modalities such computed tomography (CT) and magnetic resonance imaging (MRI) gives an added advantage with this technique.

FURTHER READING

1. Ajmani ML. Embalming Principles and Legal Aspects. New Delhi: Jaypee Brothers Medical Publishers; 2009.
2. Athavia PD. History of Anatomy and Embalming Techniques. Mumbai: Athavia PD; 2007.
3. Wikipedia. Embalming. [online] Available from http://en.wikipedia.org/wiki/Embalming. [Last accessed March, 2020].
4. Brenner E. Human body preservation: old and new techniques. J Anat. 2014;224:316-44.
5. Hagens GV. US patent 4205059. Animal and vegetal tissues permanently preserved by synthetic resin impregnation; 1980.

CHAPTER 12

Autopsy Guidelines in COVID-2019

Dhaneshwar Lanjewar

INTRODUCTION

Clinical autopsy in newly emerging infections can provide useful information of understanding pathogenesis and pathology, which serves as a very helpful tool in guiding clinicians to start effective treatment to reduce mortality. The ongoing outbreak of coronavirus disease 2019 (COVID-19) caused by the severe acute respiratory syndrome coronavirus 2 (SARS-CoV-2) has posed a significant challenge; healthcare professionals and researchers are striving hard to understand, identify and interpret the pathophysiology of COVID-19. World Health Organization have strongly recommended performing full autopsies on patients who died with suspected or confirmed COVID-19 infection, particularly in the presence of several comorbidities. It is well-known that SARS-CoV-2 spreads by a close contact (within 6 ft) with a living person via respiratory droplets. The transmission of the virus through this route is minimal while performing an autopsy. However, it is found in feces, saliva and urine and rarely in blood. In addition, CoV-2 can persist on inanimate surfaces such as metal, glass or plastic for up to 9 days. Hence, it may be possible that a person can get COVID-19 by touching a surface or object that has the virus on it. CoV-2 can be efficiently inactivated by surface disinfection procedures with 62–71% ethanol, 0.5% hydrogen peroxide or 0.1% sodium hypochlorite within 1 minute exposure time.

GUIDELINES AND PRECAUTIONS FOR PERFORMING AUTOPSY

The guidelines and precautions for performing autopsy in COVID-19 positive cadavers are outlined in order to prevent the possibility of getting infection to anyone involved in performing autopsy on COVID-19 cadavers. These guidelines will prevent or at least minimize the pathologist and the assistant from coming in direct contact with the infected tissues and body fluids.

The following facilities should be available in autopsy room:
- *Infrastructure, and engineering facility*
    - The first requirement is to install hand wash stations in the autopsy room, which is the best infection control measure.
    - Autopsy room must be separated from other parts of the building and divided into various sections such as contaminated area, semicontaminated area and buffer zone area and all these areas should be segregated by airtight doors.
    - Autopsy room should have negative pressure with no air recirculation to adjacent areas.
    - A portable high-efficiency particulate air (HEPA) recirculation unit could be placed in the room to provide further reduction in aerosols.
    - Air should not return to the building interior, but should be exhausted outdoors, away from areas of human traffic or gathering spaces and away from other air intake systems.
    - Examination table should be equipped with reverse flow air handling system and downdraft table ventilation to decrease exposure to aerosolized pathogens.
    - Sewage discharge should be equipped with filtration or disinfection devices. Infectious effluent, the waste water produced during autopsy procedure, should be treated by chemical disinfection and discharged after complete inactivation.
    - An enclosed liquid decontamination unit using high pressure 0.5% acetic acid should be available to disinfect personal protective equipment (PPE).
- Personal PPE kit and chemicals
    - Double surgical gloves interposed with a layer of cut-proof synthetic mesh gloves, fluid-resistant or impermeable gown, water-proof apron, goggle or face shield, N-95 respirators, surgical scrubs, shoe covers, surgical cap, and nitrile gloves, 0.1% sodium hypochlorite, 10% buffered formalin, 62–71% alcohol, 2–5% glutaraldehyde, 0.5% acetic acid, 0.5% hydrogen peroxide, plastic drum (60 L volume) containing buffered formalin, air disinfection, and sterile containers for collection of small bits of autopsy specimens for ancillary investigations.
- The following PPE should be worn by a pathologist and the assistant
    - Double surgical gloves interposed with a layer of cut-proof synthetic mesh gloves.
    - Fluid-resistant or impermeable gown or waterproof apron.
    - NIOSH-certified disposable N-95 respirator or higher powered, air-purifying respirators may provide increased worker comfort during extended autopsy procedures.
    - Goggles or face shield
    - Surgical scrubs, shoe covers, and surgical cap
    - Autopsy room should have a logbook that should include names, dates and time, and activities of all workers participating in the postmortem and in cleaning of the autopsy suite. Logbook is required to assist in future follow up, if necessary housekeeping staff entering during the day should also be included in the logbook.

- The number of people in the autopsy suite should be restricted to 2.
- The PPE should be preferably put on in a room separate from the autopsy suite.

Autopsy Procedure

- External examination
  - All tubes, drains and catheters on the dead body should be removed.
  - Examine skin for petechial hemorrhages and fingers and toes for gangrene.
  - After giving incision from chin to pubic symphysis skin is reflected.
- In-situ examination
  - A bone cutter should be used to cut ribs and sternum. The skull cap should be removed with the help of chisel and hammer. Use of electric saw is strictly prohibited due to risk of aerosol generation.
  - Immediately after opening the thoracic cavity, swabs from lungs are collected these swabs should be preserved in a suitable viral transport media.
  - Obtain 0.5–1 cm size tissue bits of lungs (two sections from each lobe) and preserve these bits in sterile tubes, in glutaraldehyde, and in 10% buffered formalin, for ancillary investigations.
  - En-masse technique originally described by Letulle can be adopted for removal of organs. After removal of organ bloc, 1 cm thick slices are made on all the internal organs (lungs, liver, spleen, kidneys) and the organ bloc is preserved in a drum containing 10% buffer formalin for at least 24 hours. The formalin-fixed organ bloc can be dissected after 24 hours. The brain should be suspended in the same formalin containing drum in which entire organ bloc is preserved.
- Systemic examination: This can be carried after 24 hours using the methodology outlined for the various systems, using the routine precautions.

When postmortem procedure is completed, the first layer of PPE, including every visible soiled layer should be removed in autopsy suite. PPE should be carefully removed to avoid contaminating self, the next layer of PPE should be removed in a room separate from autopsy suite. The hands should be washed with soap and water. After removing PPE, discard the PPE in the appropriate laundry or waste receptacle. Reusable PPE (e.g., goggles, face shields) must be cleaned and disinfected according to the manufacturer's recommendations.

RECOMMENDATIONS FOR GROSS CONTAMINATION AND LIQUIDS

- Large areas contaminated with body fluids should be treated with disinfectant following removal of the fluid with absorbent material. The area should then be cleaned and treated with disinfectant.
- Clean and disinfect or autoclave nonlaunderable items with detergent solution on the warmest setting. Rinse with water, decontaminate using disinfectant, and allow items to dry completely before next use.
- Keep camera, telephones, computer keyboards, and other items as clean as possible, but treat it as if they are contaminated, hence handle with gloves. Wipe the items after use.

Recommendations for Cleaning and Waste Disposal
- Do not use compressed air and/or water under pressure for cleaning, as it can cause splashing
- Keep ventilation systems active while cleaning is conducted. Wear disposable gloves. Use face shield or goggles, wear a clean, long-sleeved fluid-resistant gown to protect skin and clothing. Wear a NIOSH-certified disposable N-95 respirator
- Dispose of gloves when cleaning is completed. Never wash or reuse gloves.

Transportation of Dead Body
- After postmortem examination, the dead body should be stitched properly and washed with sodium hypochlorite solution and then it is kept in the body bag. The bag is then disinfected from the outside, after this the dead body can be handed over to the relatives for cremation

FURTHER READING
1. CDC. (2020). CDC guidelines for Collection and Submission of Postmortem Specimens from Deceased Persons with Known or Suspected COVID-19. [online] Available from: https://www.cdc.gov/coronavirus/2019-ncov/hcp/guidance-postmortem-specimens.html. [Last accessed August, 2020].
2. Kampf G, Todt D, Pfaender S, Steinmann E. Persistence of coronaviruses on inanimate surfaces and their inactivation with biocidal agents. J Hosp Infect. 2020;104:246-51.
3. Lanjewar DN. The spectrum of clinical and pathological manifestations of AIDS in a consecutive series of 236 autopsies cases in Mumbai, India. Pathol Res Int. 2011;2011:547618.
4. Ludwig J. Current Methods of Autopsy Practice, 2nd edition. Philadelphia: WB Saunders; 1979.
5. Salerno M, Sessa F, Piscopo A, Montana A, Torrisi M, Patanè F, et al. No autopsies on COVID-19 deaths: a missed opportunity and the lockdown of science. J. Clin Med. 2020;9:1472.
6. World Health Organization. Infection Prevention and Control for the safe management of a dead body in the context of COVID-19. (Interim guidance: 24 March 2020.) [online] Available from: https://apps.who.int/iris/bitstream/handle/10665/331538/WHO-COVID-19-IPC_DBMgmt-2020.1-eng.pdf. [Last accessed August, 2020].

Appendices

CASE 1

CENTRAL NERVOUS SYSTEM

Bishan Radotra

Clinical History

A 5-year-child was admitted to the hospital with a 7-day history of pain in right shoulder and upper limbs. A day later, he developed moderate grade fever, not associated with chills or rigors. This was followed by acute onset weakness in lower limbs that progressed to involve upper limbs. He complained of difficulty in swallowing and speaking a day before admission to the hospital; the difficulty was more for liquid items than solids. There was no history of bowel or bladder involvement. There was no history trauma/snakebite/toxin ingestion. The child did not complain of any neurological illness in past. There was no definite history of dog bite but the parents remembered about a possible scratch by a dog about 6 months ago. His birth and development was normal. There was no history of similar illness in family.

On general physical examination, there was no significant abnormality. His blood pressure was however, raised (130/92 mmHg). He was conscious and interacting. The central nervous system examination revealed hypotonia of all limbs—the power was 0/5, deep tendon reflexes were not elicited and the plantars did not respond. There were findings suggestive of 9th and 10th cranial nerve palsies. There were no signs of meningeal irritation and the fundus examination was normal. The examination of cardiovascular system did not reveal any abnormality. The respiratory system showed paradoxical breathing. The air entry was equal on both sides with no added sounds. The abdominal examination was normal.

His hemogram revealed normal hemoglobin levels, polymorphonuclear leukocytosis and mildly elevated blood urea. The other biochemistry including blood gases were normal. The cerebrospinal fluid (CSF) examination showed mild pleocytosis (20 polymorphonuclear leukocytes) with raised protein (90 mg/dL) and normal sugar level. The CSF culture was negative. The HIV serology was nonreactive. Blood and urine cultures were sterile. The mycoplasma serology was negative. The test for urine porphyrins was negative. The corneal impression smear for rabies was negative. MRI brain was performed, which did not reveal any specific findings. The clinical possibilities considered were paralytic rabies, Guillain–Barré syndrome with encephalopathy (Bickerstaff brainstem encephalitis) and enteroviral encephalitis.

The child went into respiratory failure and encephalopathy. He was intubated and manually ventilated. He was given intravenous immunoglobulins and antibiotics. Anti-edema therapy for raised intracranial tension and other supportive measures were taken. The patient developed coagulopathy. He suffered a cardiac arrest on day 5 of admission and expired.

Autopsy Findings

An autopsy was performed. The examination of the brain and spinal cord did not reveal any specific pathological abnormalities on external examination apart from mild congestion of meninges. The brain and spinal cord on dissection did not show any significant pathology (**Figs. 1A** to **C**). However, microscopic examination showed parenchymal and perivascular inflammation with neuronophagia, suggestive of

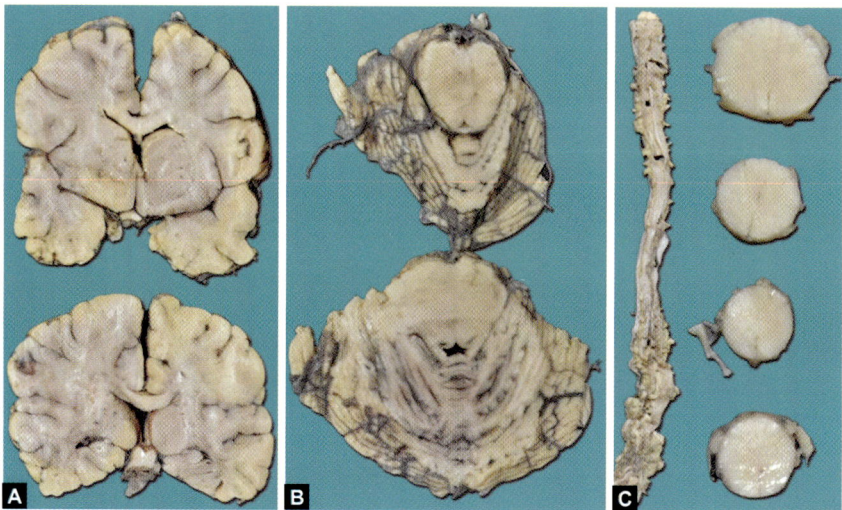

FIGS. 1A TO C: Rabies meningoencephalitis: (A) The coronal slices of the brain show only congestion. No specific lesions are noted; (B) The axial cuts of the pons and cerebellum show meningeal congestion; (C) The spinal cord on external examination and on cut sections does not show any definite pathological abnormality.

viral encephalitis. Presence of Negri bodies and the demonstration of rabies viral antigen in the neurons and axons confirmed the diagnosis of rabies encephalomyelitis (**Figs. 2A** to **D**).

This example illustrates that even with extensive investigations including imaging, the clinical diagnosis can remain obscure. It is difficult to differentiate between paralytic rabies and Guillain–Barré syndrome with encephalopathy (Bickerstaff brainstem encephalitis) particularly in view of absence of history of dog bite. About 50% cases of confirmed cases of rabies do not have history of dog bite. The reason for this is that history of dog bite not elicited during life if the diagnosis of rabies is not suspected.[1] The gross inspection of brain may not show any findings in most cases. The diagnosis of rabies encephalomyelitis is confirmed only at postmortem by demonstration of Negri bodies and rabies viral antigen and therefore autopsy is the only answer.[2,3]

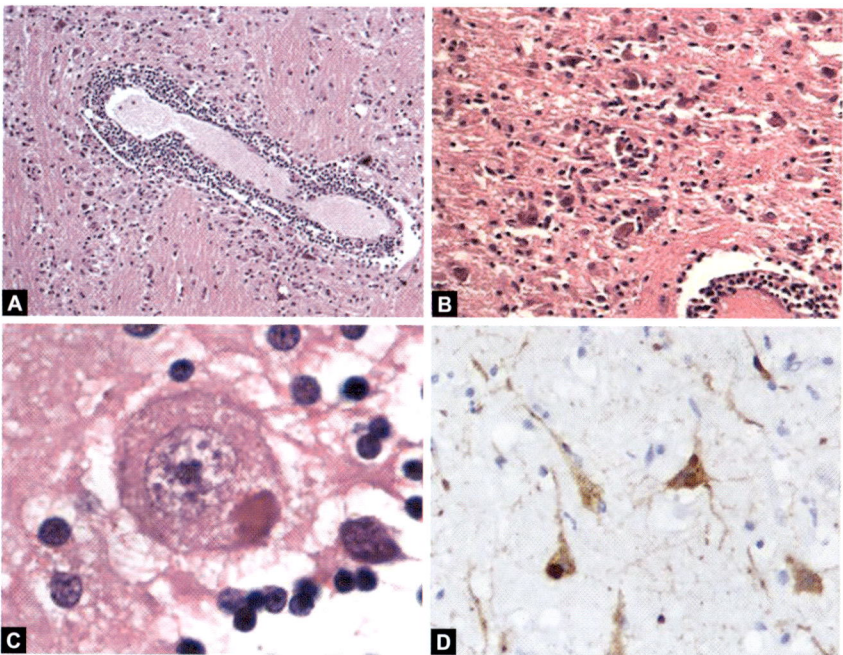

FIGS. 2A TO D: Rabies meningoencephalitis: (A) Perivascular and parenchymal lymphocytic inflammation; (B) Neuronophagia; (C) Negri body in Purkinje cell of the cerebellum; (D) Rabies viral antigen in the neurons and its processes demonstrated by immunohistochemistry using anti-rabies viral antibody.

CASE 2

CENTRAL NERVOUS SYSTEM

Bishan Radotra

Clinical History

A young man was admitted to the hospital with a history of holocranial headache and vomiting for a month without relief by any medication. He developed weakness of right upper limb followed by slurring of speech for about 20 days.

Five days prior to admission, he developed fever and altered sensorium. There was no systemic symptomatology. On examination, he was drowsy and had mild pallor. There was neck rigidity and spasticity in all four limbs but more on right side. Other systemic examination was normal.

On investigations, his routine hematological parameters, coagulation profile, liver/renal function tests were normal. The cerebrospinal fluid examination revealed glucose level of 71 mg/dL, protein 132 mg/dL and 20 lymphocytes/dL. Results of Gram and Zeihl–Neelsen staining were negative. Cryptococcal antigen test and polymerase chain reaction (PCR) for tuberculosis were negative. CT examination of the brain revealed a bulky left parietal lobe with an ill-defined hypoattenuating lesion, and another lesion right superior frontal gyrus with leptomeningeal enhancement. MR imaging revealed multiple ill-defined heterogeneous intra-axial mass lesions in both frontoparietal, left temporal, left occipital and left cerebellar hemisphere. There was mass effect with effacement of the left lateral ventricle. A provisional diagnosis of multiple brain abscesses possibly due to infective emboli was considered and he was started on parenteral vancomycin and ceftriaxone. Another possibility of tuberculous meningits with multiple space-occupying lesions was also suggested as a differential diagnosis. Anti-edema measure and steroids were also started but the patient succumbed to his illness on 3rd day after admission.

Autopsy Findings

A restricted brain autopsy was performed, which revealed edema with bilateral uncal and tonsillar herniations. Coronal slices showed multiple variable-sized hemorrhagic and necrotic lesions involving frontal and parietal lobes on both cerebral hemispheres and left cerebellum corresponding to the MRI findings (**Figs. 3A** to **C**). There was necrotizing inflammation and vasculitis causing extensive necrosis. Focal purulent meningitis and occasional giant cells were noted. Numerous amoebic trophozoites and occasional cyst form could be demonstrated (**Figs. 3A** to **C**). PCR on these sections was positive for *Balamuthia mandrillaris* and negative for *Acanthamoeba*.

This example illustrates that clinical diagnosis in this case was an infective process possibly embolic abscesses. In view of large heterogeneous masses on imaging, other possibilities considered were tuberculosis, toxoplasmosis or noninfective conditions such as malignancy. The etiological diagnosis was not possible. The definite diagnosis of amoebic meningoencephalitis is based on demonstration of amoebae

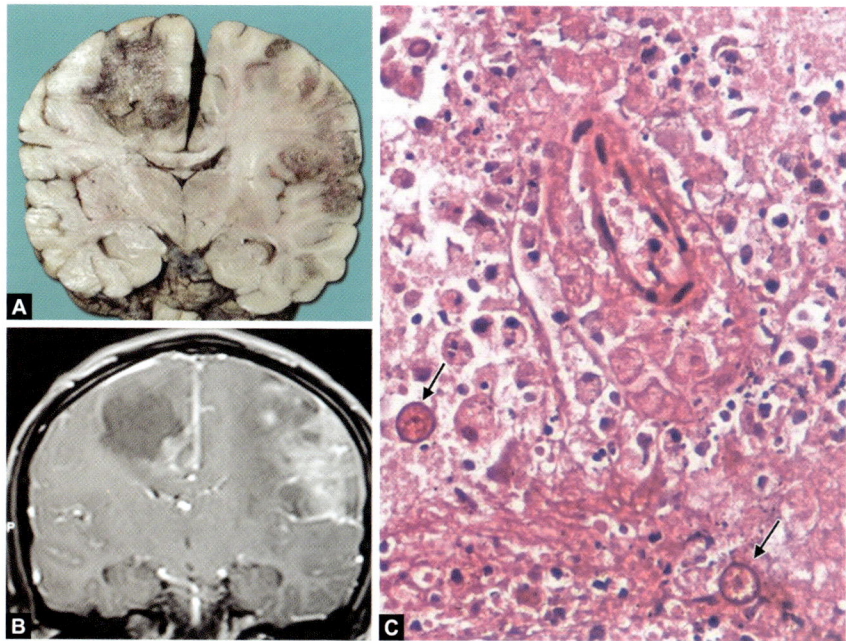

FIGS. 3A TO C: *Balamuthia mandrillaris* meningoencephalitis: (A) Coronal cut of the cerebral hemispheres shows bilateral variable-sized hemorrhagic and necrotic lesions; (B) Comparison to the MRI findings; (C) Numerous amoebic trophozoites are present in perivascular space with occasional cyst form (arrows) amidst the necrotizing inflammatory infiltrate.

on tissue examination.[4,5] Unfortunately, it is a rapidly fatal disease and these patients are in moribund state. Therefore, unless diagnosis is suspected biopsy is not taken and hence, most cases are diagnosed on postmortem. We have some experience of diagnosing amoebic meningoencephalitis during life on surgical biopsy material.[6] The exact type of organism involved can only be demonstrated from tissue as illustrated in this case and thus short of autopsy we do not know how many cases we are missing.

CASE 3

CARDIOVASCULAR SYSTEM

Pradeep Vaideeswar

Clinical History

A 57-year-old male was brought in an unconscious state to the Emergency Services Department of a tertiary-care center. As per the relatives, he had been a hypertensive for the past 7 years with irregular therapy. On examination, he was pulseless with no recordable blood pressure. The pupils were fixed and dilated. ECG also showed no cardiac activity. A medicolegal autopsy was asked for.

Autopsy Findings

A complete autopsy was performed after 3 hours of expiry. The patient had been averagely built and nourished; there was no pallor, clubbing or pedal edema. On opening the thoracic cavity, the heart appeared markedly enlarged due to marked pericardial distension. There was hemopericardium (**Figs. 4A** and **B**) with blood clots weighing 290 g. The in-situ examinations of the cranial and abdominal cavities were normal. The heart was moderately enlarged in size (weight 390 g) with moderate enlargement of the left ventricle. There was a 2 cm vertically oriented tear in the mid-portion of the posterior wall of the left ventricle, present 1 cm to the left of the posterior interventricular groove (**Figs. 5A** and **B**). The hemorrhage had tracked into the epicardial fat in not only the posterior, but also the anterior aspect of the left atrioventricular groove. Serial cross-sections at the site of tear showed the presence of a transmural fresh infarct (pale yellow and opaque) that occupied the entire posterior wall and posterior one-third of the interventricular septum. The tract was simple in nature, but forked (**Fig. 6A**) and was surrounded by hemorrhage. In addition, there was moderate hypertrophy of the myocardium. The right coronary artery had a dominant distribution and all coronaries were atherosclerotic. The posterior descending artery right from its origin was occluded by a pale brown fresh thrombus over a congested appearing eccentric atheroma for a length of 1 cm, which suggested the possibility of plaque rupture with superimposed thrombosis. Rest of the chambers and valves were normal on gross examination. Other organs were normal on gross inspection,

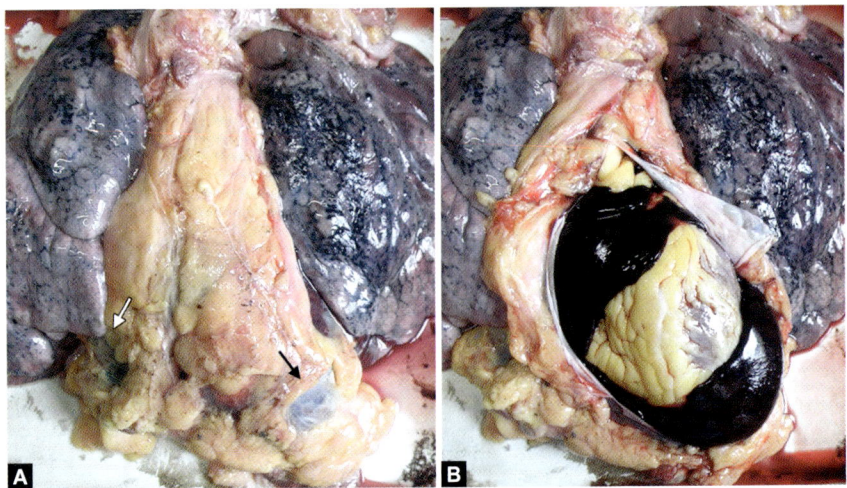

FIGS. 4A AND B: (A) Abundant adipose tissue infiltrates the parietal pericardium. The pericardial cavity is distended and at places (arrows), the outer layer appears pale red; (B) The parietal pericardium has been incised to show the heart blanketed by blood clots.

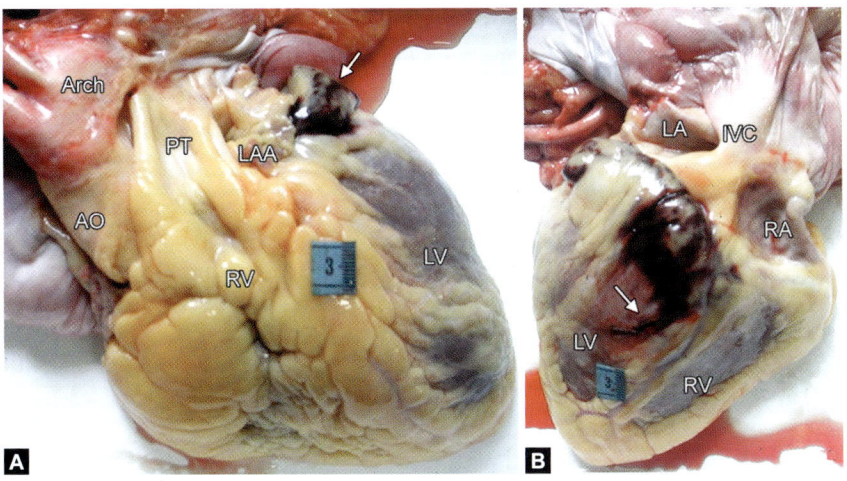

(AO: aorta; IVC: inferior vena cava; LA: left atrium; LAA: left atrial appendage; PT: pulmonary trunk; RA: right atrium; RV: right ventricle)

FIGS. 5A AND B: (A) Anterior surface of the heart, showing moderate cardiomegaly and increased epicardial adipose tissue. The fat at the left atrioventricular groove (arrow) is hemorrhagic; (B) A vertically oriented tear (arrow) is present on the posterior wall of the left ventricle (LV) below the focus of hemorrhage.

including the kidneys. An additional finding was diffuse enlargement of the entire thyroid gland.

The tract, on histology, was filled with blood and flanked by groups of myofibers showing coagulative necroses. There was extensive interstitial edema and neutrophilic infiltrate. In addition, there was fragmentation of the myofibers, histiocytic infiltrate and brisk fibroblastic proliferation indicating commencement of the repair process (**Figs. 6B** to **D**). A diagnosis of acute myocardial infarction with left ventricular free wall rupture (LVFWR) and fatal hemopericardium was made. The histology also confirmed presence of plaque rupture with superadded thrombus in the posterior descending artery. The kidneys did not show features of benign nephrosclerosis. There was Hashimoto's thyroiditis.

Left ventricular free wall rupture[7] is an example of mechanical complication of myocardial infarction. The patients are usually >60 years of age, particularly women. They often are hypertensives and manifest this complication during their first episode of transmural infarction and/or with history of delayed thrombolytic therapy. The ruptures may be late, seen in >50% of cases and occur within the first few days when the myocardium is at its softest. Sometimes, the ruptures may be early occurring within 24 hours in 13–40% of patients, explained on the basis of interstitial edema. It is important to sample the thyroid gland in all cases of ischemic heart disease to pick out cases of subclinical thyroid disease.

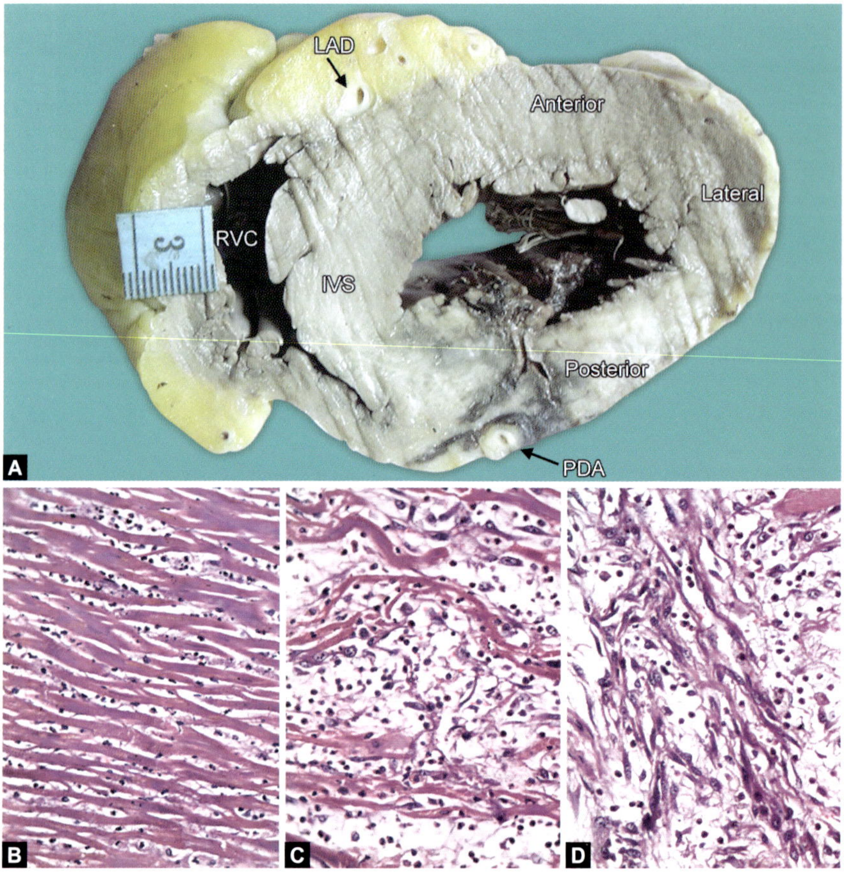

(IVS: interventricular septum; LAD: left anterior descending artery; RVC: right ventricular cavity)

FIGS. 6A TO D: (A) The transverse slice at the mid-portion shows a forked tear in the middle of the fresh infarct. The posterior descending artery (PDA) (arrow) is critically stenosed. Various histological phases of the infarct; (B) Coagulative necroses with interstitial edema and inflammation; (C) Fragmented myofibers; (D) Onset of fibroblastic proliferation (H&E ×400).

CASE 4

CARDIOVASCULAR SYSTEM

Pradeep Vaideeswar

Clinical History

A 52-year-old male, with a total ward stay of 2 hours, presented with fever with chills off and on for the last 1 month and associated loss of weight and appetite. He then developed bilateral swelling of feet with decreasing urine output for last 4–5 days. The patient had been diagnosed as a case of bleeding piles (on Ayurvedic therapy) with iron-deficiency anemia for the last 6 months; he had received regular blood transfusions. There was no history of diabetes mellitus, hypertension or any addiction.

On examination, the pulse rate was 86/min and regular; blood pressure was 100/60 mmHg. Bilateral pedal edema was noted. Systemic examination was normal; the air entry was equal on both hemithoraces and the heart sounds were also normal. The clinical impression was either a septic or cardiogenic shock. Routine investigations revealed anemia (Hb 5.8 g/dL, microcytic hypochromic picture on peripheral smear), neutrophilia (total WBC count of 18,700/mm^3 with 87% of neutrophils), normal fasting blood glucose, electrolytes and serum creatinine. Ultrasonography revealed moderate splenomegaly with wedge-shaped areas suggestive of infarctions, mild ascites, and dilated hepatic veins and inferior vena cava (possibly due to a cardiac cause). Intravenous antibiotics and hydrocortisone was started. The patient had sudden deterioration and could not be resuscitated.

Autopsy Findings

A complete autopsy was performed after 12 hours of expiry. The patient had been averagely built and nourished. There was pallor and bilateral edema feet. The in-situ examination of the cranial cavity was normal. On opening the thoracic cage, the heart appeared markedly enlarged and covered by normal appearing parietal pericardium. On opening the pericardial cavity, there was no increase in the pericardial fluid. Samples from the right atrium for blood cultures were not taken. An adhesion of the left lung apex to the thoracic cage was present. There was about 700 mL of slightly hazy amber-colored peritoneal fluid. The fluid cytology revealed neutrophils of 110 and lymphocytes of 30/mL^3. Smears also showed degenerated cells in a proteinaceous background. No organisms were identified. An enlarged liver with hemorrhagic mottling was present 3 cm below the right sub-costal margin. Coils of intestines were normal.

The heart was markedly enlarged in size and weighed 400 g. There was marked enlargement of the left ventricle with mild enlargement of the other chambers (**Figs. 7A to C**). The epicardial surface was dull all over with milk patches over the right ventricular outflow tract. The right coronary artery had a dominant distribution; all the arteries were patent with minimal focal calcific atherosclerosis in the left anterior descending artery. The heart was cut by the inflow-outflow method. The aortic annulus was markedly dilated. The entire left- and the adjoining noncoronary cusps were completely covered and destroyed by bulky yellowish-brown friable vegetations over 3 × 2.5 cm—infective endocarditis (IE, **Figs. 8A to C**). The vegetations are both flattened as well as polypoidal with distinct crater formation amidst the vegetations. This indicated a complication of the disease process in the form of a periannular abscess, substantiated by bulges noted above the anterolateral commissure of the mitral valve and above the anteroseptal commissure of the tricuspid valve (**Figs. 7B and C**). The left ventricular cavity was markedly dilated with thinning of the myocardium and mild endocardial thickening. On histology, there was extensive destruction of the semilunar cusps by large vegetations containing many clumps of bacteria. Other

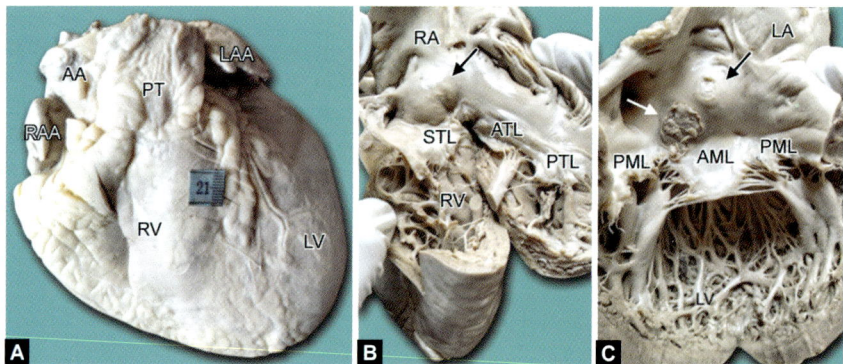

(AA: ascending aorta; AML: anterior mitral leaflet; ATL: anterior tricuspid leaflet; LAA: left atrial appendage; PT: pulmonary trunk; PML: posterior mitral leaflet; PTL: posterior tricuspid leaflet; RA: right atrium; RAA: right atrial appendage; STL: septal tricuspid leaflet)

FIGS. 7A TO C: (A) Mild cardiomegaly; (B) Opened out right ventricular (RV) inflow tract showing a pale yellow bulge just above the anteroseptal commissure; (C) Opened out left ventricular (LV) inflow tract showing presence of an ulcerated bulge (black arrow) in the mid-portion of the left atrial (LA) cavity and mural endocarditis (white arrow) above the anterolateral commissure.

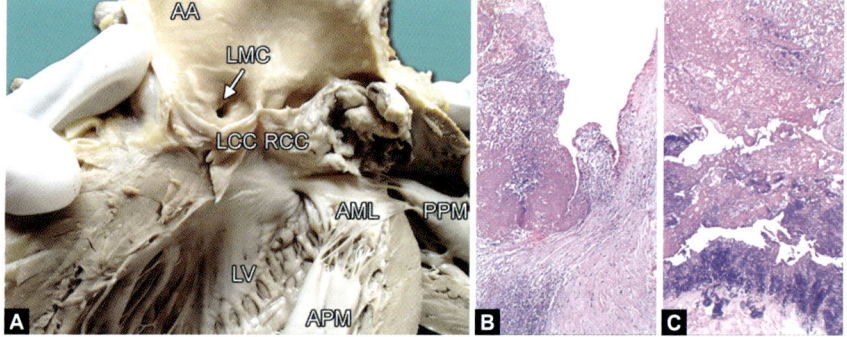

(AA: ascending aorta; AML: anterior mitral leaflet; APM: anterior papillary muscle; LCC: left coronary cusp; LMC: left main coronary artery ostium; LV: left ventricle; PPM: posterior papillary muscle)

FIGS. 8A TO C: (A) The noncoronary cusp of the aortic valve is completely obscured by large pale yellow friable vegetations, which partly extends over the right coronary cusp (RCC); (B) Vegetation adherent to the cusp composed of fibrin, platelets and clumps of neutrophils H&E ×250; (C) Granular basophilic bacterial colonies (H&E ×400).

findings at autopsy included pulmonary edema, extensive centrilobular hepatocytic hemorrhagic necroses and multiple fresh infarcts of kidneys and spleen. Since, the vegetations were seen burrowing into the adjacent tissue, the sudden death can be explained by inflammatory involvement of the atrioventricular node with consequent arrhythmia.

Infective endocarditis[8] continues to be major cause of morbidity and mortality, despite of advances in therapeutic modalities. In majority of the circumstances, IE occurs due to endothelial injury produced by turbulent blood flow, secondary to diseased valves or presence of congenital heart disease. This is followed by deposition of bland thrombi which are then colonized by microorganisms. These organisms (usually bacteria) are introduced into the bloodstream when a surface already heavily colonized is abraded or traumatized (piles in this case) and this may at times be sufficient to affect normal native valves, as was noted in the case presented. This colonization of normal valves is also aided by inherent adhesive capacities of bacteria. Apart from embolization, IE of aortic valve is often associated with intracardiac abscess, which can extend into the conduction system, causing heart block or fatal arrhythmia.

CASE 5

GASTROINTESTINAL TRACT

Anjali D Amarapurkar

Clinical History

A 50-year-male, nondiabetic, occasional alcoholic, presented with chief complaints of abdominal pain, vomiting and fever off and on. The abdominal pain was colicky, and nonradiating without localization for the past 4 days. The vomiting, present for the last 3 days, was intermittent and projectile; it contained food particles. The patient did not pass stools since then. The fever was intermittent and low grade without chills. There had been no history of diarrhea, hematemesis or jaundice. There was no family history of diabetes, hypertension, tuberculosis or malignancy.

On examination, the abdomen was distended with diffuse tenderness. The laboratory investigations revealed hemoglobin 10 g/dL, total WBC 20,500/mm^3, serum total bilirubin 5 mg/dL, aspartate aminotransferase (AST) 42 U/L, alanine aminotransferase (ALT) 50 U/L, and serum creatinine of 1 mg/dL. An abdominal ultrasonography revealed dilated bowel loops; the liver, spleen and kidneys were normal. Computed tomography showed air fluid levels suggestive of small bowel obstruction. HBsAg, HCV and HIV were negative.

The patient underwent emergency exploratory laparotomy, which showed multiple adhesions among the coils of the intestine. The adhesions were removed and intestinal obstruction was released. The surgery went uneventful. But on second postoperative day, the patient started getting pain in abdomen with fever associated with jaundice. The investigations then showed neutrophilia (total leukocyte count of count 22,500/mm^3), thrombocytopenia (platelet count of 70,000/mm^3), total bilirubin of 10 mg/dL, AST 200 U/L and ALT 180 U/L. The prothrombin time was mildly deranged. The blood culture revealed gram-negative bacteria. With above investigations working diagnosis of liver cell failure in operated case of intestinal obstruction was considered. On third postoperative day, abdominal pain and fever continued; the jaundice was pronounced and patient developed altered sensorium. The condition deteriorated and he died on fifth postoperative day.

Autopsy Findings

A complete autopsy was performed. On external examination, operative sutures were intact. Icterus and abdominal distension was noted. There was no evidence of external hemorrhages, pedal edema or signs of portal hypertension. The in-situ examination revealed 200 mL of yellowish and hazy peritoneal (ascitic) fluid (**Figs. 8A** to **C**). The microscopic examination showed 180 cells/mm^3, majority of them were polymorphs. The intestinal loops were adherent to each other and covered with yellowish exudate on serosal aspect (**Fig. 9**). There was no evidence of perforation.

On systemic examination, liver weight was 1200 g, dark green in color. Its surface was smooth without nodularity. The extrahepatic biliary tree including gallbladder were normal. The bowel loops were mildly dusky and showed serositis; their mucosal surfaces were unremarkable. The splenic capsule was also covered by exudate. The lungs, heart, kidneys and brain were unremarkable. There was no lymphadenopathy. Histopathological examination of liver showed maintained normal architecture. There was marked cholestasis within bile canaliculi (**Fig. 10**). Few bile plugs were also seen. The hepatocytes and portal tracts were normal. There was no significant inflammation, fibrosis, steatosis or bile ductular proliferation. The above features were suggestive of bland intrahepatic cholestasis. Other organs did not show specific abnormality. With above gross and microscopic examination, final cause of death was septicemia with jaundice in operated case of intestinal obstruction.

In addition to septicemia, this patient had jaundice and showed marked cholestasis on microscopic examination. Questions arise why cholestasis develops in patients with septicemia? Is there any association between the two? Is cholestasis common in sepsis? Jaundice (cholestasis) can occur in septicemia.[9] Pathogenesis of cholestasis associated with sepsis is multifactorial, which includes: Increased bilirubin load due to hemolysis, impaired liver function due to septicemia, ischemia or drugs or extrahepatic biliary tree obstruction (ligature of biliary tree, stones, stricture

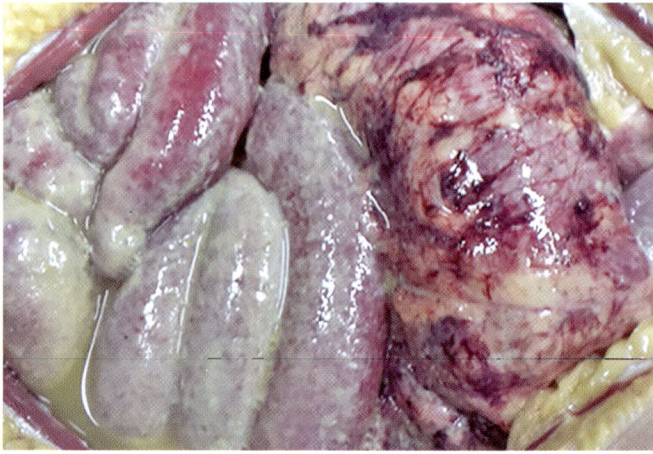

FIG. 9: The intestinal coils are covered with exudate with focal ischemic change.

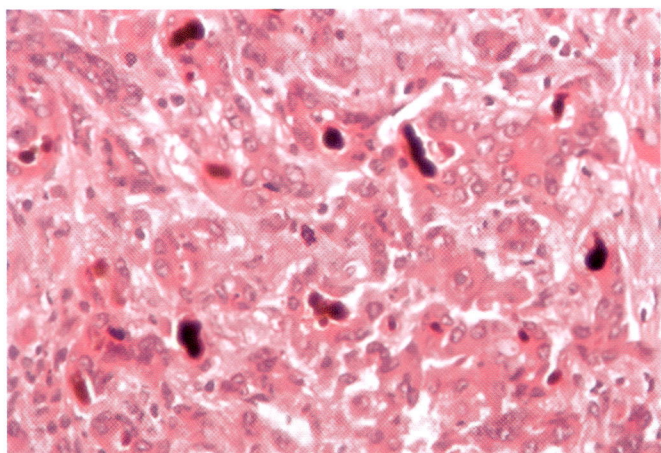

FIG. 10: Liver with marked cholestasis within canaliculi without ductular proliferation H&E ×400.

or biliary leak). Hepatic dysfunction is common in various infections especially bacterial. Bacterial products cause endotoxin mediated injury to hepatocyte canalicular membrane which affects transport of bile leading to cholestasis. Jaundice is a symptom which follows cholestasis. Prevalence of cholestasis with sepsis is not exactly known. However, it has been reported ranging from 0.6 to 54%.[10] Jaundice is commonly seen with intra- abdominal sepsis. Infections at other sites that can be associated with sepsis are hepatobiliary infections, urinary tract infection, meningitis, pneumonia or endocarditis. Liver function tests in these patients show conjugated hyperbilirubinemia between 2 mg/dL and 10 mg/dL, alkaline phosphatase not greater than 2–3 times upper limit of normal. Liver enzymes are mildly elevated. Prognosis depends upon the severity of sepsis. If septicemia is controlled, liver functions can be normalize with disappearance of jaundice.[11,12] Hence, jaundice in sepsis is not uncommon, may not be always due to biliary obstruction and is reversible if septicemia is treated appropriately.

CASE 6

URINARY TRACT

Vinaya Shah

Clinical History

A 58-year-old male was admitted with history of pain in the left knee and inability to walk over a period of 3 months, which apparently developed after lifting weights. There was also loss of weight and appetite. There was no significant past history.

The local examination showed enlargement of left knee with tenderness. Chest radiography showed multiple radiopacities in bilateral lungs suggestive of metastases with associated mild pleural effusions. Ultrasonography of left knee revealed a mass lesion arising from end of femur most probably malignant origin. The patient expired within 3 days of hospital stay.

Autopsy Findings

The patient appeared cachectic. There was swelling at the left knee joint with stretching of the overlying skin. Significant findings were observed in kidneys and lungs. The right kidney was enlarged with nodular external surface. On cut surface, a large mass 18 × 17 × 16 cm mass was seen to replace the whole parenchyma; a thin rim of renal tissue was seen at the periphery. The tumor was gray white with a variegated appearance due to areas of necrosis, hemorrhage and cystic changes. The pelvicalyceal system was distorted due to tumor infiltration (**Fig. 11A**). The left kidney is normal. The lungs showed multiple firm white well demarcated nodules, measuring 1-5 cm in diameter (**Fig. 11B**). The other organs, such as brain, spleen adrenal and gastrointestinal tract were unremarkable. The sections from kidney tumor revealed the classic features of renal cell carcinoma (RCC) with nests of clear cells supported by fine vascular septa (**Fig. 11B**, inset). There were few foci showing spindling of tumor cells. The diagnosis of RCC was given. The lung nodules also showed features of renal cell carcinoma. The cause of death was given as disseminated RCC with cachexia.

Renal cell carcinoma is the most frequent urological malignancy in adults, occurring most frequently in fifth and sixth decades of life. The classic presentation of RCC comprising pain, flank mass and hematuria occurs in only 10% of cases.[13] Many patients with RCC (20-40%) are asymptomatic, and the diagnosis is made incidentally from a radiologic study obtained for other reasons.[14] In some, the RCC is characterized by varied and sometimes obscure manifestations, which include unusual metastatic sites and paraneoplastic/vascular syndromes. Regional lymph nodes, lungs, bones

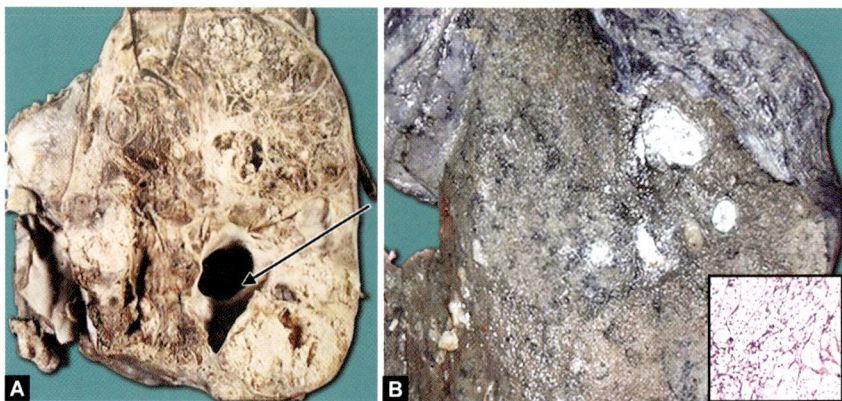

FIGS. 11A AND B: (A) Tumor replacing the entire renal parenchyma with distortion of the pelvis (arrow); (B) Multiple firm white lung nodules. Inset shows kidney tumor composed nests of clear cells separated by slender fibrous septa.

and liver are the most common sites. The bones are favored targets; however, sole presentation as joint swelling/fracture of long bones is distinctly uncommon. There is nothing characteristic about these renal cancers clinically or radiologically that would aid in differentiating the neoplasm from primary malignant bone tumors. Metastatic sarcomatoid RCC to bone can occasionally stimulate intense reactive host woven bone or osteoid and may be mistaken for fibrosarcoma or osteosarcoma. Patients with osseous metastases of RCC have an unfavorable prognosis. In some studies, >50% of patients die within the 1st year.[15] The paraneoplastic syndromes include fever, hypercalcemia, anemia or erythrocytosis, hypertension, nonmetastatic hepatocellular enzyme elevation (Stauffer syndrome), polyneuromyopathy, amyloidosis, or even dermatomyositis.

CASE 7

AUTOPSY IN INFECTIOUS DISEASE

Dhaneshwar Lanjewar

Clinical History

The story of this case began in February 2006, in the village Jaikheda near Nawapur town of Nandurbar district, Maharashtra state wherein 55,000 poultry birds died within 1 week. Subsequently bird flu virus (H5N1) was detected in them. The state government culled 1,95,124 poultry birds and 14,669 domestic birds and around 3.6 lakh eggs were destroyed in Nawapur town. Mumbai city was put on guard after confirmed report of bird flu in the state and health officials were posted at all check points to ensure no infected poultry gets into Mumbai. All the restaurants in Mumbai were asked to instruct kitchen staff to be extra careful while handling poultry meat.

During this time period, a 12-year-old boy residing in that village presented with fever without chills and rigors and bodyache for 7 days, followed by breathlessness with chest pain and altered sensorium for 3 days. He was treated by private practitioner in Nawapur; however, there was no improvement. A provisional diagnosis of bird flu was made and the boy was referred to tertiary care hospital in Mumbai. Clinical examination revealed that the boy was febrile and delirious with heart rate of 160/min, respiratory rate of 60/min; blood pressure was not recordable. There was decreased air entry on both sides of chest. The laboratory investigations showed hemoglobin, 7.3 g/dL and total leukocyte count of 19,400/mm^3 (predominantly neutrophilic). The X-ray chest showed features of bilateral patchy pneumonia and presence of slightly increased fluid in pleural space; the examination of pleural fluid showed numerous pus cells. The cerebrospinal fluid (CSF) examination showed 900 cells/mm^3, with differential count of neutrophils 90% and lymphocytes 10%. The patient did not respond to treatment and died within 24 hours due to severe respiratory distress. A clinical postmortem was requested to know cause of death and to confirm whether the death was caused by H5N1 infection.

From the clinical and laboratory findings, following are possibilities:
- The significant disease is in both lungs and there is also a possibility of involvement of brain.
- Laboratory findings of increased total leukocyte count above normal and increase in neutrophil percentage above normal favors the possibility of bacterial infection. Presence of neutrophils in pleural fluid and CSF also confirms the presence of bacterial infection of lung and brain. There is also a possibility that the boy initially suffered from viral infection which is complicated by bacterial infection.
- The infectious diseases likely to be identified in this case will be in the lungs (lesions of bacterial/viral bronchopneumonia) and also in the brain (pyogenic meningitis).
- The autopsy should answer whether death is caused by avian influenza virus.

Before proceeding for the postmortem examination, it is necessary to have some understanding of influenza virus, its pathogenesis and pathology.[16] Based on core protein influenza virus is divided into 3 types: A, B, and C. Type A affects humans, animals and birds, Type B affects humans only and Type C affects humans and pigs only. On the basis of presence of hemagglutinin (HA) protein, influenza virus A is sub typed as H1 to H15 and on the basis of presence of nuclear (N) protein, it is subtyped as N1 to N9. These subtypes demonstrate species specificity. For example, H1 to H15 infect birds, H1, H2, H3 infect human beings and H5, H7, and H9 usually infect birds and also humans. There are no subtypes of influenza virus B and C. The outbreaks of human disease due to avian influenza are described since 1997 and human deaths have been reported and nearly 85 million chickens, ducks, geese, turkeys have been died or destroyed. If human disease due to H5N1 continues to occur, global epidemic is likely to erupt because current world population does not have immunity to this new virus subtype. This influenza produces pleural and parenchymal hemorrhages in lung, focal necrosis of alveolar walls and hyaline thrombosis within arterioles and capillaries, hyaline membrane formation, and hemorrhagic encephalitis in central nervous system. Secondary bacterial infections are common in influenza. In this case, a postmortem investigation needs to be done to confirm or rule out diagnosis of avian influenza. These investigations would be:
- Virus culture,
- Reverse transcription-polymerase chain reaction (RT-PCR),
- Immunofluorescence using monoclonal antibody to H5N1, and
- Serological test (ELISA) for detection of specific antibody.

Autopsy Findings

Since this case is from avian influenza region; universal safety precautions need to be taken before starting postmortem, the following materials should be made available:
- Gloves, masks, protective dress, protective goggles, N-95 masks (which have 25% capability of preventing transmission of particles <0.3µ), sterile syringes and needles, sterile throat swab, blood culture broth, slides, culture media, etc. (**Fig. 12A**).

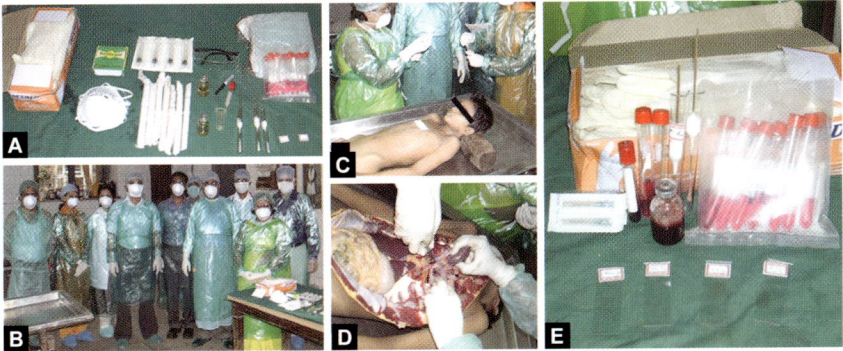

FIGS. 12A TO E: (A and B) Preparation for an infectious diseases autopsy; (C) Collection of nasal swab; (D) Collection of blood from right atrium; (E) Blood collected in broth and smears made from nasal swab and pleural exudate.

- The postmortem should be performed by a team of doctors comprising pathologists, microbiologists, and their assistants (**Fig. 12B**). The microbiologists are needed to collect appropriate samples for postmortem investigations. The samples are collected from nose with the help of nasal swab (**Fig. 12C**). Blood is collected from posterior surface of right atrium for blood culture (**Fig. 12D**).
- Blood is collected in broth, smears are prepared on slides from nasal swab, and nasal swabs are also collected for bacterial and viral culture and blood is also collected in plain bulb (**Fig. 12E**).

The external examination did not show any significant findings. In-situ examination showed yellowish patchy exudates and reddish black hemorrhagic areas on pleural surfaces (**Fig. 13A**). The brain showed widening of gyri and narrowing of sulci (features of edema) and the inferior surface of brain showed minimal hazy exudates (**Fig. 13B**). The liver, kidneys and spleen were slightly enlarged, while the heart was normal. The cut surfaces of both the lungs showed extensive parenchymal hemorrhages and focal yellowish abscesses (**Fig. 13C**), which on histology showed extensive intra-alveolar hemorrhages, purulent exudates within the airways with ulceration of their linings and aggregates of bluish bacterial colonies (**Fig. 13D**) and hyaline membrane formation (**Fig. 13E**). The brain showed neutrophilic infiltration in subarachnoid space (pyogenic meningitis, **Fig. 13F**). Microscopic hemorrhages were also identified focally in gastrointestinal tract, adrenals, and heart. Postmortem investigations confirmed growth of *Staphylococcus aureus* in pleural swab and blood. Postmortem samples were tested by RT-PCR and was negative for avian influenza virus. This rules out avian influenza virus infection in this case. The cause of death was staphylococcal hemorrhagic bronchopneumonia with multiple pulmonary abscesses and diffuse alveolar damage[17] with pyogenic meningitis.

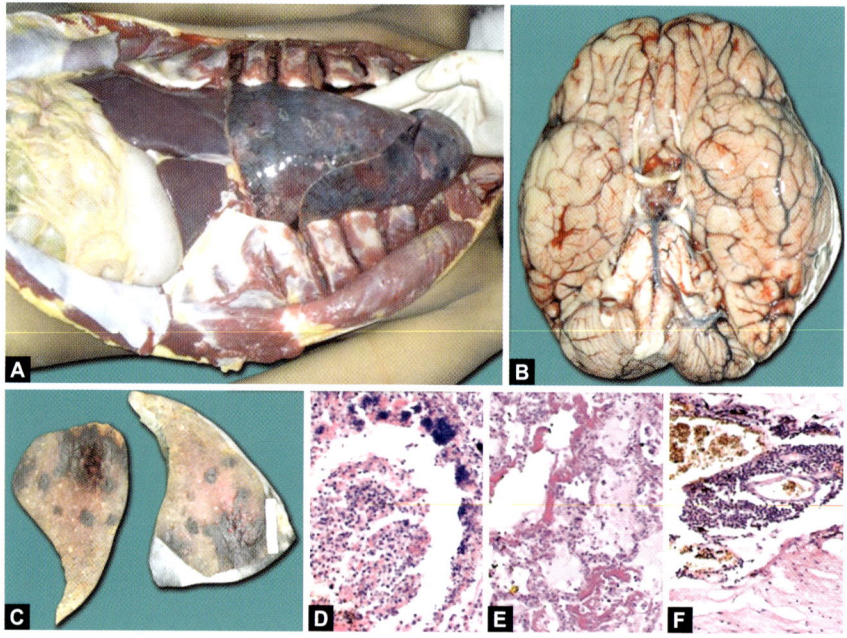

FIGS. 13A TO F: (A) In-situ examination of the thorax shows presence of focal yellowish pleural exudate multiple hemorrhages within the parenchyma; (B) Striking brain edema with faintly purulent exudates at the base; (C) Cut slices of the lung showing small yellowish-white abscesses along with the dark red foci of hemorrhage; (D) Basophilic bacterial colonies clinging to the ulcerated bronchiolar lining (H&E ×400). Note presence of luminal exudate; (E) Alveolar septa lined by ribbon like pink hyaline membranes (H&E ×400); (F) Neutrophils in the subarachnoid space (H&E ×400).

Case 8

MATERNAL MORTALITY

Kusum Jashnani

Clinical History

A 23-year-old woman (primigravida with 5 months amenorrhea) was admitted in a tertiary-care center with a history of deviation of angle of mouth, weakness of left hand and both lower limbs with increased somnolence for past 10–20 days, fever with chills, vomiting and giddiness for the past 5 days and loss of vision since 2 days. She was a known case of hypertension and hypothyroidism, but not on regular treatment. She had two antenatal visits but she had not been co-operative with immunization and nutritional requirements. On examination, she was drowsy and disoriented with proptosis, bilateral rectus palsy and left upper motor neuron palsy. Her blood pressure was 200/130 mmHg. The pupils were dilated and sluggishly reacting to light. The uterus was 20 weeks' size and relaxed; per vaginal examination revealed a closed os. The clinical impression had been eclampsia with altered sensorium. On fundoscopy, there was no evidence of papilledema and changes of hypertensive or diabetic retinopathy. The pelvic ultrasonography showed a live single fetus (17 weeks, cephalic presentation) with adequate amniotic fluid. Apart from neutrophilia and elevated transaminases (SGOT/SGPT-356/675), all routine hematological, biochemical (including the thyroid hormones) and serological investigations had been normal. The cytological examination of the cerebrospinal fluid revealed 190 cells/mm^3 with 95% lymphocytes and 5% polymorphonuclear leukocytes. The computed tomography (CT) and magnetic resonance imaging (MRI) showed dilated ventricular system with thick exudates in sulcal spaces of both cerebral hemispheres and other brain parts, suggesting a diagnosis of tuberculous meningitis. Unfortunately, she succumbed within 48 hours of hospital admission.

Autopsy Findings

The general examination had been normal. The brain had been edematous and weighed 900 g with the presence of prominent basal gray white thick exudates. On histology, the subarachnoid spaces showed very dense mononuclear cell infiltrate without a granulomatous reaction (**Fig. 14**). The arteries had fibrin thrombi. The pituitary gland appeared enlarged (1.1 × 0.7 × 0.4 cm) and weighed 2 g. Surprisingly, the histology revealed an adenoma (confirmed by loss of reticulin network) that produced compression of the adjacent parenchyma. Areas of coagulative necroses, hemorrhage and focal neutrophilic infiltrate were also seen within the adenoma (**Figs. 15A** to **D**). The uterus was had a 130 g sized fetus with crown-rump length of 12 cm. The placenta was implanted on anterior surface of uterine fundus and was 10 cm in diameter. The myometrium showed physiologic hypertrophy without preischemia on histopathologic examination. Focal areas of acute tubular necrosis were seen in

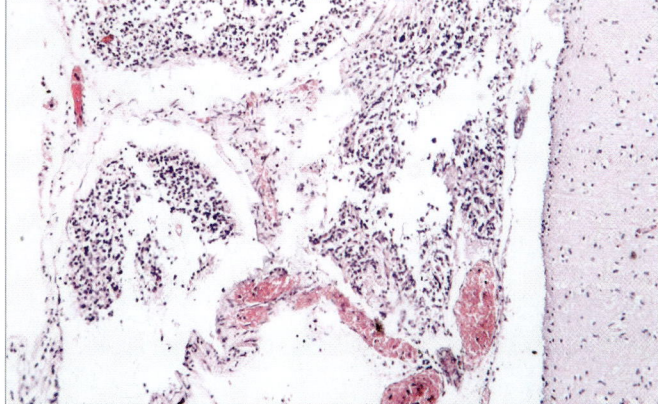

FIG. 14: Subarachnoid space showing mononuclear cell infiltrate and congested meningeal vessels (H&E ×100).

the kidneys; other organs were normal. The cause of death was related to pituitary adenoma with apoplexy in a case of chronic lymphocytic meningitis.

Though the exact chronology of events is not known, the symptoms of the patient point toward CNS involvement. CT/MRI of the brain gave a picture of tuberculous meningitis with hydrocephalus and the clinical presentation can be explained by this diagnosis. Somewhere along the line, nonfunctioning pituitary adenoma had developed with intratumoral necroses and bleeding during pregnancy leading to apoplexy. Pituitary apoplexy is a rare but potentially life-threatening condition with an incidence of about 0.6–10.5% among cases of pituitary adenoma. It is caused by a hemorrhage or infarction in patients with pituitary adenoma.[18] The main clinical features are headache, cranial nerve palsy, decreased visual acuity and visual field defects, nausea or vomiting, an altered level of consciousness and some degree of pituitary insufficiency. The cavernous sinus also contains the carotid artery, which supplies blood to the brain; occasionally, compression of the artery can lead to one-sided weakness and other symptoms of stroke. Because of the overlap of clinical symptoms with other common medical conditions especially infectious meningitis, misdiagnosis of pituitary apoplexy or meningitis with one another is well known resulting in delay in management. Literature is full of case reports such as where intracranial tuberculoma has presented with pituitary apoplexy syndrome or cases where pituitary apoplexy has masqueraded as acute meningitis.[19,20] In the present case both pathologies have developed in the patient, though the exact chronological event is not known. Since there is overlap in the clinical presentation of these two pathologies, importance has been given to infectious meningitis both clinically as well as radiologically. It has been reported that the patients who presented with histological features of pituitary tumor infarction alone had less severe clinical features on presentation, a longer course prior to presentation, and a better outcome than those presenting with hemorrhagic infarction or frank hemorrhage. The endocrine replacement requirements were similar in both groups.

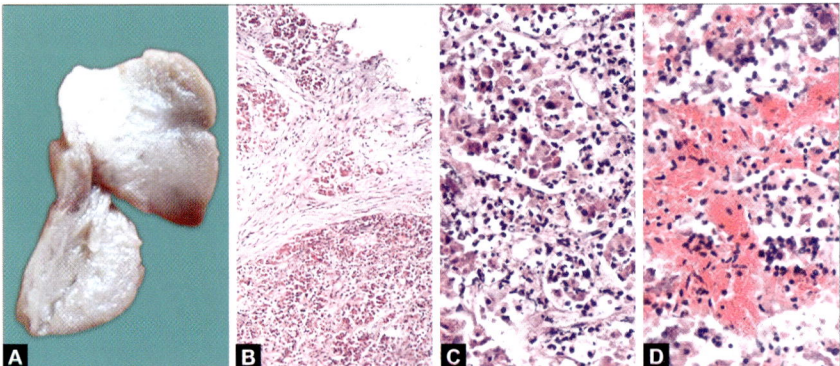

FIGS. 15A TO D: (A) Gross specimen of the enlarged pituitary; (B) Junction between the well circumscribed adenoma and normal compressed pituitary at the periphery (H&E ×100); (C) Area of necrosis showing neutrophils and loss of cells in the adenoma (H&E ×400); (D) Hemorrhage in the adenoma (H&E ×400).

Case 9

PEDIATRIC AUTOPSY

Pragati Sathe

Clinical History

A 15-minute-old female child was born vaginally to a 19-year-old primigravida by vertex presentation. The child was full term and weighed 2.6 kg. The baby did not cry immediately after birth. The heart rate was 10 beats/min and there was no spontaneous respiration. The baby was intubated and given bag and mask ventilation. However, these measures were not successful and the neonate succumbed. The antenatal ultrasonography performed at 34 weeks of gestation showed severe oligohydramnios, enlarged hyperechoic polycystic kidneys and mega cisterna magna. There was no contributory past or family history or history of consanguinity.

Autopsy Findings

A complete autopsy was performed. The abdominal circumference, chest circumference, crown-rump length and crown-heel length was 35, 34, 33 and 50 cm, respectively. The shape of the skull was distorted with a conical protuberance posteriorly. The anteroposterior diameter was 25 cm and the lateral diameter, 22 cm. On opening of cranial cavity, 100–150 mL straw colored clear cerebrospinal fluid oozed out. Meninges appeared hazy. There was a kink in the cervicomedullary junction that was suggestive of Arnold-Chiari malformation (**Fig. 16**). Serial coronal

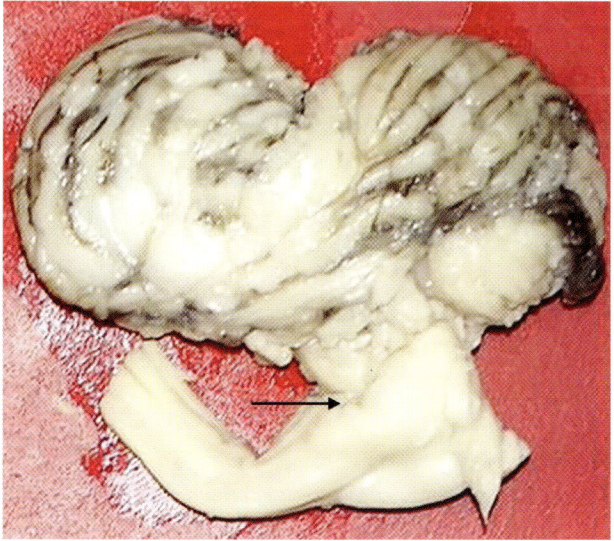

FIG. 16: Arrow points to the kink in the cervicomedullary junction.

slices revealed hydrocephalus. On opening of thoracic cavity, the pleurae were thin and shiny. Bilaterally, the lungs were small in size (the lower borders not reaching the lower border of the heart, **Fig. 17**) and rubbery to feel. The heart was normal. On opening of abdominal cavity, there was no free fluid. The liver, spleen and gastrointestinal tract did not reveal any abnormality. The kidneys weighed 100 g each. The reniform shape was maintained but the surface was bosselated and also showed the fetal lobulations. On cut surface, corticomedullary junction was not well-defined with distortion of the pelvicalyceal system and multiple cysts, linear in the cortex and more spherical in the medulla.

On microscopy, kidneys showed a disorganized parenchyma. There were dilated tubules (**Fig. 18A**) lined by flattened to cuboidal epithelium with luminal eosinophilic fluid. Occasional glomeruli were seen. The intervening parenchyma showed fibrosis, thick nerve bundles, lymphocytic collections and foci of calcification. Few tubules were surrounded by mesenchymal collars and lined by dysplastic epithelium. Microscopy was suggestive of autosomal recessive polycystic kidney disease (ARPKD) with focal dysplasia. The lungs showed irregularly expanded parenchyma. The line drawn from the terminal bronchiole to the pleural surface showed <4 and half alveolar spaces suggestive of lung hypoplasia. The liver showed multiple foci of extramedullary hematopoiesis. The portal tracts are expanded due to proliferation of bile ductules at the periphery (**Fig. 18B**) and hepatic arteriole and portal venules in the center. No cystic dilatations of bile ductules were seen. The features were suggestive of congenital hepatic fibrosis (CHF). The cause of death was related to multiple congenital anomalies.

Autosomal recessive polycystic kidney disease[21] has four subgroups as follows: (1) Perinatal; (2) Neonatal; (3) Infantile; and (4) Juvenile depending on their age of presentation. This case belongs to the first subgroup which presents around birth with the kidney disease and lung hypoplasia. The CHF is an incidental finding

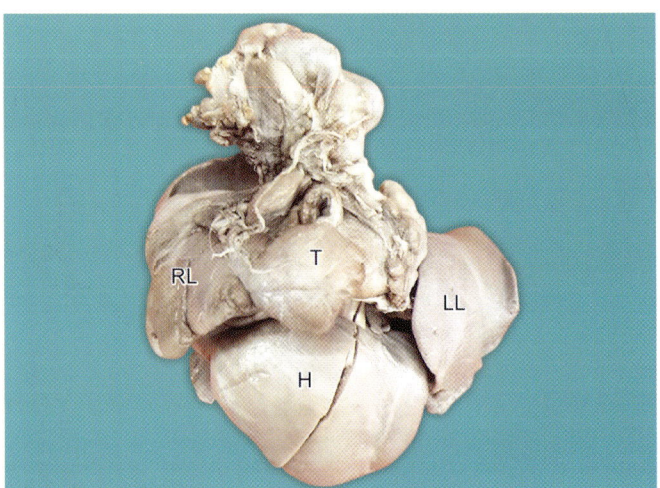

(H: heart; LL: left lung; RL: right lung; T: thymus)

FIG. 17: The heart and lung block showing bilateral lung hypoplasia.

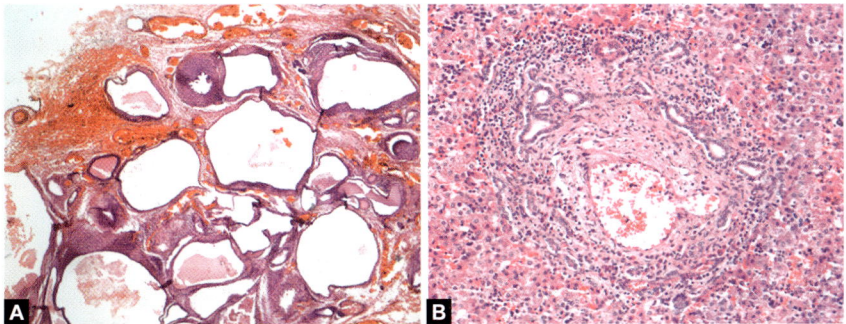

FIGS. 18A AND B: (A) Dilated tubules lined by cuboidal epithelium with luminal pink fluid; (B) Proliferation of bile ductules in the portal tract (H&E ×400).

without manifestation of portal hypertension in this age group. ARPKD and CHF have been grouped under fibrocystic diseases with "ciliopathy" being the underlying pathogenesis.[22] Oligohydramnios is one of the most common factors leading to lung hypoplasia. Due to polycystic renal disease there is decreased formation of urine. Urine is the main contributor to the volume of the amniotic fluid. Thus, there is an absence of good amount of amniotic fluid. For normal development of the lung, the main physical force is the breathing movements of the fetus leading to stretching of the chest cavity. Oligohydramnios leads to reduction in the size of thoracic cavity thus hampering the normal lung development leading to pulmonary hypoplasia. The severity of lung hypoplasia usually decides the prognosis. At least 40% of lung volume is needed for survival. So, in an autopsy showing any one of these findings, one has to look for abnormalities in other organs as well. The importance of an autopsy in cystic renal diseases is mainly to know the type and thus the pattern of inheritance. This helps in genetic counseling for future pregnancies.

Case 10

URINARY SYSTEM AND GASTROINTESTINAL TRACT

Dhaneshwar Lanjewar

Clinical History

A 55-year-old male presented with swelling over upper and lower extremities, abdominal distension, and difficulty in micturition of 15 days' duration. There was no history of chest pain, dyspnea/orthopnea, cough, palpitation, fever, skin rashes, pain in abdomen, and neck rigidity. There was no history of hypertension, diabetes mellitus, chronic obstructive lung disease and tuberculosis. The clinical examination revealed that the patient was moderately built conscious and well oriented to time, place and person with pitting edema of the extremities. His pulse was 84/min, blood pressure 160/110 mmHg and respiratory rate of 19/min. Chest auscultation revealed normal heart sounds and clear chest. His abdomen was distended. Significant laboratory investigations were hemoglobin (Hb) 4.6 g/dL, serum creatinine 7.9 mg/dL and blood urea 239 mg/dL. A provisional diagnosis of chronic renal failure (CRF) was made. On 6th day of admission, the patient suddenly collapsed, became pulseless and died. A clinical autopsy was advised to know cause of sudden death.

Autopsy Findings

External examination showed edema of upper and lower extremities, and of the scrotum. Severe pallor was noted; the skin did not show petechial hemorrhages. In-situ examination showed normal dura and leptomeninges. The heart was enlarged in size (cardiomegaly). The lungs and pleurae were normal. The peritoneal cavity showed 500 mL of clear watery fluid. The stomach, liver and spleen were normal. The serosa of small intestine and large intestine had cyanotic bluish appearance. There was no evidence of peritonitis.

Systemic examination showed that the heart was enlarged due to left ventricular hypertrophy. The anterior surface of heart, 3 cm proximal to the apex showed a grayish-white irregular milk patch measuring 2.5 × 1.5 cm in size. The right-sided chambers and valves and the left atrium and mitral valve were normal. The left ventricular myocardial thickness was 2 cm with a small sized cavity-concentric hypertrophy (**Fig. 19**). There was no evidence of recent or old infarct; the endocardium was also smooth. The aortic valve was thin and shiny. The left anterior descending (LAD) and left circumflex (LCA), arteries showed about 50% luminal narrowing by a yellow atheromatous plaque. The esophagus and stomach showed normal walls. The serosal

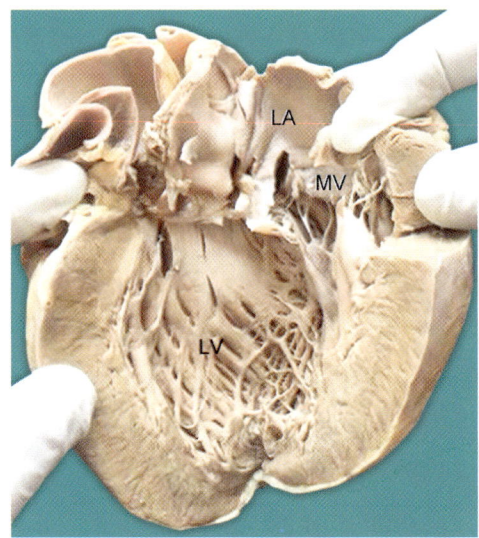

(LA: left atrium; MV: mitral valve)

FIG. 19: Opened out left ventricular (LV) inflow tract showing moderate concentric hypertrophy.

surface of small and large intestines showed slightly bluish tinge. The lumen of entire small and large intestine showed presence of blood clots (**Figs. 20A** and **B**). There was no evidence of ulcer and or tumor. The left kidney measured 6 × 4 × 3 cm and the right kidney measured 5 × 4 × 3 cm in size. Both kidneys were small contracted with coarse granularity and 2–3 irregular depressed scars (**Figs. 20C** and **D**). The cortex was narrow and indistinct; medulla and pelvicalyceal system appeared normal. The gross examination of other organs showed normal features.

The microscopic findings of heart showed hypertrophic cardiomyocytes. The histology of the LAD and LCA showed presence of atherosclerosis. The histology of small intestine and large intestine showed presence of blood clots. The histology of both kidneys showed hyalinization and periglomerular fibrosis of 90% of the glomeruli. The tubules were small and atrophic, and few tubules were dilated and showed pink secretion (thyroidization). The interstitium showed interstitial fibrosis and intense mononuclear cell infiltration. The walls of the arterioles were thickened due to concentric fibrosis with luminal narrowing. The microscopic examination of other organs did not show any specific findings.

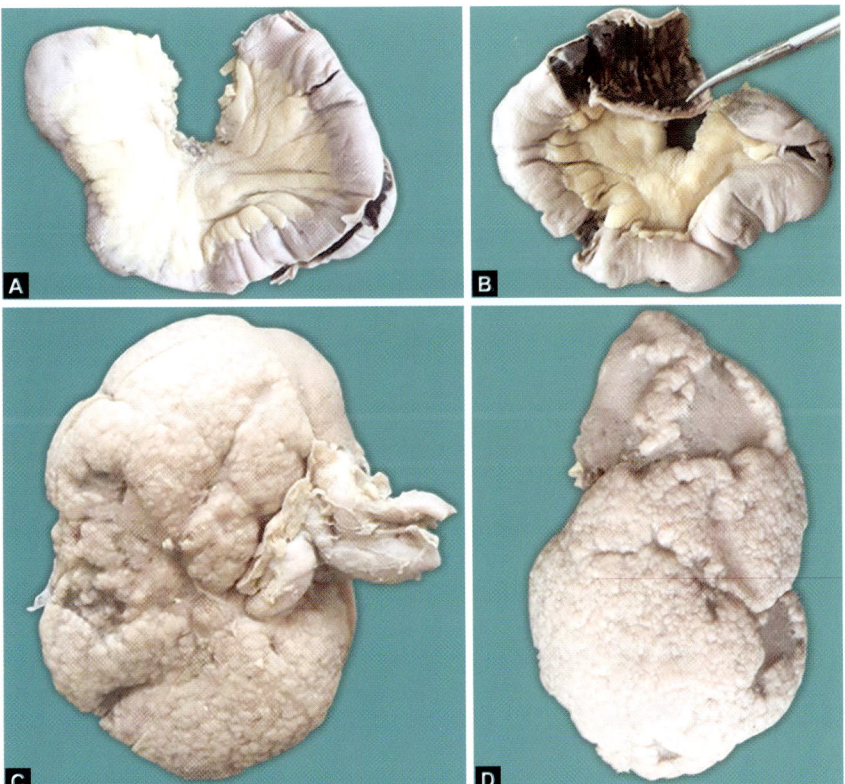

FIGS. 20A TO D: (A) Slight bluish discoloration of the serosal aspect of a loop of the small intestine; (B) Presence of luminal blood clot; (C and D) Both right and left kidneys are contracted with coarse granularity and broad scars.

Cause of death: Immediate cause of death—hypovolemic shock due to bleeding in small and large intestines. The secondary cause is—CRF due to chronic interstitial nephritis.

The clinical presentation in this case would have begun with the urinary tract infection. This infection progressed to bilateral chronic interstitial nephritis due to which patient developed CRF. In CRF, there is retention of sodium along with retention of water, explaining the development of generalized anasarca in the present case. Increased level of serum creatinine and blood urea is also explained on the basis of CRF. In renal failure, hypertension is produced by increase in sympathetic activity and increase in vasoconstriction. The cardiomegaly due to left ventricular hypertrophy is produced due to hypertension. At admission this patient had Hb value of 4.9 g/dL, which in renal disease is caused by decrease erythropoietin. In addition, CRF shows increase concentration of factor VIII-related antigen (VIII-RA), increase factor VIII procoagulant activity and decrease in factor VIII-von Willebrand factor activity.[23,24] This functional abnormality of the factor VIII protein may partly explain the prolonged bleeding time commonly found in patients with CRF. In addition platelets aggregation and adhesion defect are observed in patients with CRF. The blood clots in small and large intestine found in this patient were secondary to CRF. The gastrointestinal tract bleeding is found in 1-3% patients with CRF.[25]

Case 11

RESPIRATORY SYSTEM

Pradeep Vaideeswar, Saranya Singaravel

Clinical History

A 40-year-old postmenopausal woman presented with intermittent fever, chills, bodyache, easy fatigability and generalized weakness for 2 months. She had been admitted in a private hospital, where she was given symptomatic treatment and was transfused with packed red cells. On examination, she was afebrile with a pulse rate of 94/min, blood pressure of 140/90 mmHg and extreme pallor. Systemic examination had been normal. Her complete blood counts were as follows: Hb 5.2 g/dL, total leukocyte count 1500/mm^3, platelet count 84000/mm^3. The peripheral smears showed very few leukocytes with marked anisopoikilocytosis, hypochromasia and few nucleated red cells. Buffy coat smears were prepared, which revealed few atypical cells of myeloblast morphology (myeloperoxidase positive). There was mild elevation of the transaminases (SGOT/SGPT–159/564 U/L) and bilirubin (total/direct–1.49/0.51 mg/dL); rest of the biochemical investigations had been normal. She was started on intravenous antibiotics. Subsequently, she became drowsy with bradycardia and hypotension. She did not respond to resuscitative measures.

Autopsy Findings

A complete autopsy was performed. There was moderate cardiomegaly (weight 290 g) with mild biventricular dilatation and a thin film of fibrinous exudate. The atria, atrioventricular and arterial valves were normal. Both the lungs were of normal size and shape. The visceral pleura showed multiple foci of congestion with pale granular exudates, below which were present multiple soft hemorrhagic foci of consolidation (**Fig. 21**). Smaller foci were also seen in the rest of the parenchyma. Cavitation was not present. The arteries within and adjacent to these foci showed the presence of fresh thrombi. On histology, there was coagulative necrosis of the alveolar septa (**Fig. 22A**), which focally were lined by prominent hyaline membranes. The arteries showed fresh thrombi within which were the fungal elements (**Fig. 22B**). The spaces contained pale pink wispy to granular eosinophilic material. The parenchyma was traversed by lightly basophilic slender septate fungal hyphae (**Fig. 22C**) suggesting *Aspergillus* species. There was hardly any inflammatory reaction around these areas. Blasts were seen within the bone marrow, liver and spleen.

This was an example of angioinvasive pulmonary aspergillosis developing in a setting of aleukemic acute myeloid leukemia. *Aspergillus* is a ubiquitous fungus that can produce a wide spectrum of clinical features depending on the immune status of the host and the presence of underlying structural lung disease. The sinonasal tract and lungs are the most commonly involved sites, reflecting the portals of entry of the infectious asexual spores (conidia). The gastrointestinal tract and skin are less commonly involved. The term pulmonary aspergillosis[26] encompasses allergic bronchopulmonary aspergillosis (a hypersensitivity reaction to fungi in asthmatic individuals), aspergilloma (noninvasive colonization of a pre-existing pulmonary cavity by a fungus ball), chronic necrotizing aspergillosis (semi-invasive fungal infection accompanied by necrotizing granulomatous inflammation), and invasive/angioinvasive aspergillosis (invasion of blood vessels by fungal hyphae).

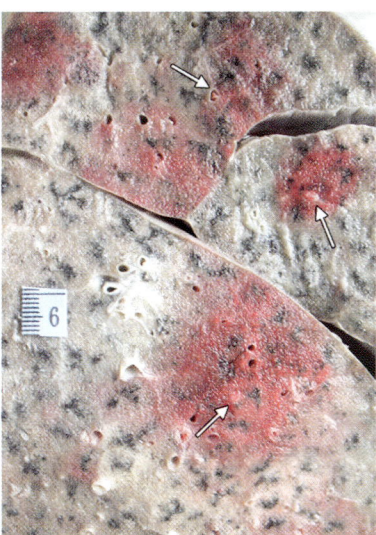

FIG. 21: Pale red foci of consolidation with arterial thrombi (arrows).

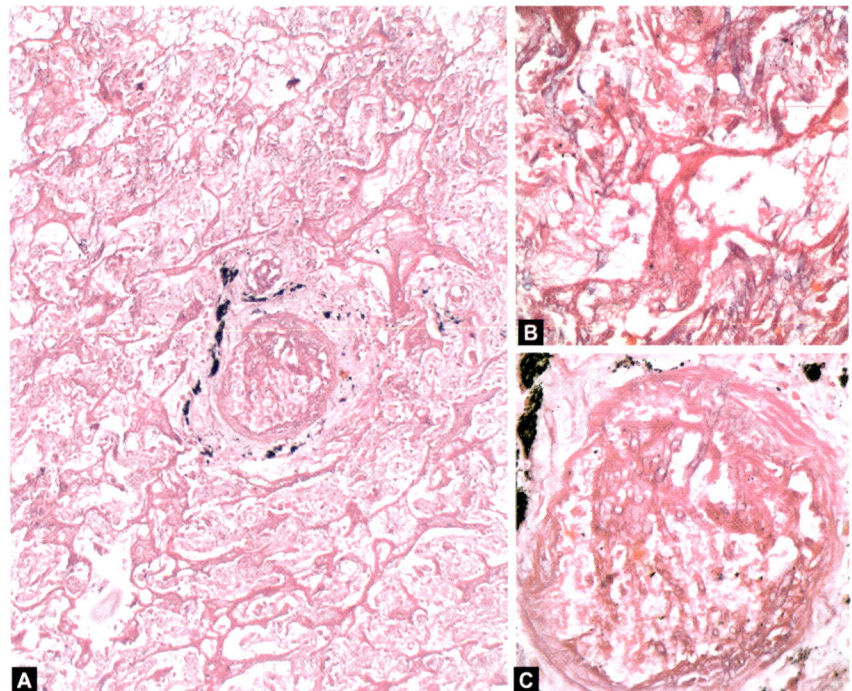

FIGS. 22A TO C: (A) An artery in the center is occluded. The surrounding parenchyma shows coagulative necrosis with deposits of fibrin over the septa (H&E ×100); Fungal hyphae are present in the (B) Necrotic parenchyma (H&E ×400) and (C) Artery (H&E ×400).

Neutrophil NADPH oxidase and activation of antimicrobial proteases constitute the most important host defenses against fungal hyphae. Neutropenia (absolute neutrophil count <500/μL) for >10 days is the most classic high-risk factor for invasive aspergillosis.[27] Other factors may be intermediate risk (prolonged treatment with corticosteroids or immunosuppressives; solid organ and lung transplantation; autologous bone marrow transplantation; HIV infection; solid organ cancer) or low-risk (intensive care unit stay; chronic obstructive pulmonary disease; hepatocellular and/or renal failure; steroid treatment of short duration; malnutrition; postcardiac surgery status; construction activity in or around hospital premises; contamination with ventilation systems).[27]

The key pathologic finding in invasive aspergillosis (and other invasive fungal pneumonias) is invasion of blood vessels by fungal hyphae, often accompanied by thrombosis, which produces areas of hemorrhage and infarction.[28] Grossly, target lesions (zone of necrosis surrounded by a hemorrhagic rim) are characteristic of invasive aspergillosis. Microscopically, they are comprised of a central zone of ischemic necrosis, surrounded by a zone of fibrinous exudate and a zone of parenchymal hemorrhage; neutrophils were absent in this case.

Although the majority of septate fungal hyphae with narrow-angle branching in the lung represent *Aspergillus*, this organism cannot be distinguished from morphologically similar fungi such as *Pseudallescheria* and *Fusarium* species; cultures are required for definitive identification.[29] Serum galactomannan is a useful laboratory test for invasive aspergillosis, and voriconazole is the antifungal agent of choice.[29]

Case 12

CENTRAL NERVOUS, CARDIOVASCULAR AND RESPIRATORY SYSTEMS

Bishan Radotra

Clinical History

A middle aged man was diagnosed as a case of myasthenia gravis about 13 years back. He was investigated and found to have a mediastinal mass which turned out be a cortical thymoma (**Figs. 23A** and **B**). Since then he was under neurology follow-up. He was being treated with prednisolone, neostigmine, pyridostigmine and azathioprine, without any crisis till date. Currently, he presented with fever for 2 months, which was moderate to high grade, intermittent and associated with chills and rigor. He also had holocranial headache, which was associated with nausea. There was no diurnal variation. There was no blurring of vision, diplopia, focal deficit or seizure. There was history of anorexia and significant weight loss. He was a nonsmoker and nonalcoholic. He had no skin rash, cough, expectoration, chest pain, dyspnea, abdominal pain,

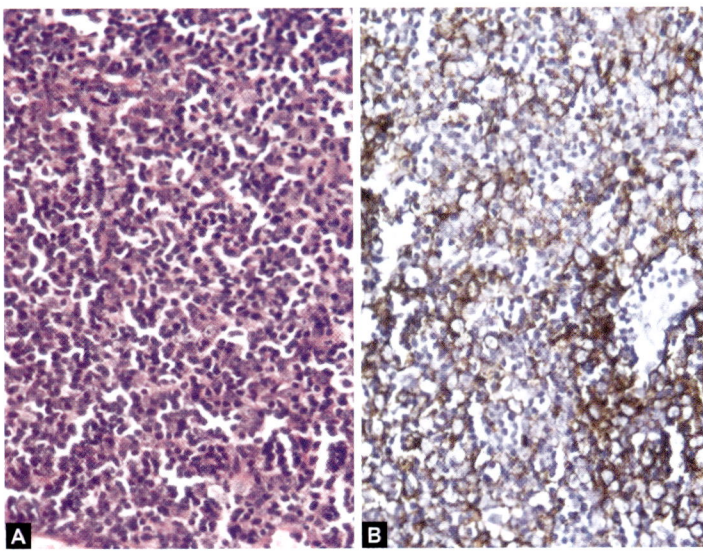

FIGS. 23A AND B: Cortical thymoma: (A) H&E ×400; (B) Cytokeratin immunohistochemistry (×400).

diarrhea, jaundice or joint pain. On examination, he had Cushingoid facies with a pulse rate of 98/min and blood pressure of 130/90 mmHg. Examination of the thorax was normal. Striae were present on lower abdomen. The central nervous system examination revealed normal fundus. There was terminal neck rigidity and right VI nerve palsy. The Kernig's sign was negative and power was 5/5 in all limbs. All his reflexes were 2+ and planter was down.

Hemogram revealed normal hemoglobin, platelets, total and differential leukocyte counts. The peripheral smear for malarial parasite was negative; card test for malarial parasite was also negative. The coagulogram was normal. The liver function tests, renal function tests and serum electrolytes were within normal range. The cerebrospinal fluid (CSF) examination revealed raised protein 258 mg/dL and reduced sugar level 9 mg/dL (corresponding blood sugar 154 mg/dL). Cytology of CSF revealed 90 cells with 70% neutrophils. The CSF adenosine deaminase level was 6 U/L. The polymerase chain reaction for *Mycobacterium tuberculosis* was negative. The India ink preparation did not reveal any *Cryptococcus*; however, *Cryptococcus* latex agglutination was positive. The multiple blood cultures were sterile and blood fungal serology for *Candida* and *Aspergillus* species were negative. The serology for HBV/HCV/HIV was all negative. At admission, the urine routine examination was normal. The urine culture grew *Enterococcus*, which was sensitive to vancomycin but resistant to ampicillin, ciplox and nitrofurantoin on one occasion. Subsequent urine culture after 4 days grew *Pseudomonas* sensitive to cephalosporin but resistant to ciplox. Urine cultures at other three occasions were sterile.

Computed tomography (CT) of paranasal sinuses was normal. Magnetic resonance imaging of the brain revealed multiple T2 and flair hyperintensities in bilateral basal ganglia and subcortical white matter of right parietal region, suggestive of ischemic changes. CT chest and abdomen revealed lung nodules and consolidation in bilateral lower lobe, suggestive of infective etiology. A compression ultrasonogram did not reveal any deep venous thrombosis.

In view of *Cryptococcus* latex agglutination positivity in CSF, the patient was started on ceftriaxone and amphotericin B. The patient initially improved for 1 week. But there was recurrence of fever with generalized tonic clonic seizures. As urine culture grew enterococcus, teicoplanin was added. The patient developed leukopenia and elevated transaminases. On day 34 of hospital stay, patient developed high-grade fever and diarrhea. Subsequently he developed hypovolemic shock and altered sensorium. He ultimately succumbed to his illness and an autopsy was requested.

Autopsy Findings

A complete autopsy was performed. The brain weighed 1,350 g. The external examination revealed thin meningeal exudate over both cerebral convexities, the base, the brain stem and the cerebellum. There was no herniation. The blood vessels of the circle of Willis were of medium caliber, with no atheroma. On coronal slicing of the brain, the right putamen showed about 0.8 cm granular cavitating lesion (**Fig. 24**); similar lesions were also seen in the thalamus. On microscopic examination, chronic meningitis with lymphomononuclear inflammation (**Fig. 25A**) admixed with multinucleate giant cells. Many cryptococci were noted under higher magnification in the exudate and in the giant cells (**Figs. 25B** and **C**). Foci of necrosis and ill-formed

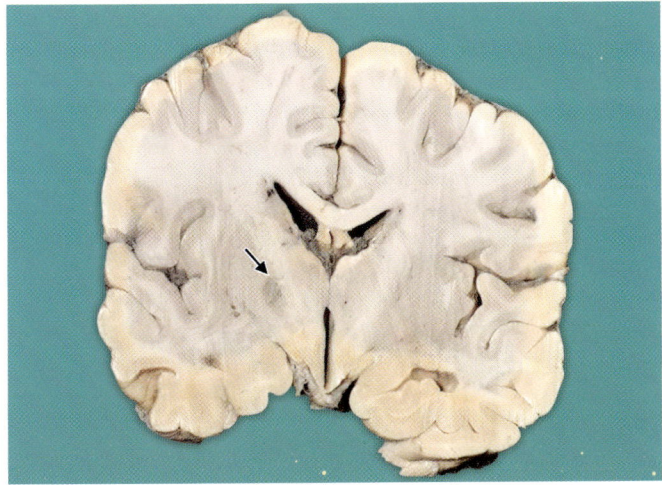

FIG. 24: Coronal slice of brain showing a small cavitary lesion in putamen (arrow).

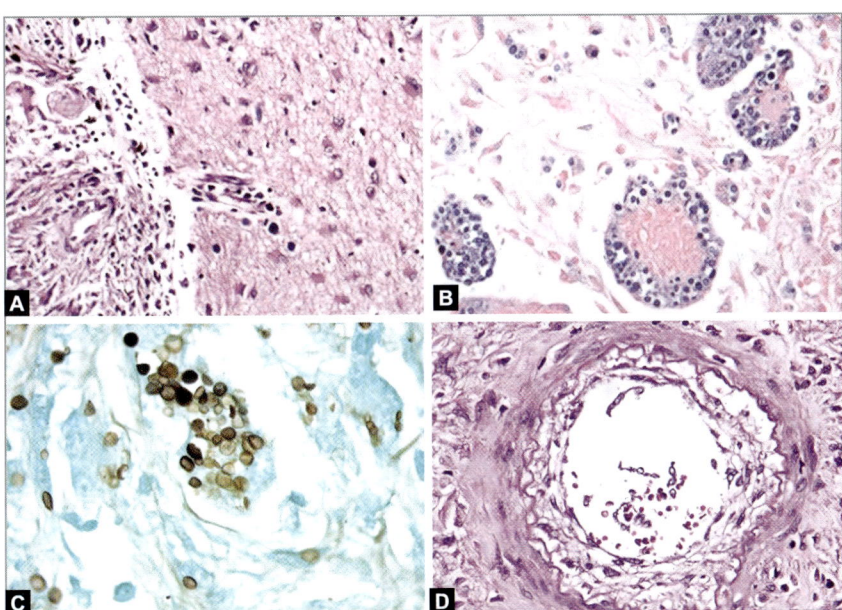

FIGS. 25A TO D: (A) Chronic leptomeningeal exudates; (B) Numerous Cryptococci within the multinucleated giant cells (Alcian blue ×400); (C) Many cryptococci in the leptomeningeal exudates (Gomori methenamine silver ×400); (D) Endarteritis and periarteritis of the leptomeningeal arteries in subarachnoid space (H&E ×400).

granulomas were present. The inflammatory exudate extended to the Virchow–Robin spaces with periarteritis and endarteritis (**Fig. 25D**), resulting in small infarcts. Few parenchymal cryptococcomas, marked choroid plexitis and ventriculitis were present.

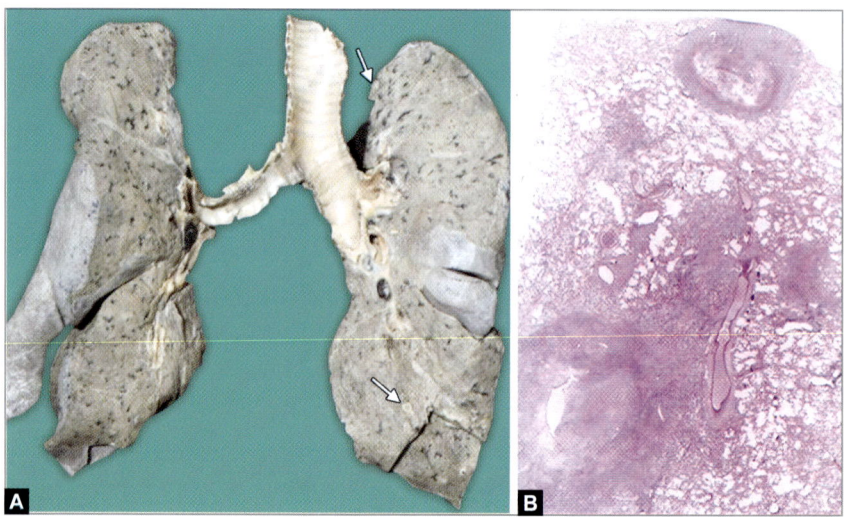

FIGS. 26A AND B: (A) Cut surface of the lungs shows normal tracheobronchial tree and a few subpleural and intraparenchymal nodules (arrows); (B) Scanned slide (H&E) showing subpleural and parenchymal necrotic lesions surrounded by fibrosis.

The pleural cavities contained about 500 mL fluid. The lungs were 950 g with few pleural adhesions. Subpleural and parenchymal nodular yellowish-white lesions (0.5–1.0 cm) were present (**Figs. 26A** and **B**). Histology revealed well-defined granulomatous lesions, some with central necrosis and some with organization and fibrosis. Multinucleated giant cells containing cryptococci were demonstrated (**Figs. 27A** and **B**).

The heart weighed 370 g. There was concentric left ventricular hypertrophy. The heart valves were normal. The left atrium contained partially adherent thrombus. The arch of aorta showed many ulcerated grade III atheromatous plaques. A large thrombus was sticking to one of the atheromas area and had extended into the aortic arch branches (**Figs. 28 A** and **B**). The left atrial and aortic thrombi contained fungal hyphae consistent with the morphology of *Aspergillus* (**Fig. 28C**) causing pericarditis, rupture of aortic wall and periaortitis. Large blood clots surrounded and encircled the great vessels and periaortic area (**Fig. 28D**).

The liver weighed 1350 g. It was mildly enlarged and soft in consistency. Mild portal inflammation and focal fatty change were present. The spleen weighed 150 g and revealed only congestion. The gastrointestinal tract, kidneys, adrenals, and testes did not show any significant pathology. The bone marrow was normally cellular representing all three components.

The final autopsy diagnosis was:
   In a known case of myasthenia gravis due to cortical thymoma on immunosuppressive therapy treatment:
- Disseminated cryptococcosis: Cerebromeningeal and pulmonary.
- Left atrial *Aspergillus* mural endocarditis and grade III complicated atherosclerosis with *Aspergillus* aortitis and aortic arch rupture.

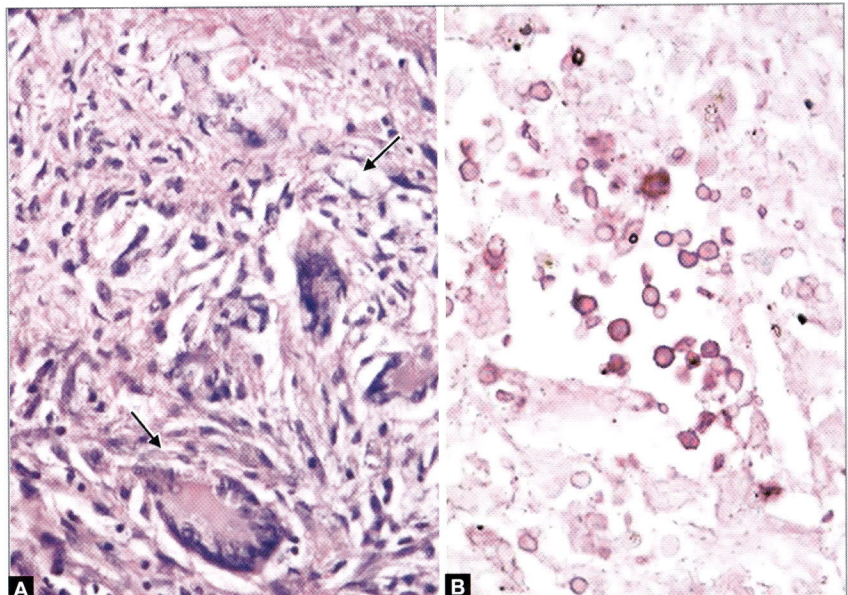

FIGS. 27A AND B: (A) Lung showing granulomatous inflammation with multinucleate giant cells containing cryptococci (arrows); (B) The organisms are better appreciated in mucicarmine stain (× 400).

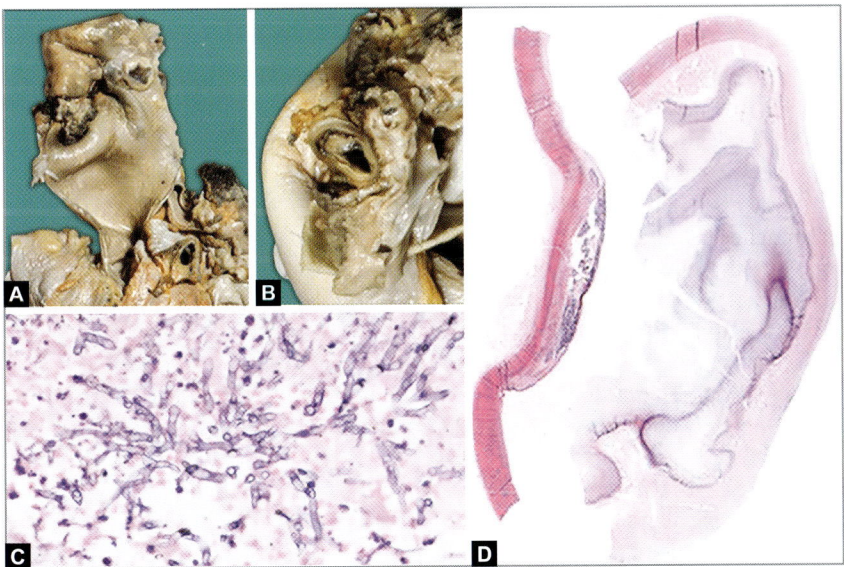

FIGS. 28A TO D: (A) The ascending aorta shows atheroma and a large thrombus; (B) The thrombus was extended to right brachiocephalic artery; (C) Slender, septate, lightly basophilic fungal hyphae resembling those of the *Aspergillus* species; (D) Scanned slide (H&E) showing calcified atheroma in the ascending aorta and periaortic blood clots.

This autopsy case demonstrates that autopsy is an essential approach to help our clinicians comprehend their uncertainties. It is an illustration of mortality in a patient of thymoma associated myasthenia gravis, who was doing well after surgery and during chemotherapy. He developed cryptococcal meningitis disseminating from a primary source in lungs and was treated with amphotericin B and showed partial improvement. During his hospital stay, patient developed high-grade fever, hypovolemic shock and altered sensorium and he suddenly succumbed to his illness. The cause of his sudden demise even when he was improving initially with amphotericin was a surprise and unexplained for the treating unit and hence an autopsy was requested.

At autopsy, cryptococcal meningitis was confirmed. The meningeal exudate was very thick at places and revealed multinucleate giant cells containing numerous cryptococci indicating it to be chronic meningitis. Giant cell reaction is an unusual feature of cryptococcal meningitis as generally this infection evokes a sparse inflammatory response mainly with histiocytes and lymphocytes. In this case because of presence of cryptococci predominantly in giant cells and only a few in the circulating CSF may be the cause of negative CSF India ink preparation of this patient. The bilateral subcortical white matter and basal ganglia hyperintensities seen on MRI brain were due to multiple small cryptococcomas as well as distended Virchow–Robin spaces due to extension of exudate along the vessels.

The surprise in this case was fungal left atrial mural endocarditis and aortic fungal arteritis which caused necrosis of the aortic wall leading to aortic rupture; large blood clots compressed the root of aorta. The aortic rupture explains the sudden cause of death in this patient. The disseminated cryptococcosis in this case was not the immediate cause of death. Both the fungi, i.e., *Cryptococcus* and *Aspergillus* in this case were due to immunosuppression caused by long-term treatment with prednisolone and azathioprine. The former was a chronic infection and the latter was an acute event and acquired during his hospital stay. The isolated involvement of left atrium by fungus can occur rarely. The involvement of ascending aorta and its root by *Aspergillus* has been reported but again it is extremely rare.[30] Most cases of fungal aortitis have been reported postsurgery for aortic valve replacement or other manipulations or even on prosthetic valves.[31] Even large homogeneous floating mass, athrombus/vegetation in the aortic archas a part of systemic aspergillosis is also reported.[32] In this case, the fungal mass occurred on areas of aorta which were involved by atheromatous plaques. There was no valvular endocarditis in this case. Although the autopsy on this patient explains the sudden demise of this patient, however, there are still limitations. Firstly, the entire length of aorta was not kept by the prosector and one does not know whether rest of aorta was involved by fungus or not. Secondly, the primary source of *Aspergillus* infection is not known in this case. Although it was acquired in the hospital, but a primary focus has not been demonstrated in the lungs which is usual route of infection. The primary mural endocarditis or aortitis is very rare. Extensive sampling of the lungs could have possibly solved this problem. Thirdly, CSF culture and sample from atrial or aortic thrombus were not taken at autopsy which could have given us the exact type/subtype of both fungi involved such as *Cryptococcus neoformans* or *gattii*. The morphologically of the *Aspergillus* resembles *Fusarium* and therefore it could be an odd presentation by a rare fungus, which we usually not encounter.

Case 13

MULTI-SYSTEM INVOLVEMENT

Bishan Radotra

Clinical History

A 42-year-old male with no previous comorbidities presented with history of fever and blood-mixed loose stools for 10 days. He also complained of vomiting and reduced urine output for 2 days. The fever was low-grade (100°F), 2–3 spikes/day and was not associated with night sweats; it was relieved with antipyretics. The frequency of loose stools was 6-7 times/day, small in volume, mucoid and associated with abdominal pain. The vomiting (3-4 times/day) was nonbloody, nonbilious and contained undigested food particles. There was history of loss of appetite. The urine output was reduced. The urine was high colored, but there was no history of hematuria or flank pain. There was no history of focal neurological deficit or seizure. There was no past history of diabetes mellitus, hypertension or contact with tuberculosis. He was a smoker and alcohol consumer.

At admission, the patient was conscious, oriented, with pulse rate of 72/min, respiratory rate of 18 per minute and blood pressure 80/60 mmHg. On systemic examination, the chest, cardiovascular system, abdomen and central nervous system were essentially normal. Subsequently during hospital stay, patient developed altered sensorium.

On hematological investigations, he had normal Hb of 12.4 g%, which declined to 5.6 g% during hospital stay over 2 weeks. There was leukopenia at admission which persisted till the last few days when he had leukocytosis. The differential count revealed initially neutropenia which gradually reversed and there was neutrophilia terminally. The platelet count also declined during hospital stay (137,000-58,000/mm^3 over 13 days). The peripheral film showed normocytic normochromic picture with few macrocytes; no spherocytes or schistocytes were present. His bone marrow trephine biopsy revealed necrotizing granulomatous inflammation (**Fig. 29**); however stain for AFB was negative.

His renal function test was normal initially, which subsequently worsened (urea 151 mg/dL and creatinine 3.9 mg d/L). The liver function tests did not show significant abnormality. Thyroid profile was normal and the cortisol level was 925 nmol/L. The C3 and C4 levels were 58.6 (normal range 90-180) and 26.0 (normal range 10-40), respectively. The other biochemical investigations and blood gas analysis were normal. The urine and stool routine examination were normal. The cerebrospinal fluid (CSF) examination revealed raised proteins 151 mg/dL, sugar 83 mg/dL (corresponding blood sugar 146 mg/dL) and 10 neutrophils. The AFB/GeneXpert/cryptococcal antigen tests on CSF were negative. The blood cultures were sterile throughout his hospital stay. The urine and stool cultures did not yield any organism. The endotracheal (ET) aspirate culture showed *Aspergillus fumigatus*. His Widal test was positive (1:320). The dengue serology (NS1/IgM/IgG) was negative. The tests

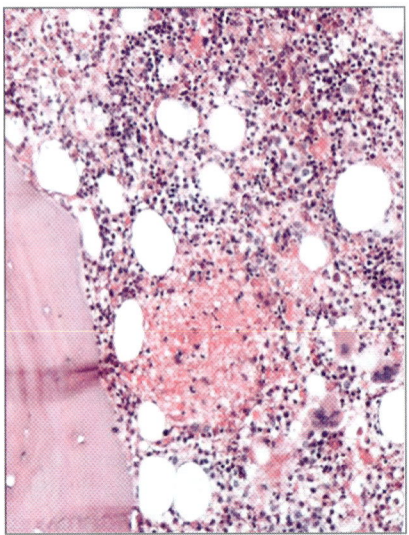

FIG. 29: Antemortem bone marrow trephine biopsy showing a necrotic granuloma (H&E ×400).

for HBsAg, HCV, EBV (IgM), CMV (IgM), leptospira/ scrub typhus and IgM/IgG for chikungunya were all negative. The IgM/IgG for Leishmania donovani was negative and malaria antigen test was negative.

His radiological investigations revealed a normal X-ray chest at admission (**Fig. 30A**). His subsequent X-ray (**Fig. 30B**) and computed tomography (CT) scan of the chest showed mild right pleural effusion as well as multiple small nodules progressing to fluffy alveolar opacities and consolidation in both lungs over the next 2 weeks. An abdominal ultrasonography a day after admission revealed a moderate fatty liver and prominent small bowel loops, suggestive of subacute intestinal obstruction. The CT of abdomen showed bilateral renal parenchymal disease with mild splenomegaly and mild ascites a week after admission. The echocardiography did not show any significant abnormality. His CT scan of head was normal (**Fig. 30C**).

This patient was treated with ciprofloxacin, metronidazole, doxycycline, ceftriaxone and azithromycin. Over the next 3 days, the patient developed paralytic ileus, which was attributed to hypokalemia and managed conservatively. On day 4, the blood cultures grew *Escherichia coli* and he was started on imipenem. As his ET aspirate showed septate hyphae and fungal culture revealed *Aspergillus fumigatus*, the patient was started on amphotericin on day 7. Later on the ET aspirate GeneXpert was positive for *Mycobacterium tuberculosis* and antituberculous therapy was started. Eventually, he developed refractory septic shock and succumbed to his illness after 13 days of hospital stay. At the time of his death, his final clinical diagnosis was considered as disseminated tuberculosis involving lung, bone marrow, central nervous system and gastrointestinal tract (GIT) with ventilator-associated colistin-resistant *Klebsiella/ Acinetobacter* pneumonia with sepsis-related acute kidney injury. The cause of death was considered as septic shock and an autopsy was requested.

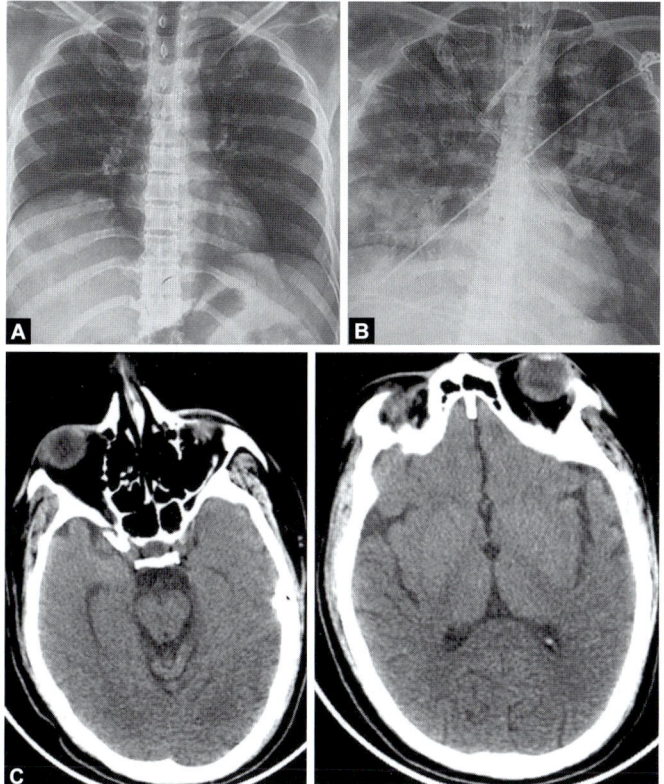

FIGS. 30A TO C: Chest X-ray—(A) Normal at admission; (B) Development of fluffy shadows during hospital stay; (C) CT scan of the head after admission did not show any abnormality.

Autopsy Findings

A complete autopsy was performed by a thoracoabdominal incision and brain was removed by a bitemporal incision. At autopsy, the serous cavities contained 210 mL of pleural fluid and 800 mL of peritoneal fluid. The bone marrow biopsy from vertebrae was cellular with all types of marrow elements (**Fig. 31A**). There were no granulomas; however, hemophagocytosis was prominent (**Figs. 31B** and **C**).

The brain weighed 1,220 g. External examination showed a 2 cm patch of subarachnoid hemorrhage in left temporal lobe. Multiple 0.1–0.2 mm hemorrhages were seen in the coronal slices, predominantly in the white matter on both sides of cerebral hemispheres; the involvement of the corpus callosum was noteworthy (**Fig. 32A**). Similar hemorrhages involved mid-brain, pons, medulla and cerebellum. Microscopically, most of these hemorrhages were fresh (**Fig. 32B**) and centered on a small vessel containing fibrin thrombus (**Figs. 32C** and **D**). Some of them were accompanied by a microglia reaction indicative of some duration. There was myelin loss in these hemorrhages and the axons were preserved.

The lungs were heavy (1,720 g) and firm to feel. The pleura was dull and fibrinous at many places. The tracheobronchial tree was congested and ulcerated. On cutting

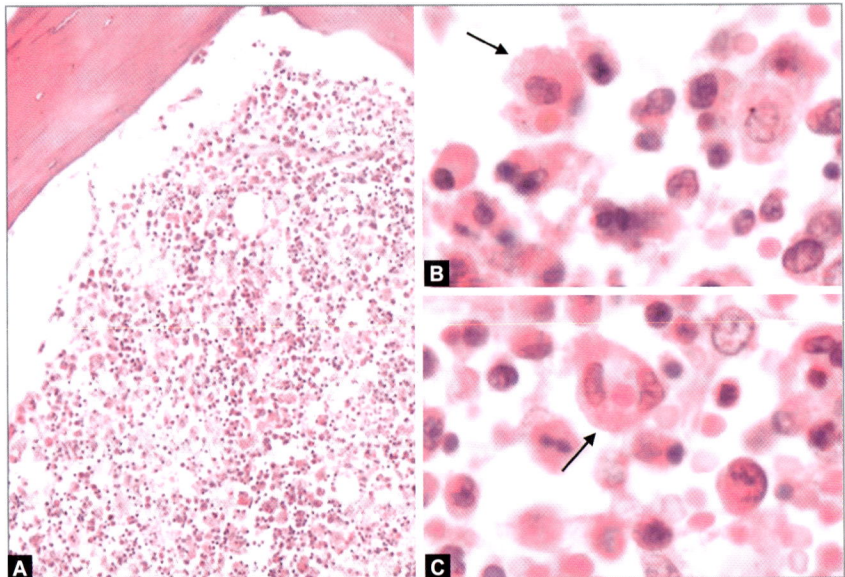

FIGS. 31A TO C: (A) Postmortem bone marrow biopsy showing all cell types, but there were more macrophages; there are no granulomas; (B and C) Prominent hemophagocytosis (arrows, H&E ×400).

the lungs, edema fluid could be exuded. The cut surface revealed consolidated and hemorrhagic areas with prominent well-demarcated necrotic areas and bronchocentric consolidations (**Fig. 33**). Histologically, the necrotic areas were surrounded by acute inflammatory cells response were confirmed (**Fig. 34A**). Bronchial destruction due to septate, dichotomously acute angle fungal hyphae consistent with morphology of *Aspergillus* was a prominent feature (**Figs. 34B** and **C**). There was alveolitis, alveolar hemorrhages and edema fluid. In other areas, organization of the alveolar exudate was noted in the form of Masson bodies. The gross examination of the GIT showed multiple variable-sized ulcers in the ileum, round to oval and mostly occurring along the longitudinal axis (**Fig. 35A**). Histological examination showed that many of these were submucosa deep with an underlying hypertrophied lymphoid tissue (**Fig. 35B**). The ulcers were covered over by inflammatory exudate which consisted of lymphohistiocytic cells; there was paucity of neutrophils. There was no fibrosis. A few large ulcers showed transmural inflammation, necrosis of the both muscle layers and significant organizing serositis. There was no significant mesenteric lymphadenopathy.

The liver was enlarged (weight 1,530 g) and appeared fatty (**Fig. 36A**). The microscopic examination revealed portoportal bridging with formation of incomplete nodules (**Fig. 36B**) with macrovesicular steatosis, centrilobular venular fibrosis (**Fig. 36C**), mild portal/lobular inflammation and numerous Mallory hyaline bodies (**Fig. 36D**). The sinusoids contained fibrin in many areas. The spleen was enlarged (280 g) and was markedly congested. The pancreas was normal. Both kidneys (weight 30 g each) were congested and showed superficial scars (**Fig. 37A**). Histologically,

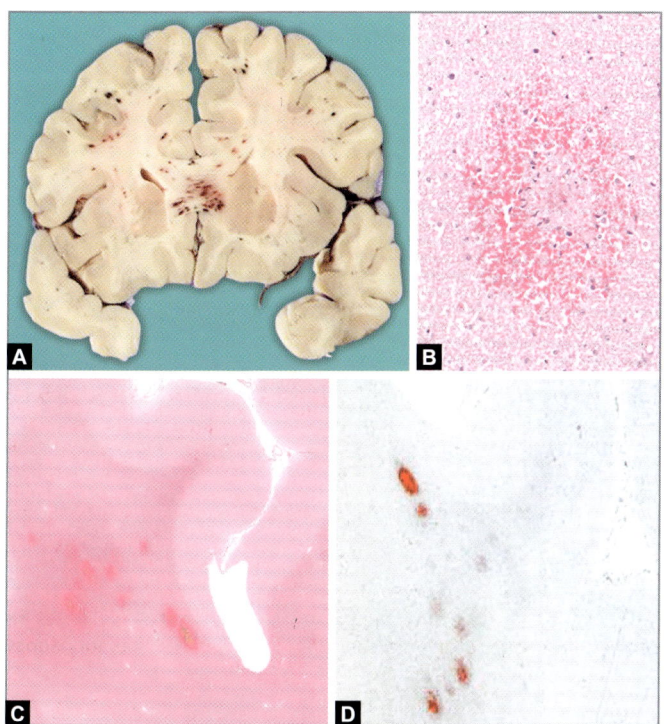

FIGS. 32A TO E: (A) Numerous pin-head sized hemorrhages involving central white matter and genu of the corpus callosum; (B and C) Fresh ring hemorrhages centered around a venule of the white matter; Scanner view of cortical sections showing D. Multiple hemorrhages in white matter (H&E) and E. Fibrin in the vessels (Martius scarlet blue).

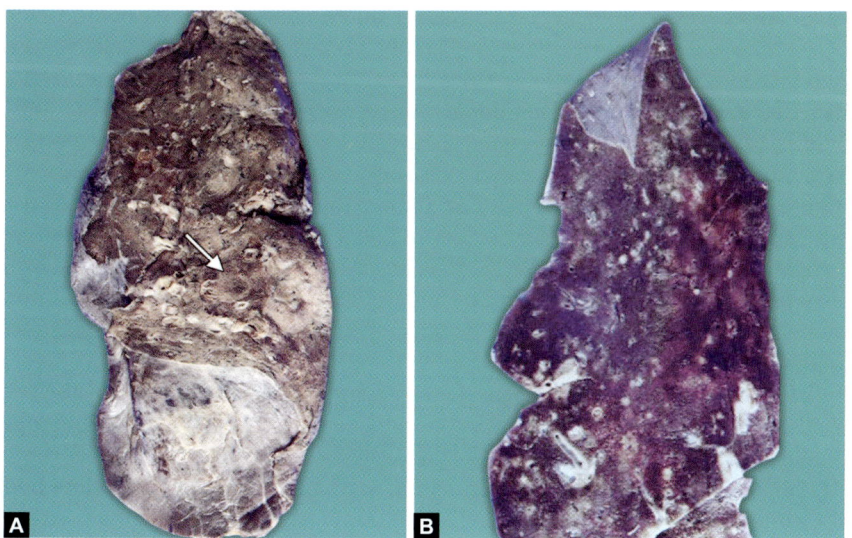

FIGS. 33A AND B: (A) Consolidated lung with areas of necrosis (arrow); (B) Bronchocentric distribution of small whitish areas of necrosis.

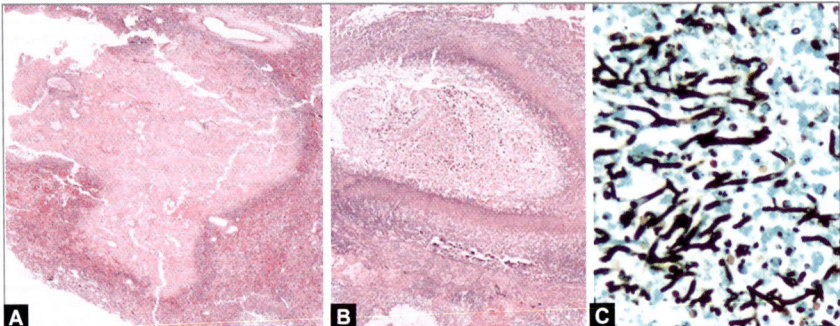

FIGS. 34A TO C: (A) Scanned slide (H&E) showing large necrotic area in pulmonary parenchyma involving some bronchi and surrounded by dense inflammatory reaction; (B) Scanned slide (H&E) showing necrotic wall with large fungal invasion into surrounding pulmonary parenchyma; (C) Dichotomously acute angle branching fungi (Gomori methenamine silver ×400).

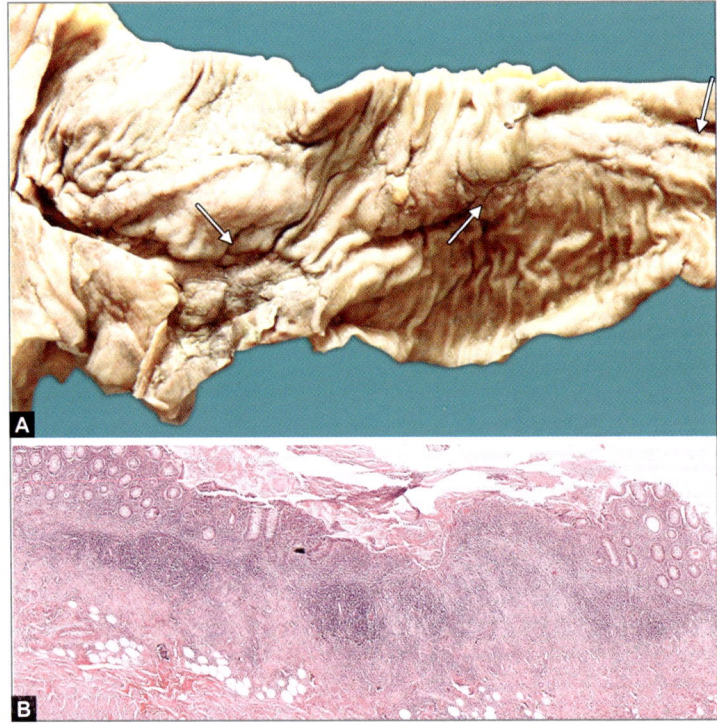

FIGS. 35A AND B: (A) Many variable sized longitudinal ulcers in the terminal ileum (arrows); (B) Large ulcer in the ileum over a Peyer's patch.

there was mesangiolysis in the glomeruli (**Fig. 37B**), venular fibrin thrombi (**Fig. 37C**) and granular and pigmented casts in the tubules (**Fig. 37D**). The urinary bladder was contracted and showed submucosal hemorrhages. The heart, thyroid and adrenals were normal.

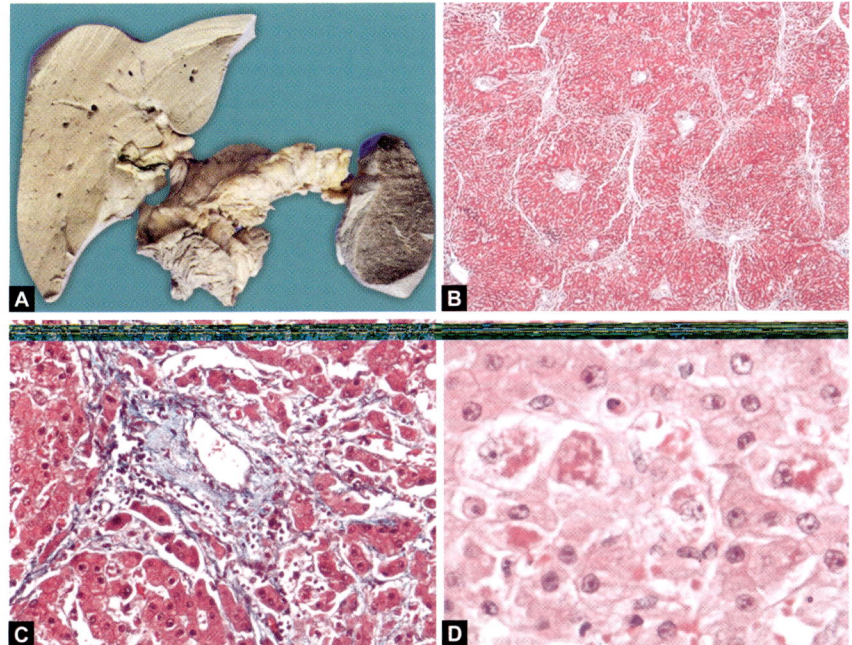

FIGS. 36A TO D: (A) The organ complex showing enlarged mild fatty liver, congested enlarged spleen and normal pancreas: (B) Portoportal bridging with appearance of incomplete nodule formation. (Masson trichrome ×100); (C) Centrivenular sclerosis seen as blue-green collagenic fibrosis (Masson trichrome ×400); (D) Numerous Mallory hyaline in hepatocytes (H&E ×400).

The final autopsy diagnosis was:
- Acute ileitis with multiple ulcers and perforation—*Salmonella* infection
- Alcohol-related steatohepatitis with bridging necrosis
- Invasive pulmonary aspergillosis
- Disseminated intravascular coagulation
- Pigmented cast nephropathy

This case was extensively investigated during life in the hospital; however the diagnosis of enteric perforation was missed. This patient had all the clinical symptoms and signs of an enteric fever and possible perforation including sluggish bowel sounds and sonographic findings of prominent small bowel loops suggesting of subacute intestinal obstruction.[33,34] The Widal test was also positive (1:320), although a rising titer was not demonstrated. The autopsy showed organizing serositis and myonecrosis of muscle wall of small gut indicative of an earlier sealed perforation. The finding of a necrotic granuloma in bone marrow trephine biopsy (although negative for AFB) misled the clinicians for diagnosis of tuberculosis. Such necrotic foci in bone marrow may be seen in any severe infection including typhoid and are not be a specific finding. To complicate further, GeneXpert on tracheal aspirate came out to be positive and therefore it substantiated the clinical diagnosis of tuberculosis. Presence of these two findings led to the diagnosis of disseminated tuberculosis and antituberculous therapy was started. False positivity of GeneXpert is well-known and should be kept in mind. This patient did not have any tuberculous focus anywhere in the body.

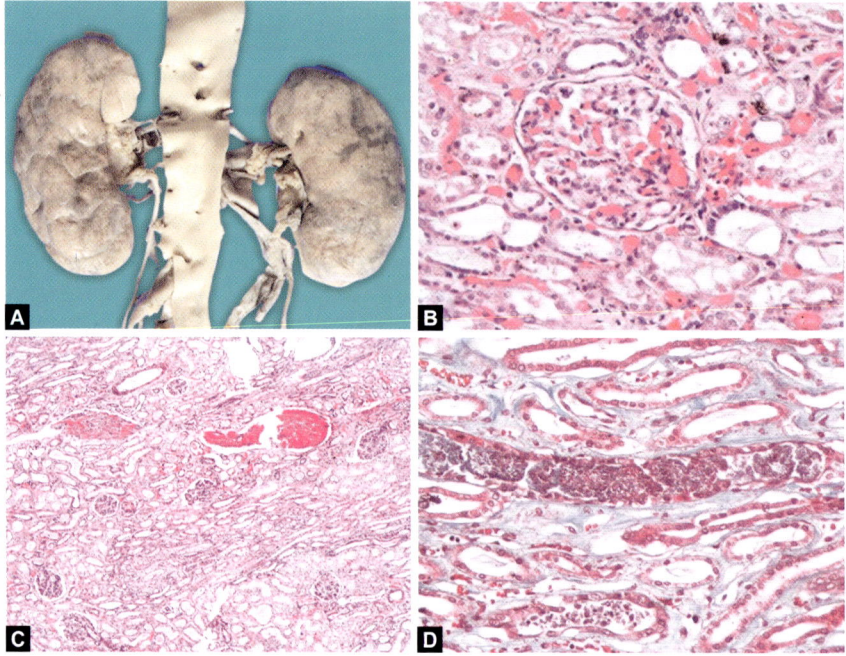

FIGS. 37A TO D: (A) Both kidneys show congestion and small superficial scars; (B) The glomeruli showed mesangiolysis (H&E ×400); (C) The small veins in the kidney were occluded with fibrin thrombi (H&E ×250); (D) Pigmented casts seen in the kidney tubules (Masson trichrome ×400).

During hospital stay, the patient acquired heavy fungal infection involving both lungs, which led to septicemia culminating into disseminated intravascular coagulation in which the brain was severely affected besides other organs.[35] The gradual fall in hemoglobin and platelets during hospital stay is attributed to disseminated intravascular coagulation, lung hemorrhages and secondary hemophagocytosis. The patient was alcohol consumer and revealed steatohepatitis with bridging necrosis. This patient died of acquired fungal infection with its accompanying complications.

Case 14

GASTROINTESTINAL TRACT

Dhaneshwar Lanjewar, Saroj Bolde

Clinical History

A 40-year-old female presented with pain in abdomen since 1 month and vomiting since 5 days. The abdominal pain was in the umbilical region. There is no history of fever, chills, cough, chest pain, hematemesis, or melena. The patient was non-hypertensive and nondiabetic mellitus. About 2 months ago, she was diagnosed as abdominal tuberculosis for which antituberculosis treatment was advised. On examination, her general condition was poor. She was conscious, afebrile, and cachectic with pulse rate was 80/min and blood pressure of 112/84 mmHg. There was moderate distension of the abdomen with mild tenderness; cardiovascular and respiratory systems did not show any abnormal findings. Significant laboratory investigations showed Hb 7.2 g/dL, blood sugar 63 mg/dL, serum lipase 920 U/L; the HBsAg was negative and HIV was nonreactive. Abdominal ultrasonography showed moderate ascites, diffuse circumferential thickening of terminal ileum and cecum with clumping of mesentery and enlarged pre-/para-aortic, and peripancreatic lymph nodes. The patient was diagnosed as abdominal tuberculosis and was given antituberculous treatment. On the 11th day of hospitalization, she became disoriented and breathless with bradycardia (heart rate of 50/min) and hypotension (60/30 mmHg). She was resuscitated but did not respond and died. A clinical autopsy was performed to know the cause of death.

Deduction

The patient's symptomatology of pain in abdomen and vomiting suggested the possibility of gastrointestinal pathology, mostly intestinal tuberculosis. It is important to note that despite antituberculosis treatment for last 2 months and 11 days, her clinical condition did not improve. The abnormal investigations of decrease in blood sugar of 63 mg% and increase value of serum lipase, 920 U/L cannot be explained in intestinal tuberculosis.

Autopsy Findings

External examination showed distension of abdomen. In-situ examination revealed approximately 300 mL of yellow colored fluid in the peritoneal cavity (**Fig. 38A**). The peritoneal fluid was collected for further investigations. The serosal surface of stomach was smooth, and the gastroesophageal junction showed enlarged lymph node (**Fig. 38B**). The stomach showed prominent rugal folds (**Fig. 39A**), with markedly thickened and grayish-white wall. The coils of small intestine and pancreas were entangled in mesentery, the mesenteric lymph nodes were enlarged and showed grayish-white appearance; suggestive of metastatic deposits (**Fig. 39B**). The pleural surfaces of both the lungs showed grayish-white nodularity (**Fig. 40A**). The lower lobes of both lungs showed subpleural hemorrhagic infarcts (**Fig. 40B**) with grayish-white metastatic deposits in pulmonary parenchyma and in hilar lymph nodes. Paratracheal lymph nodes were enlarged and their cut surface showed grayish-white metastatic tumor deposits (**Fig. 40C**). The liver and spleen were enlarged. Metastatic deposits were seen in the liver, spleen, right kidney (**Figs. 41A to C**), right ureter and right adrenal and cut surface of it showed grayish-white subcapsular tumor deposit (**Fig. 41A**). Both ovaries were enlarged and solid with yellowish cut surfaces (**Fig. 42A**). Examinations of brain and heart did not show any significant findings.

The cytology of the peritoneal fluid showed round to oval tumor cells having hyperchromatic nuclei and abundant cytoplasm; few of them showed peripherally placed nuclei (**Fig. 42B**). The microscopic examination of the stomach showed

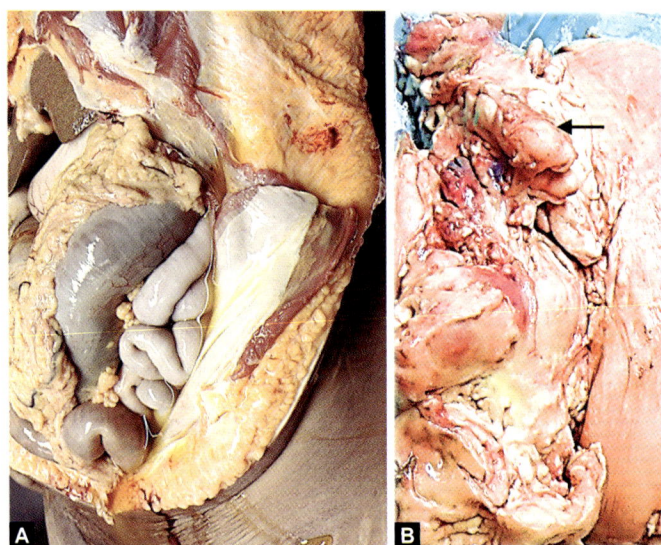

FIGS. 38A AND B: (A) Peritoneal cavity containing yellow colour serous fluid; (B) Gastroesophageal junction shows enlarged lymph node (arrow).

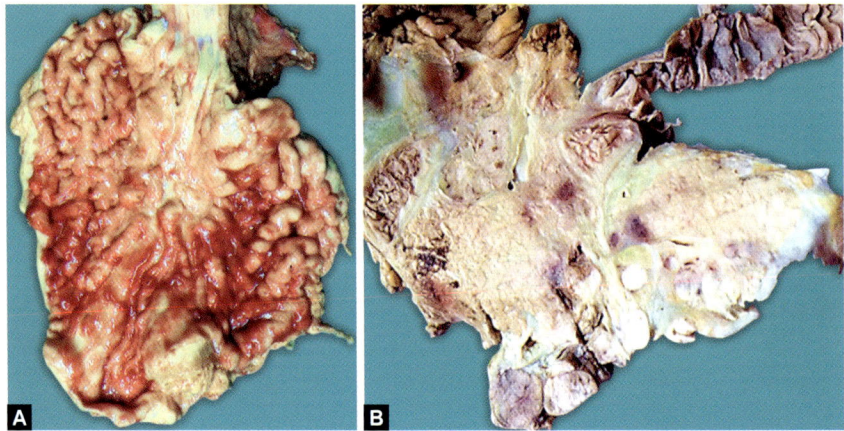

FIGS. 39A AND B: (A) Stomach shows prominent rugal folds and congested mucosa; (B) Entrapped lumens of small intestine, pancreas and mesenteric lymph nodes.

presence of tumor cells in submucosa, muscle coat and serosa. The tumor cells showed abundant cytoplasm and eccentrically displaced nuclei that formed crescent shapes, a feature of signetring cell carcinoma (**Fig. 42C**); the cytoplasm was strongly PAS positive (**Fig. 42D**). The histology of lungs showed metastatic tumor deposits, infarcts and vascular tumor emboli. The microscopic examinations of liver, spleen, right kidney, right ureter, right adrenal gland, ovaries (Krukenberg tumor), and mesenteric lymph nodes showed metastatic tumor deposits. The pancreas showed

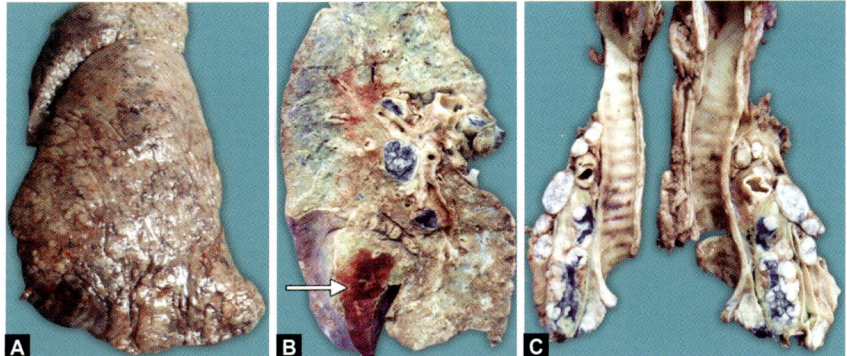

FIGS. 40A TO C: (A) Lungs show focal grayish-white nodularity on pleural surface and raised hemorrhagic areas in the lower lobes; (B) Cut surface of left lung shows grayish-white tumor deposits, metastases in hilar lymph nodes and hemorrhagic infarct in lower lobe (arrow); (C) Metastases in paratracheal group of lymph nodes.

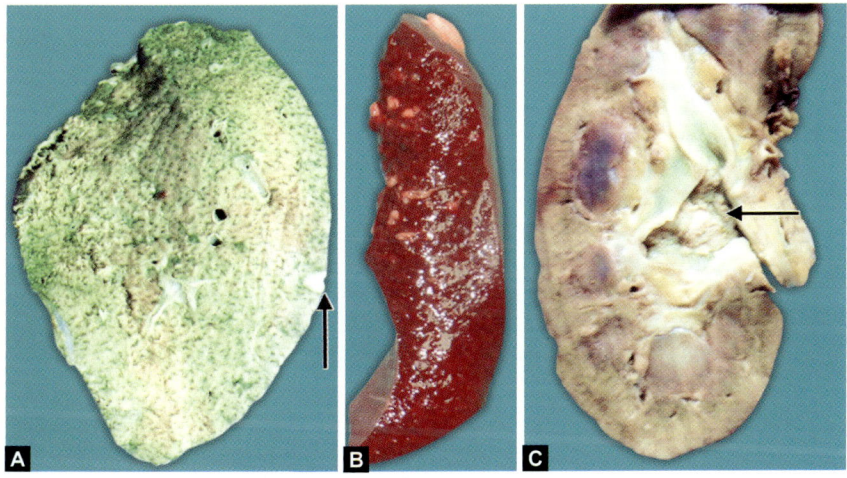

FIGS. 41A TO C: (A) Cut surface of liver shows subscapular grayish-white metastasis (arrow); (B) Cut surface of spleen shows focal grayish-white tumor deposits; (C) Cut surface of right kidney shows tumor deposit in renal pelvis (arrow).

interstitial infiltration by tumor cells. The gross and microscopic examination of small and large intestine did not show any evidence of tuberculosis.

Postmortem diagnosis: Signet ring cell carcinoma of stomach with widespread metastasis. The tumor stage of the carcinoma stomach is T4N3M1.

Between 2 and 10% of all gastric carcinoma are diagnosed in patients younger than 40 years of age.[36,37] Female predominance has been reported in young patients with gastric carcinoma. In advanced gastric carcinoma, the tumor invades the gastric wall beyond submucosa. Clinically, symptoms include epigastric pain, dyspepsia, anemia and weight loss. Some patients, particularly the young, have intra-abdominal dissemination at presentation. This patient presented with pain in abdomen and

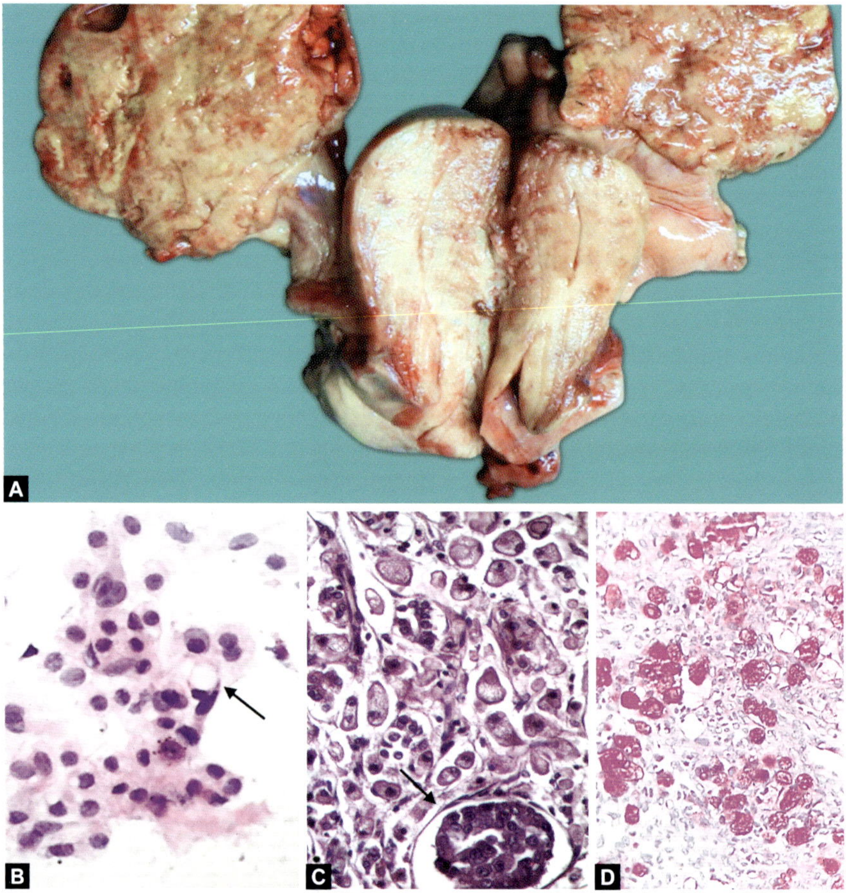

FIGS. 42A TO D: (A) Uterus, cervix and bilaterally enlarged ovaries with yellowish tumor; (B) Peritoneal fluid cytology showing tumor cells, some with a signet ring cell (arrow) appearance (H&E ×400); (C) Histology of stomach shows diffusely infiltrating tumor, the tumor cells contain abundant cytoplasm and peripherally pushed nucleus. Vascular tumor emboli (arrow) are also seen (H&E ×400); (D) The cytoplasm shows PAS positive globules (PAS ×400).

vomiting, which are characteristic clinical manifestations of gastric carcinoma. The vomiting in the present case can be explained by: (1) Pressure effect of enlarged metastatic lymph nodes in the gastroesophageal junction; and (2) Intestinal obstruction due to entrapped loops of small intestine. The increase in serum lipase[38] level found in this case can be explained due to infiltration of pancreatic tissue by metastasis of carcinoma of stomach. Gastric carcinoma per se can cause increase in lipase levels.[38] Hypoglycemia is an uncommon but well recognized complication of many tumors including carcinoma of stomach; this explains low blood sugar level (63 mg/dL) in the present case. The possible mechanisms of hypoglycemia are: (1) Secretion of insulin or insulin-like substances by tumor cells; and/or (2) Glucose consumption by tumor cells.

Sixty-five percent of patients with gastric cancer are diagnosed at an advanced stage. The abdominal tuberculosis is a great mimicker of pancreatic tumors, colonic cancer, gastric cancer, and lymphomas.[39,40] Even in countries where tuberculosis is prevalent, a correct clinical diagnosis of abdominal tuberculosis is made in only half of the patients.[41] A simple cost-effective diagnostic laboratory test that can be used routinely for abdominal tuberculosis is not yet available. The diagnosis of abdominal tuberculosis should be reached by a combination of clinical, laboratory, radiographic, and pathological findings.

REFERENCES

1. Jogai S, Radotra BD, Banerjee AK. Immunohistochemical study of human rabies. Neuropathology. 2000;20:197-203.
2. Jogai S, Radotra BD, Banerjee AK. Rabies viral antigen in extracranial organs: a post-mortem study. Neuropathol Appl Neurobiol. 2002;28:334-8.
3. Solanki A, Radotra BD, Vasishta RK. Correlation of cytokine expression with rabies virus distribution in rabies encephalitis. J Neuroimmunol. 2009;217:85-9.
4. Singh P, Kochhar R, Vashishta RK, Khandelwal N, Prabhakar S, Mohindra S, Singhi P. Amebic meningoencephalitis: spectrum of imaging findings. Am J Neuroradiol. 2006; 27:1217-21.
5. Vyas S, Jain V, Goyal MK, Radotra BD, Khandelwal N. Granulomatous amoebic meningoencephalitis. Neurol India. 2013;61:530-31.
6. Khurana S, Hallur V, Goyal MK, Sehgal R, Radotra BD. Emergence of *Balamuthia mandrillaris* meningoencephalitis in India. Indian J Med Microbiol. 2015;33:298-300.
7. Vaideeswar P, Chaudhari JP, Butany J. Mechanical complications of myocardial infarction. Diagn Histopathol. 2012;19:13-9.
8. McDonald JR. Acute infective endocarditis. Infect Dis Clin N Am. 2009;23:643-64.
9. Nguyen KD, Sundaram V, Ayoub WS. Atypical causes of cholestasis. World J Gastroenterol. 2014;20:9418-26.
10. Chand N, Sanyal AJ. Sepsis-induced cholestasis. Hepatology. 2007;45:230-41.
11. Whitehead MW, Hainsworth I, Kingham JG. The causes of obvious jaundice in South West Wales: perceptions versus reality. Gut. 2001;48:409-13.
12. Moseley RH. Sepsis and cholestasis. Clin Liver Dis. 1999;3:465-75.
13. Curti BD. Renal cell carcinoma. JAMA. 2004;292:97-100.
14. McLaughlin JK, Lipworth L. Epidemiologic aspects of renal cell cancer. Semin Oncol. 2000;27:115-23.
15. Lin PP, Mirza AN, Lewis VO, Cannon CP, Tu SM, Tannir NM, Yasko AW. Patient survival after surgery for osseous metastases from renal cell carcinoma. J Bone Joint Surg Am. 2007;89:1794-801.
16. Korteweg C, Go J. Pathology, molecular biology, and pathogenesis of Avian Influenza (H5N1) infection in humans. Am J Pathol. 2008;172:1155-70.
17. Gillet Y, Issartel B, Vanhems P, Fournet J, Lina G, Bes M, et al. Association between *Staphylococcus aureus* strains carrying gene for Panton-Valentine leucocidin and highly lethal necrotizing pneumonia in young immunocompetent patients. Lancet. 2002;359:753-9.
18. Semple PL, De Villiers JC, Bowen RM, Lopes MB, Laws ER Jr. Pituitary apoplexy: do histological features influence the clinical presentation and outcome? J Neuro Surg. 2006;104:931-7.
19. Verma R, Patil TB, Lalla R. Pituitary apoplexy syndrome as the manifestation of intracranial tuberculoma. BMJ Case Rep. 2014;2014.
20. Wang SY, Chuang CS. Pituitary apoplexy resembling acute meningitis without visual defect and ophthalmoplegia. Int J Case Rep Imag. 2012;3:26-9.
21. Guay-Woodford LM. Autosomal recessive polycystic kidney disease: the prototype of the hepato-renal fibrocystic diseases. J Pediatr Genet. 2014;3:89-101.

22. Wen J. Congenital hepatic fibrosis in autosomal recessive polycystic kidney disease. Clin Transl Sci. 2011;4:460-5.
23. Kazatchkine M, Sultan Y, Caen JP, Bariety J. Bleeding in renal failure: a possible cause. Br Med J. 1976;2:612-5.
24. Warrell RP, Hultin MB, Coller BS. Increased factor VIII/von Willebrand factor antigen and von Willebrand factor activity in renal failure. Am J Med. 1979:66:226-8.
25. Boyle JM, Johnston B. Acute upper gastrointestinal bleeding in patients with chronic renal disease. Am J Med. 1983;75:409-12.
26. Kosmidis C, Denning DW. The clinical spectrum of pulmonary aspergillosis. Thorax. 2015;70:270-7.
27. Kousha M, Tadi R, Soubani AO. Pulmonary aspergillosis: a clinical review. Eur Respir Rev. 2011;20:156-74.
28. Vaideeswar P, Prasad S, Deshpande JR, Pandit SP. Invasive pulmonary aspergillosis. A study of 39 cases at autopsy. J Postgrad Med. 2004;50:21-6.
29. Patterson KC, Strek ME. Diagnosis and treatment of pulmonary aspergillosis syndromes. Chest. 2014;146:1358-68.
30. Ramchandani M, Motomura T, David E, Kurrelmeyer K, Shah D, Garami Z. Fungal mycotic vegetation in the ascending aorta. Methodist Debakey Cardiovasc J. 2011;7:41-5.
31. Calcaterra D, Bashir M, Gailey MP. Ascending aortic graft thrombosis and diffuse embolization from early endoluminal *Aspergillus* Infection. Ann Thorac Surg. 2012;94:1337-9.
32. Grothues F, Welte T, Grote HJ, Roessner A, Klein HU. Floating aortic thrombus in systemic aspergillosis and detection by transesophageal echocardiography. Crit Care Med. 2002;30:2355-8.
33. Nuhu A, Dahwa S, Hamza A. Operative management of typhoid ileal perforation in children. Afr J Paediatr Surg. 2010;7:9-13.
34. Dunne JA, Wilson J, Gokhale J. Small bowel perforation secondary to enteric *Salmonella* paratyphi A infection. BMJ Case Rep. 2011;2011.
35. Lai CC, Liaw SJ, Lee LN, Hsiao CH, Yu CJ, Hsueh PR. Invasive pulmonary aspergillosis: high incidence of disseminated intravascular coagulation in fatal cases. J Microbiol Immunol Infect. 2007;40:141.
36. Koea JB, Karpeh MS, Brennan MF. Gastric cancer in young patients: demographic, clinico-pathological, and prognostic factors in 92 patients. Ann Surg Oncol. 2000;7:346-51.
37. Kokkola A, Sipponen P. Gastric carcinoma in young adults. Hepatogastroenterology. 2001;48:1552-5.
38. Hameed AM, Lam VW, Pleass HC. Significant elevations of serum lipase not caused by pancreatitis: a systematic review. HPB (Oxford). 2015;17:99-112.
39. Macdougall IC, Fleming S, Frier BM. Hypoglycemic coma associated with gastric carcinoma. Postgrad Med J. 1986;62:761-4.
40. Kahn CR. The riddle of tumour hypoglycaemia revisited. Clin Endocrinol Metab. 1980;9:335-60.
41. Debi U, Ravisankar V, Prasad KK, Sinha SK, Sharma AK. Abdominal tuberculosis of the gastrointestinal tract: revisited. World J Gastroenterol. 2014;20:14831-40.

Index

Page numbers followed by *f* refer to figure and *t* refer to table.

A

Abdominal aorta, part of 39*f*
Abdominal cavities 17*f*, 18, 24, 103*f*
Abdominal incision 76
Abdominal pain 62
   acute 62
   chronic 62
Abortion
   criminal 116
   unsafe 116
Abrasion 12
Abscess 23, 103
   large 72
   multiple 72*f*
   periannular 167
Abundant adipose tissue 164*f*
Acanthamoeba 162
Acanthosis nigricans 11
Acinetobacter pneumonia 194
Acquired immunodeficiency syndrome 10, 15, 150
Acromegaly 11
Acute respiratory syndrome, severe 15
Adenosine
   diphosphate 11
   triphosphate 11
Aerosols, limiting generation of 138
Ague cake spleen 92
Air embolism, method for 57*f*
ALC see anterolateral commissure
Alcoholic cirrhosis 74
Alcoholic liver cirrhosis 12*f*
Alcoholic micronodular cirrhosis 71*f*
Ambiguous genitalia 101*f*
Amebic liver abscess 72
Amenorrhea 176
AML see anterior mitral leaflet
Amniotic fluid embolism 108
Ampulla of Vater 103
Amyloidosis 89
Anasarca 14, 108
Anesthetic deaths 116
Angiodysplasia 68
Angioinvasive aspergillosis 185
Anorexia nervosa 10

Antemortem bone marrow trephine biopsy 194*f*
Anterior tricuspid leaflet 51, 52
Anterolateral commissure 51, 53, 167
Anthrax 138
Antiseptics 133
Antituberculous therapy 199
Aorta 39, 42, 43, 46, 48, 54, 165
   abdominal 76*f*
   ascending 23, 39, 42, 46, 48*f*, 52, 168, 191*f*
   examination of 11
Aortic valve 52, 54, 168*f*
   cusps 52
Aplasia 97
APM see anterior papillary muscle
Appendicitis 62
Arachnodactyly 11
Arrhythmia 168
Arterial embalming 151
Arterial thrombi 185*f*
Aspergilloma 185
Aspergillus 185, 186, 192, 196
   aortitis 190
   fumigatus 193, 194
   mural endocarditis 190
   species 188
Asphyxia, cases of 100
Asplenia 92
Atelectasis 103
Atheromatous plaques 45*f*, 49*f*
ATL see anterior tricuspid leaflet
Atrial appendages, morphology of 42
Atrophy 37
Autopsy 1-3, 7, 15, 16, 69
   adult 100, 140
   and law 118
   audit of 16, 145, 147
   before 140
   beginning of 2
   biosafety, general rules for 137
   brain at 31
   clinical audit monitors 147
   complete 2, 17, 167
   contributions of world leaders in 4*t*
   designing of 135

diagnosis 199
equipment for 139
external examination at 10
guidelines for performing 154
history of 2, 5
isolation room for high-risk 133
negative 116
partial 2
pathological 1
pediatric 99, 100, 179
precautions for performing 154
procedure 1, 156
quality, aspect of 145
role of 108
room 40, 132
   design of 130
   size of 131
safety precautions 136
second 124
services, dimensions in 15
special situations 99
staff 133
   care of 135
suites 130
table 131, 145
techniques of 15, 20
types of 1
   high-risk 138
use of 15
AV see aortic valve
Avian influenza 174
   virus infection 175
Axillary lymph nodes 13
Ayurvedic therapy 167

B

Bacteria, clumps of 167
Balamuthia mandrillaris 162
   meningoencephalitis 163*f*
Basic functional areas 130
Betadine 150
Bickerstaff brainstem encephalitis 160
Bicuspid aortic valve 52
Biliary obstruction 62
Biliary system, xamination of 11
Biliary tract, normal 69*f*
Biliary tree, ligature of 170
Biowaste disposal 141
Bird flu virus 173
Bird-headed dwarfism 5
Bisected left lung 60*f*
Bladder mucosa 84*f*

Bleeding piles 167
Blood 141
   cells 89
   collection of 175*f*
Blood-borne antigens 89
Blunt dissection 19, 28
Blunt trauma 84
Body
   fluid 141
   restoration of 134
Bone marrow
   biopsy, postmortem 196*f*
   examination 97
Bowel gangrene 68
Bowel perforation 64
Brain 177, 178
   after fixation, examination of 33
   before fixation, examination of 31
   coronal slice of 189*f*
   examination of 27
   fixation of 32
   growth, greatest 100
   knife 132
   removal procedure 28
   slices of 35*f*
Breast carcinoma 13, 22
Bronchial arterial diseases 58
Bruises 12
Budd–Chiari syndrome 70
Buffered formalin 40

C

CA see celiac artery
Cachexia 10, 12*f*
Cadaver
   handling of 140
   injector 150
Candida species 188
Capsular surface, examination of 70
Carbolic acid 149
Cardiac dissection 48*f*
Cardiac pathology 38
Cardiac size 46
Cardiac surfaces 41
Cardiovascular diseases 38
Cardiovascular system 38, 110, 163, 166, 187
Carotid artery, left common 39, 46
Cavity embalming 152
Cavity-concentric hypertrophy 182
Celiac artery 76
Cellular pathology 5
Central nervous system 27, 110, 159, 162, 187

Cerebral malaria 23
Cerebral venous thrombosis 110
Cerebrospinal fluid 31, 105, 160, 173
Cervical canal 86
Cervical cancer, disseminated 12*f*
Cervicomedullary junction 179*f*
Cervix 204*f*
Chest
    pain 201
    X-ray 195*f*
Cholangiocarcinoma 73
Cholecystitis 62
Cholelithiasis 62
Choroid plexitis 35
Chronic diseases 10, 56
Circle of Willis 33
    examination of 31
Circulatory system, anatomy of 148
Cirrhosis indicates, background of 71
Cirrhotic liver, assessment of 70
Clinical autopsy 118*t*, 154
Clinical Autopsy Program 7
Coagulative necroses 80
Coagulopathies 99
Coccidioidomycosis 138
College of American Pathologists 16
Colonic ulcers 68
Common congenital anomaly 52
Common iliac arteries 47
Complete abruptio placentae 114*f*
Concentric hypertrophy, moderate 182*f*
Conception, examination of products of 116
Congenital anomalies 99
Congested meningeal vessels 177*f*
Congestive heart failure 13
Coronary arterial
    anatomy 44
    dissection 44
    ostia 40
Coronary artery, left 44, 52, 168
Coronary cusp, left 52, 168
Coronary sinus 49, 51
Coronavirus disease 2019 154
Coroner's autopsy 1
Cortical thymoma 187*f*
COVID-19
    autopsy guidelines in 154
    cadavers 154
    infection 154
Cranial bones 101
Cranial cavity, examination of 22
Cranial nerves 30

Cribriform plates 31
Crista supraventricularis 52
Crohn's disease 67, 68
Cryptococcal meningitis 192
Cryptococcus 188, 192
CS see coronary sinus
CSV see crista supraventricularis
Custodial deaths 127
Cystic fibrosis 74
Cystic lesions 103
Cysts, small 78*f*
Cytokeratin immunohistochemistry 187*f*
Cytomegalovirus 105

D

De Humani corporis fabrica 1
Dead body, transportation of 157
Dehydration 22
Demyelination 37
Deoxyribonucleic acid 105
Dermatomyositis 173
Descending thoracic aorta 39, 46
Diabetes mellitus 38, 99
Diaphragmatic hernia, congenital 25*f*
Diarrhea 188
Diarrheal disease 105
DIC see disseminated intravascular
    coagulation
Dieulafoy's lesion 68
Dissection, alterations in 53
Disseminated intravascular
    coagulation 107, 109
Disseminated tuberculosis, diagnosis of 199
Diverticular disease 62
Diverticulitis 67
Donated bodies 2
Down's syndrome 101*f*
Down-draught ventilation 144
Dowry deaths 121
DTA see descending thoracic aorta
Duodenojejunal junction 63
Dwarfism 11
Dyspepsia 203
Dysplasia 97

E

Ear infection, middle 22
Early pregnancy bleeding 107
Ebola virus infections 15
Eclampsia 99
Edema feet 108
Electron microscopy 31

Embalming 148
　machine 150
　methods of 151
　principle of 149
Embolism 109
Employee health 141
Encounters 127
Endocardium, thickened 51
Endocrine disorders 11
Endometrial cavity 86
Engorged abdominal veins 69
Eosin solution 149
Epicardial surface, appearance of 41
Epidural hemorrhage 22
Epigastric pain 203
Equipment required for embalming 150
Escherichia coli 194
Esophageal atresia 103
Esophageal carcinoma 65
Esophageal perforation 65
Esophageal varices 68
Esophagitis 62
Esophagus 65, 66*f*
　carcinoma 62
Ethanol 149
Ethyl alcohol 149
Ethylene glycol 152
Eventual pyelonephritis 83
Evisceration, techniques of 19
Exophthalmoses 13
Extradural hematoma 34*f*
Extradural hemorrhage 22
Extrahepatic biliary atresia 73
Extraintestinal diseases 63
Eyes 2

F

Face 2
　shields 156
Facial appearance, abnormal 100
Fallopian tube 87
Fatal pulmonary thromboembolism 58*f*
Fatty liver
　discoloration in 70*f*
　mild 199*f*
Female genital tract, examination of 86
Femoral vein drainage 151
Fetal lobulations 78*f*
Fetal squamous cells 109*f*
Filariasis 14
First systematic cadaveric dissection 1
First-aid supplies 133

FO see fossa ovalis
Foci of scars and cysts 77
Fog spraying machine 139
Fogging machine 139
Foramen magnum 30
Forensic autopsy 118, 118*t*
Formaldehyde 149
Formalin acts 149
Fossa ovalis 51
Founder of Pathologic Anatomy 3
Fractures 100
Frontal lobes 30*f*
Fully-developed thymus 96
Fungal infection 13
Fusarium species 187

G

Gallbladder 69*f*
　lumen 74
　status of 74
Gamna–Gandy bodies 92
Gangrene 14, 64
　absence of 13
Gastric carcinoma 204
Gastroenteritis 4
Gastroesophageal junction 66
Gastroesophageal reflux disease 62
Gastrointestinal bleeding 68
Gastrointestinal gastrinoma, small 73*f*
Gastrointestinal perforation 67
Gastrointestinal symptoms 62
Gastrointestinal system 111
Gastrointestinal tract 62, 181, 169, 200
　examination of 68
Gastrosplenic ligament 88
Gaucher disease 89
General medical autopsy 27
Generative organs 88
Genital tract infection 108
Genital trauma 116
Gestational age babies 100
Ghon's method 20
Gigantism 11
Glomerulonephritis, chronic 78, 79
Glutaraldehyde 139
Glycerin 149, 152
Goggles 156
Granulomatous inflammation 193
Gravity tank method 150
Gray-white tissue 26*f*
Great arterial relations 44
Great arteries 23

Gross contamination and liquids 156
Growth factor-β, transforming 115
Guillain-Barré syndrome 160

H

Hairy cell leukemia 89
Hand-sanitizers, alcohol-based 133
Handwashing 139
Hashimoto's thyroiditis 165
Heart 38
   and lung block 39*f*, 180*f*
   anterior surface of 41
   diseases, congenital 11, 102
   external examination of 41
   fixation of 38
   internal examination of 48
   rate 179
Helicobacter pylori 66
HELLP see hemolysis, elevated liver
    enzymes, and low platelet count
Hemagglutinin protein, presence of 174
Hematemesis 201
Hematopoiesis 88
Hemoglobin 182, 188
Hemolysis, elevated liver enzymes, and low
    platelet count 107
Hemorrhage 37, 100, 116
   antepartum 107
   extensive intrauterine 114*f*
   intra-alveolar 175
   multifocal 36*f*
   pneumonia 103
   postpartum 107, 109
Hemorrhagic cystitis 84*f*
Hemorrhagic fever viruses 136
Hemorrhagic gastritis 111
Hemorrhagic ulcers 68
Hepatic amebiasis 72*f*
Hepatic outflow tract obstruction 73
Hepatic veins, examination of 73
Hepatitis
   A 69
   B 69
     virus 136
   C 69
     virus 136
   D 69
   E 69
Hepatobiliary system 112
Hepatocellular carcinoma, development
    of 71*f*
Hereditary anemias 11

Herpes simplex 105
Heterotaxy syndromes 102
High-efficiency particulate air 133, 155
His hemogram 160
Homocystinuria 22
Horse-shoe shape 104
Hospital wards 130
Household bleach 139
Human brain tissue repository 15
Human immunodeficiency virus 12, 130, 136
Human nervous tissues 15
Humani corporis fabrica 3
Hydrocele 14
Hyperechoic polycystic kidneys 179
Hyperplasia 97
Hypersensitivity reactions 62
Hypertension
   malignant 77
   pregnancy-induced 115
Hyperthermia 116
Hypodermic embalming 152
Hypoglycemia 204
Hypoplasia 79, 103, 104
Hypothyroidism, congenital 11

I

Icterus 108
Ileal tuberculosis, transverse ulcers of 104*f*
Ileoileal intussusception 64*f*
Immunological tests 105
In situ examination 22, 63, 109
Infected peripartum 108
Infection 62, 64, 116
   congenital 105
Infectious autopsies 130
Infectious disease, autopsy in 173, 175*f*
Infectious organisms 136
Infective endocarditis 23, 168
Inferior vena cava 14, 40, 43, 165
Influenza 133
   virus A 174
Internal carotid arteries 30
Internal systemic examination 110
Interstitial edema 77
Interstitial lung diseases 61
Interstitial pneumonitis 61, 61*f*
Interventricular septum 54, 166
Intestinal coils 170*f*
Intestine
   large 63
   small 63, 202*f*
Intrahepatic cholangiocarcinoma 72, 73*f*

Intrauterine ischemic 102
Ischemia 64
Ischemic heart disease 38, 41*f*
Ischemic ulcers 65*f*
Isolation room 138
IVC see inferior vena cava
IVS see interventricular septum

J

Jaundice 188
   color of skin for 69
   disappearance of 171
Joint pain 188

K

Kayser–Fleischer ring 13
Kidney 79, 175
   consistency of 77
   cortex of 77
   cut surface of 79
   disease 180
   external examination of 76
   external surface of 78*f*, 80*f*
   right and left 183*f*
Koilonychias 13
Kyphosis 13

L

LAA see left atrial appendage
LAD see left anterior descending artery
Law related to medicolegal postmortem 122
LBCA see left brachiocephalic artery
LCC see left coronary cusp
LCCA see left common carotid artery
Left anterior descending artery 50, 166
Left atrial appendage 39, 42, 43, 43*f*, 46, 48, 51, 54, 165
Left brachiocephalic artery 46
Left bronchus 58
Left lung, bronchiectasis of 61*f*
Left pulmonary
   artery 40, 43, 52, 58*f*
   vein 40, 43
Left renal artery 76
Left subclavian artery 39*f*, 46*f*
Left superior pulmonary 46
   vein 39, 48
Left ventricular
   apex 54*f*
   free wall rupture 165
Legionellosis 138
Leprosy 133

Leptomeningeal exudates, chronic 189*f*
Leptomeninges 29
Leukoderma 12
Levocardia 41
Lienorenal ligament 88
LIPV see left inferior pulmonary vein
Liver 175
   and intestine, examination of 3
   color of 70
   cut surface of 203*f*
   enlarged 103*f*
   examination of 11
   parenchyma 104*f*
   problems 69
   slice of 113*f*
      normal 69*f*
LMC see left main coronary artery
Lobular pneumonia 5
Lower limbs 176
Lower segment cesarean section 114
LPA see left pulmonary artery
LPV see left pulmonary vein
LRA see left renal artery
LSA see left subclavian artery
LSPV see left superior pulmonary vein
Luminal blood clot 183*f*
Lung 38
   carcinomas of 22
   diseases, chronic 19
   dissection 57
   examination of 59
   hypoplasia, bilateral 180*f*
   in fresh state 59*f*
   tissue 102
Lyme disease 15
Lymph node 88
   autopsy from enlarged 96*f*
   enlarged 202*f*
   examination of 93
   mediastinal 95*f*
Lymphoid organ 88
   largest 88
   primary 88
Lymphoma 23
Lymphoreticular organs 88
Lymphoreticular system 88
   examination of 88

M

Maceration, grades of 101*t*
Macronodular cirrhosis-autoimmune hepatitis 71*f*

Malabsorption syndromes 11
Malignant tumors 10
Mallory–Weiss tears 68
Massive splenomegaly 90*f*
Masson's trichrome 54
Mastoiditis 22
Maternal death
  autopsy in 107
  causes of 107*t*
Maternal medical disorders 99
Maternal mortality 107, 176
  ratio 108
Medicolegal autopsy 118, 124, 164
Melena 201
Meningitis 22, 35
  acute 178
Meningococcal meningitis 133, 136
Meningococcemia 138
Mesenteric lymph nodes 202*f*
Mesocardia 47
Metabolic diseases 103
Metabolism, inborn errors of 99
Metastasis 13, 22
Metastatic adenocarcinoma 96*f*
Metastatic deposits 24
Metastatic liver 73*f*
  disease 73*f*
Metastatic nodes 95
Metastatic tumors 22
Mimic multicystic disease 82
Mitral leaflet, anterior 48, 51-53, 168
Mitral valve 54
Modern embalming 148
Molluscum contagiosum, tumors 14
Mononuclear cell infiltrate 177*f*
Mortuary technician, countersignature
    of 134
Mouth 2
Mucoid inspissated secretions 93*f*
Multicystic dysplastic kidney 82
Multicystic renal dysplasia 104*f*
Multidrug resistant bacteria 133
Multinucleate giant cells 191*f*
Multiple pulmonary abscesses 175
Multiple tiny cysts 104*f*
Multi-system involvement 193
Muscular interventricular septum 52
MV see mitral valve
Mycobacteria 140
Mycobacterium tuberculosis 130, 136, 188
Myelofibrosis 89
Myeloid leukemia, chronic 89
Myocardial ischemia 62

Myocardial pathology 47
Myocardium 54
Myocyte caliber 110

N

Nasal swab, collection of 175*f*
National Human Right Commission 121
Necrotic granuloma 194*f*
Necrotic parenchyma 186*f*
Necrotizing aspergillosis, chronic 185
Necrotizing papillitis 82
Negri body in purkinje cell 161*f*
Nephritic syndrome, causes of 77
Nephritis, end stage of 79
Nephronophthisis 81
  benign 78, 78*f*, 82
Nephrotic syndrome 80
Neurofibromatosis 11
Neuromuscular causes 62
Neuronophagia 161*f*
Neutrophils 167
Nitabuch's layer 113
No objection certificate 150
Nodular enlargement 13
Nodular hyperplasia and carcinomas 86
Nodule
  abnormally sized 71
  texture of 71
Noncirrhotic liver, assessment of 72
Normal anatomy 2
Nutritional requirements 176

O

Obstetric haemorrhage, causes of 107*t*
Obstetric hysterectomy 116
Obstructive lung disease 181
Ochronosis 11
Oligohydramnios 181
One-point injection 151
Opening heart and heart weight 47
Opsis 1
Organs
  abdominal 19
  demonstration of 141
Otitis media 23
Oxalate 149

P

Pampiniform plexus 85
Panchanama 126
Pancreas 69*f*, 112, 202*f*
  cystic fibrosis of 11
  examination of 11, 75

Pancreatic disease 62
Pancreatic neoplasms 62
Pancreatitis
  acute 62
  chronic 62
Papillary muscles 51, 52
  anterior 51, 52, 168
  posterior 51-53, 168
Paralytic rabies 160
Parenchyma 185
Parenchymal lymphocytic inflammation 161f
Parenchymal tumors, benign 82
Parietal pericardium 23, 42f
Passive venous congestion, chronic 70
Patchy pneumonia, bilateral 173
Pathogenic microorganisms 136
Pathologia indica 7f
Pathology museums 6
Pelvic mucosa 79
Pelvic ultrasonography 177
Pelvis, distortion of 172f
Peptic ulcer disease 67, 68
Perfumes 149
Pericardial cavity 23
Pericardial effusion, moderate 42f
Peripheral cyanosis 11
Peripheral lymphoid organs 88
Perirenal fat, normal 77
Perirenal tissue 76
Peritoneal adhesions 67
Peritoneal cavities 132
  peritoneum or 67
Peritoneal fluid, cytology of 201
Peritoneal nodules metastasis 25
Peritoneum covers 86
Peritonitis 67, 182
Periventricular leukomalacia 102
Personal protective
  attire 139
  equipment 155
Petechial hemorrhages 13, 78f
Peutz-Jeghers
  polyp 103
  syndrome 11
Peyer's patch 198f
Phenol 149, 152
Pituitary disorders 11
Pituitary gland
  enlarged 178f
  necrosis 110
Placenta penetrates myometrium 113

Placenta previa 113
Plague 133, 136, 138
Plastination 152
Platelets 188
Pleural cavities 190
  and lungs 24
Pleural effusion, pre-existing 24
Pleural mesothelioma 24
Plumbing 132
  related leakages 132
PMC see posteromedial commissure
PML see posterior mitral leaflet
Pneumonia 4, 23
Pneumonitis 62
Pneumothorax 56, 61, 109
  demonstration of 55f
Polycystic kidney disease 81f, 180
Polycythemia 22
Polymerase chain reaction 27, 162
Polyvalent alcohol 152
Porphyria 11
Portal veins, examination of 73
Postanalytical phases 145
Posterior descending artery 166f
Posterior mitral leaflet 48, 51, 53
Posteromedial commissure 51, 53
Postexposure prophylaxis 138
Postmortem 1
  examination 1
  second 125
  investigations 105
PPM see posterior papillary muscle
Preeclampsia 72, 115
  development of 115
  syndrome 72
Pregnancy, acute fatty liver of 112, 112f
Preliminary anatomic diagnosis 147
Preliminary skin incisions 17
Prematurity, common signs of 101t
Prion disease 133
Prostate 76
  carcinomas of 22
  examination of 86
  middle lobe of 84
Protozoal infections 24
Proximal duodenum 62
Pseudallescheria 187
Pseudomembranes 64
Pseudomembranous colitis 65f
Pseudomonas 188
PT see pulmonary trunk
PTL see posterior tricuspid leaflet

Puerperal sepsis 115
Pulmonary arterial
　bifurcation 42
　diseases 58
Pulmonary arteries 40f, 56
Pulmonary aspergillosis 185
Pulmonary embolism 23
Pulmonary thromboembolism 109
Pulmonary trunk 23, 39, 42, 46, 48, 52, 165
Pulmonary tuberculosis 144
Pulmonary valve 52
Pulmonary vein, left inferior 39, 46, 48
Purified protein derivative 141
PV see pulmonary valve
Pyelonephritis 77
　acute 81f
　chronic 78f
Pyemic abscess 77
Pyogenic meningitis 23, 175

R

RAA see right atrial appendage
Rabies 133, 136, 138
　meningoencephalitis 160f, 161f
Rapes 127
RBCA see right brachiocephalic artery
RCA see right coronary artery
RCC SE Right coronary cusp
RCCA see right common carotid artery
Recordkeeping 133
Refrigeration 134
Regional lymph nodes 172
Relation with relatives 135
Renal agenesis 104
Renal arterial
　ostia 76
　ostium, right 76f
Renal cell carcinoma 82, 82f, 172
Renal diseases 79
Renal function test 193
Renal injury 80
Renal parenchyma 172f
Renal pelvis 203f
Renal rickets 11
Renal sinus 79
Resection anastomosis 116
Respiratory complications 99
Respiratory syndrome coronavirus 2,
　acute 154
Respiratory system 110, 187
　examination of 55
Retention cyst 81, 81f

Retroperitoneal hematomas 25
Rheumatic mitral stenosis 53f
Rib markings 56
Rickettsioses 138
Right atrial appendage 39, 42, 43, 43f, 46, 54, 168
Right atrium 51
Right brachiocephalic artery 39, 46
Right bronchus 58
Right common carotid artery 46
Right coronary
　artery 44f, 52
　cusp 52
Right inferior pulmonary vein 39, 46
Right lenticular hemorrhage with
　edema 36f
Right pulmonary
　artery 40, 52
　vein 40
Right renal artery 76
Right subclavian artery 46
Right superior pulmonary vein 39
Right ventricle leads 51
Right ventricular cavity 166
Rigor mortis 11
RIPV see right inferior pulmonary vein
Rokitansky method 20
RPA see right pulmonary artery
RPV see right pulmonary vein
RRA see right renal artery
RSA see right subclavian artery
RSPV see right superior pulmonary vein
Rubella 105
RVC see right ventricular cavity

S

Saddle-shaped thromboemboli 56
Saliva 62
Saphir's method 20
Scars, small superficial 200f
Sella turcica, diaphragm of 31
Seminal vesicles 83
　examination of 86
Sepsis 116
Septal band 51
Septal tricuspid leaflet 51
Septic spleen 92
Septicemia 68
Serum creatinine 167
Sharp instruments, safe use of 138
Sheehan's syndrome 110
Shock 11

Sickle cell anemia 22
Signet ring cell 204*f*
  carcinoma 203
Sinoatrial node 43*f*
Sinus, sagittal 110
Sinuses-of-valsalva 52
Skeletal development 100
Skin
  abdominal 18
  changes in 11
  infection 12, 23
  reflection 55
  tests 141
Skull
  cap 29*f*
  cavity 100
  cut edges of 29*f*
Slender fibrous septa 172*f*
SMA see superior mesenteric artery
Small intestine
  coils of 201
  loop of 183*f*
Sodium
  borate 149
  citrate 149
  hypochlorite 139
    solution 157
Solitary cyst 93*f*
Specimen
  handling 144
  storage of 130
Spinal cord 160
  examination 27
    and sampling 36
  removal of 32
Spleen 69*f*, 88, 89, 175
  absent 92
  cut surface of 93*f*
  enlarged 91*f*
  examination of 74, 89
  hilum of 91
  removal of 89
Splenic lesion 94*f*
Splenic touch imprint 93
Splenomegaly 89
Splinter hemorrhages 13
Split injection 151
Staphylococcus aureus 175
Stauffer syndrome 173
Sternoclavicular joints 18
STL see septal tricuspid leaflet
Stomach content, collection of 66

Stryker saw 28
Subclinical thyroid disease 165
Subcutaneous tissue 56
Subdural empyema 31
Superior mesenteric artery 76
Superior vena cava 42, 43, 51
  left 46
Supraclavicular lymph nodes 13
Surface embalming 152
SVC see superior vena cava
Syphilis 105
Systemic examination 27, 63, 102

T

Tap water 149
TC see terminal crista
Terminal crista 51
Testes
  examination of 85
  size of 14
  test for normal 85*f*
Tetanus 136
Thick gallbladder with choledocholithiasis 75*f*
Thoracic and abdominal viscera 19*f*
Thoracic cavity 102, 156
  left 101*f*
Thoracic organs, block of 19
Thorax, in-situ examination of 176*f*
Thrombophlebitis 14
Thymic abnormality 97
Thymic dysgenesis 97
Thymic lesions 97*t*
Thymus 96
  normal 97*f*
Thyroid
  carcinomas of 22
  gland 13
Thyrotoxicosis 22
Tiny blood vessel in lung 109*f*
Tiny ligaments 88
Tissues
  microscopic examination of 105
  transport of 140
Torsion 93
Toxoplasma 105
Trabeculo septomarginalis 52
Trachea 58
Tracheal bifurcation 58*f*
Tracheoesophageal fistula 65, 103
Transmissible spongiform encephalopathy 143

Transmural myocardial infarction, acute 50*f*
Tricuspid leaflet, posterior 51, 168
Tricuspid valve 54
Trophoblastic invasion 115
Tropical ulcers 14
TSM see trabeculo septomarginalis
Tuberculosis 4, 10, 67, 133, 181
    particularly 56
Tubular necroses, acute 77, 80
Tumor
    absence of 13
    cells 204
TV see tricuspid valve
Typhoid 4
    pulmonary complications of 5

U

Ulcerative colitis 68
Ulcers, absence of 13
Unilateral edema 14
Upper motor neuron palsy 176
Uremia 62
Uremic medullary cystic disease 81
Ureters 83
    examination of 83
Urinary bladder, examination of 83
Urinary system 181
Urinary tract 171
    anomalies of 104
Urogenital system 112
Urogenital tract 76
Urothelial carcinoma 23, 84*f*
Urticaria pigmentosa 11
Uterine atony 113
Uterine perforation 116
Uterus 204*f*

V

Vaginal discharge 108
Valvular heart diseases 38
Vascular endothelial growth factor 115
Venous thrombosis 33
Ventilation 132
    system 133
Ventriculitis 35
Vertebral column 32, 100
Vesicocutaneous 85
Vesicointestinal fistulas 85
Vesicovaginal 85
Viral encephalitis and rabies 31
Viral hemorrhagic fevers 138
Virchow triad 5
Virchow's method 20, 53
Virchow's node 95
Virtual autopsy 2
Visceral layers 56
Visceral pleura 56
Vitiligo 12

W

Wandering spleen 93
Waste disposal, cleaning and 157
Waterproof bandages 133
Wilm's tumor 82, 104*f*
    large 104*f*

Y

Yersinia 67
Y-shaped incision 23

Z

Ziehl-Neelsen stains 94f